NEW RESEARCH ON PARKINSON'S DISEASE

New Research on Parkinson's Disease

Timothy F. Hahn

And

Julian Werner

Editors

Nova Biomedical Books
New York

NOTICE TO THE READER

The Publisher has taken reasonable care in the preparation of this book, but makes no expressed or implied warranty of any kind and assumes no responsibility for any errors or omissions. No liability is assumed for incidental or consequential damages in connection with or arising out of information contained in this book. The Publisher shall not be liable for any special, consequential, or exemplary damages resulting, in whole or in part, from the readers' use of, or reliance upon, this material.

Independent verification should be sought for any data, advice or recommendations contained in this book. In addition, no responsibility is assumed by the publisher for any injury and/or damage to persons or property arising from any methods, products, instructions, ideas or otherwise contained in this publication.

This publication is designed to provide accurate and authoritative information with regard to the subject matter covered herein. It is sold with the clear understanding that the Publisher is not engaged in rendering legal or any other professional services. If legal or any other expert assistance is required, the services of a competent person should be sought. FROM A DECLARATION OF PARTICIPANTS JOINTLY ADOPTED BY A COMMITTEE OF THE AMERICAN BAR ASSOCIATION AND A COMMITTEE OF PUBLISHERS.

Library of Congress Cataloging-in-Publication Data
New Research on Parkinson's disease/Timothy F. Hann and Julian Werner,editors.
    p. ; cm.
Includes bibliographical references and index.
ISBN 978-1-60456-601-7(hardcover)
1.Parkinsons's disease. I. Hann, Timothy F. II. Werner,Julian.
[DNLM: 1. Parkinson Disease.WL 359 N5328 2008]
RC382.N486 2008
616.8'33—dc22   2008013802

Published by Nova Science Publishers, Inc. ✦ New York

3/9/09

Contents

Preface

Parkinson's disease (PD) is characterized by an insidious onset with slowing of emotional and voluntary movement, muscular rigidity, postural abnormality and tremor. Parkinson's disease was first described in 1817 by James Parkinson. It is a progressive, neurological disease mainly affecting people over the age of 50, although at least 10% of cases occur at an earlier age. It affects people of either sex or all ethnic groups. In the normal brain, some nerve cells produce the chemical dopamine, which transmits signals within the brain to produce smooth movement of muscles. In Parkinson's patients, 80 percent or more of these dopamine-producing cells are damaged, dead, or otherwise degenerated. This causes the nerve cells to fire wildly, leaving patients unable to control their movements. This new book examines new research results from around the world.

Chapter I - Recently the authors developed gene manipulated mice to determine the therapeutic potential of metallothioneins (MTs) in Parkinson's disease. Metallothioneins transgenic (MT_{trans}) mice were genetically resistant to 1-methyl, 4-phenyl, 1,2,3,6-tetrahydropyridine (MPTP) parkinsonism as compared to metallthioneins 1 and 2 gene knock out (MT_{dko}) mice. Furthermore MPTP-induced α-synuclein nitration was significantly inhibited in MT_{trans} mice. The striatal coenzyme Q_{10} was significantly reduced upon chronic intoxication of MPTP in MT_{dko} mice as compared to MT_{trans} mice. This was confirmed by the observation that MT-1_{sense} oligonucleotides transfected human dopaminergic (SK-N-SH) neurons were resistant where as MT1$_{antisense}$ oligonucleotide-transfected neurons were susceptible to MPP^+ apoptosis. A potent peroxynitrite ion generator, 3-morpholinosydnonimine (SIN-1)-induced oxidative and nitrative stress and apoptosis were also attenuated in MT-1_{sense} oligonucleotides transfected SK-N-SH neurons. As such MT_{dko} mice did not exhibit typical Parkinsonism however they were highly susceptible to MPTP, 6-hydroxy dopamine, salsolinol, and rotenone neurotoxicity. We developed a rare colony of α-synuclein-metallothioneins triple knock out (α-Syn-MT_{tko}) mice by crossbreeding α-synuclein knock out male mice with MT_{dko} females. The litter size of α-Syn-MT_{tko} mice was significantly reduced and these genotypes exhibited increased head size, reduced body weight, and reduced life span. The striatal coenzyme Qs could not be detected by conventional procedures. Therefore the authors developed a sensitive method of coenzyme Qs determination from these genetically susceptible mice. Furthermore weaver mutant (wv/wv) mice exhibited typical Parkinsonism characterized by severe body tremors and postural irregularities. The striatal coenzyme Q_{10} and MTs were significantly reduced in wv/wv mice and they exhibited progressive nigrostriatal dopaminergic neurodegeneration as seen in Parkinson's disease. The striatal ^{18}F-DOPA uptake was significantly reduced in wv/wv mice. Progressive reduction in the striatal ^{18}F-DOPA uptake was correlated with the depletion in coenzyme Q_{10}. Cross-breeding wv/wv female mice with MT_{trans} male mice produced a rare colony of metallothioneins over-expressing wv/wv (wv/wv-MTs) mice. wv/wv-MTs mice possessed significantly increases striatal dopamine and mitochondrial bioenergetics as determined by microPET neuroimaging with ^{18}F-DOPA and ^{18}FdG respectively. The striatal coenzyme Q_{10} and dopamine synthesis were also significantly augmented in wv/wv-MTs mice, suggesting that MTs provide neuroprotection by acting as potent free radical scavengers, by augmenting brain regional coenzyme $Q_{10,}$ and dopamine synthesis in Parkinson's disease. Since MTs provide neuroprotection by ameliorating the brain regional mitochondrial bioenergetics and dopaminergic neurotransmission, therapeutic interventions augmenting brain regional MTs may provide neuroprotection in Parkinsons's disease.

Chapter II - Parkinson disease *(PD)* is primarily an age-related progressive neurodegenerative disorder affecting as many as 1,500,000 people in the United States alone. Clinically, PD is characterized by bradykinesia, muscular rigidity, resting tremor, and gait abnormalities with later postural instability [1]. Pathologically, PD results in dopaminergic neuronal cell loss in the substantia nigra pars compacta *(SNpc)*, axonal terminal loss in the caudate/putamen (striatum), oxidative stress *(OS)*, dopamine depletion, increased iron levels, increased lipid peroxidation, and decreased mitochondrial complex I activity [2, 3]. The mechanisms underlying the interplay between the rise in oxidative stress and dopaminergic neuronal cell loss are poorly understood. More critically, very little is known regarding the transcriptional changes that occur in Parkinson's disease and its relation to oxidative stress and dopaminergic cell loss. Epidemiological studies suggest an association with pesticides and other environmental toxins [4]. In particular, the toxin 1-methyl-4-phenyl-1,2,3,6-tetrahydropyridine *(MPTP)* and its active metabolite MPP+, are selectively imported into dopaminergic neurons by the plasma membrane dopamine *(DA)* transporter. Once imported, MPP+ induces parkinsonian-like patterns of degeneration [5]. MPTP effects have been extensively studied in vivo using well developed ferritin heavy chain *(FtH)* transgenic mouse models [6, 7]. Recent studies in FtH deficient mice have shown that iron and the iron storage protein FtH, are two major key players in PD disease mechanisms [8]. Both iron and FtH levels are elevated in PD [7, 9]. As iron becomes required for vital biological reactions like dopamine production [10], FtH is degraded through lysosomal activities to release its stored iron [11]. Nevertheless, when iron homeostasis is disturbed, excess iron becomes involved in Fenton reactions producing highly reactive oxygen species *(ROS)* [10]. Excess iron can react with hydrogen peroxide H_2O_2 to produce hydroxyl radicals *(·OH)* [12]. Excess ·OH and other ROS species leads to lipid peroxidation, DNA breakage, and bio-molecular degradation that eventually lead to neuronal death [10]. FtH is known to sequester Fe^{+2} thus it plays a protective role against substantia nigra, gloubus pallidus, and striatum cell death [10]. In this view, it is the authors' hypothesis that the therapeutic potentials of FtH in vivo and in combination with embryonic stem *(ES)* cells would yield greater benefits in understanding and treating PD. ES cells have extensive self-renewal capacity and high potential in differentiating to dopaminergic neurons [13-15]. They also have been extensively cultured in-vitro and shown to successfully differentiate into dopaminergic neurons for Parkinson's mice models [15]. On another level, glutathione S-transferase p1 *(GSTP1)* has been shown to mediate protection against H_2O_2 induced cell death [16, 17] and affects the clinical manifestation of PD [18]. Also, NF-E2 related factor 2 *(Nrf2)* is known to bind ARE activators like tert-butylhydroquinone *(tBHQ)* and many antioxidant genes with high relevance to PD [19, 20].

Chapter III - Parkinson's disease (PD) prevalence various significantly globally and its etiology remains unknown. Both genetic and environmental factors as well as their interactions are believed to be important in the etiology of PD. Published epidemiological studies indicate that the prevalence of PD in Asian and African population is much lower than in the Caucasian population. This suggests that the incidence of PD may vary by race. Migration studies indicate that environmental exposures potentially mediated or modified by ethnicity-related lifestyle exposures may also be important. Efforts to characterize gene-environment interactions have intensified in the last decade. For example, genetic studies show that the MAO B G/A genotype frequency in Asian population differ from frequencies in Caucasians and the prevalence of the LRRK2 G2019S mutation is rare in Asian population. Recently, a common genetic variant (LRRK2 G2385R) has been found to be associated with a two-fold increased risk of sporadic PD in ethnic Chinese populations in Singapore and Taiwan. Epidemiological and genetic studies suggest that race/ethnicity effects should be considered in the context of new genetic breakthroughs and haplotype mapping given the extensive population heterogeneity due to genetic admixture. In this article the authors review the available data and discuss the possible contributions of race and ethnicity to the epidemiological, clinical and pathological features, and genetics of PD.

Chapter V - Recent theoretical accounts of the brain's construction of the sense of Self have described widely distributed neural networks which participate in support of various aspects of the sense of self. In this paper, the authors suggest that right frontal cortex is a key node in these distributed networks which supports the sense of an enduring Self. Independent evidence suggests that patients with Parkinson's disease (PD) exhibit impairment on cognitive tasks that depend on both the right and left frontal lobes. If the sense of Self requires intact frontal function, then the sense of Self should be impaired in PD, particularly in those patients with right frontal dysfunction. In this paper, the authors review a series of studies they conducted to examine links between changes in the sense of Self/personality to changes in mood, neuropsychologic and dopaminergic function in PD patients. The authors used sentence completion tests of identity development ('self-test'), personality inventories and measures of mood, memory and neuropsychologic functioning to assess the sense of Self in PD. They found that Self and personality test responses significantly correlated with performance scores on tests of frontal function but not parietal or temporal lobe function. Patients with predominantly left-sided onset/involvement exhibited a different personality profile and performed poorly on tests of autobiographical memory recall relative to patients with right-sided onset/involvement. The authors conclude that a healthy autonomous sense of Self depends on intact right frontal function.

Chapter VI - Sympathetic neurocirculatory failure in Parkinson`s disease is common. Orthostatic hypotension is the most frequent symptom. Cardiovascular disturbances have so far been met with the highest degree of clinical and scientific interest. Histological studies have proven the presence of Lewi`s bodies in sympathetic and parasympathetic neurons and also in central structures associated with the autonomic regulation.

Extrasystoles occur in normal subjects, but are more frequently seen in Parkinson patients. Heart rate variability is a useful non-invasive test to assess autonomic dysfunction in PD. It allows a differentiation of the sympathetic and parasympathetic activation, which are related to a low-frequency (0.05 - 0.15 Hz; LF) and a high-frequency (0.15-0.5Hz; HF) component of the heart rate variability (HRV) signal, respectively. The resulting LF/HF ratio is a quantitative index of the sympatho-vagal balance. The physiological function of HRV is commonly known to be to buffer changes in blood pressure. In the PD-patients group (n=107, mean age 71 years, mean PD-duration 7.0 years, Hoehn and Yahr 3.0 ± 0.9) the LF/HF ratio was lower than in the control group in rest (2.19 vs. 1.25, $p < 0.05$); in deep respiration (3.3 vs. 2.4, $p < 0.01$) and in tilt-table testing (2.6 vs 1.9, $p < 0.01$). The LF/HF ratio in tilt-table testing was significantly more reduced in PD with OH than without (2.1 vs. 1.3, $p < 0.05$). Scintigraphy with ^{123}I-Metaiodobenzylguanidine (MIBG) appears to be a highly sensitive and useful in demonstrating sympathetic postganglionic cardiac nerve disturbances. In the heart, MIBG uptake in all examined 57 Parkinson's (PD) patients was decreased (H/M-Ratio: 1.14 ± 0.16). Loss of sympathetic innervation of the heart seems to occur independent of orthostatic hypotension and baroreflex failure in PD. We found no correlation between myocardial MIBG uptake and sympathovagal balance, blood pressure or other autonomic findings. This results could be explained by different time course of loss of intact postganglionic sympathetic cardial innervation and disturbed baroreflex response or the involvement of central autonomic pathways in PD.

The significance of the abnormalities in cardiovascular regulation among PD patients is not fully known yet. It is possible that the dysbalance of the sympathetic and parasympathetic tone is connected with heart arrhytmias. The connection between autonomic dysregulation and arrhythmia related death has recently been considered in PD. The mortality of PD patients is almost twice that for age and sex-matched healthy control groups.

Chapter VII - Parkinson's disease is a neurodegenerative disorder characterized by a progressive loss of dopaminergic neurons of the substantia nigra pars compacta, followed by dopamine depletion in the striatum. Cellular death takes place in a well-defined group of neurons, this fact becomes Parkinson's disease in a perfect target for the development of gene therapy. A variety of methods have been used in order to delivery genes into the Central Nervous System and they can be contained into two approaches. The first, *in vivo* gene therapy, includes the delivery of a therapeutic gene directly into host cells using viral vectors. Each one of these viral vectors has advantages and disadvantages but the most suitable, up to date, seem to be adeno-associated viruses and lentiviruses. For application of the second approach, *ex vivo* gene therapy, cells should be genetically modified *in vitro* and implanted into a recipient host. A great variety of cellular sources have been used as vehicle of gene delivery, but the ideal cells to be employed in gene therapy seem to be stem cells due to its capacity to differentiate and generate an unlimited number of cells. Gene therapy carried out in Parkinson's disease includes delivery of genes encoding biosynthetic enzymes for dopamine synthesis and neurotrophic factors. However, protective therapy using GDNF, with the aim to prevent neuronal death, is the most promising approach. Gene therapy is a powerful tool in the treatment of neurodegenerative disorders and it has potentiality to be applied in Parkinson's disease.

Chapter VIII - Excessive manganese exposure may induce a neurological syndrome similar to Parkinson's disease (PD), called manganism. However, close observation of manganism patients reveals a clinical disease entity different from PD, not only in the clinical manifestation and therapeutic response, but also in the neuroimaging studies, such as magnetic resonance images (MRI), positron emission tomography (PET), and dopamine transporter images (DAT), and in the neuropathological findings. The differences in the clinical manifestations between manganism and PD include in the former less-frequent resting tremor, more frequent dystonia, gait en bloc, and a wide-based and characteristic cock-walk gait. In PD, a persistent focal asymmetry is noted, whereas in manganism there is a high degree of symmetry. However, a unilateral cock-walk gait and asymmetric dystonia are also found in chronic manganism. Therefore, symmetry is not a good differential clue between manganism and PD. A failure to achieve a sustained therapeutic response is noted in manganism. Neuroimaging studies may distinguish manganism from PD. The findings in manganism are hyperintensity in the basal ganglia on T1-weighted MRI scans, and normal 6-fluorodopa PET and DAT scans. Neuropathologically, PD is associated with neuronal loss in the substantia nigra pars compacta and locus ceruleus, and the presence of Lewy bodies, whereas in manganism, gliosis mainly is limited to the globus pallidum and substantia nigra pars reticularis, with an absence of Lewy bodies. Furthermore, manganism has a clinical course different from PD; in long-term follow-up, manganism patients show a prominent deterioration in the parkinsonian symptoms in the initial 5-10 years, followed by a plateau in the following 10 years.

In the most recent few years, the possible potential risk of inhaling welding fumes to accelerate the onset of PD or induce PD has been raised. Previous studies have not provided adequate evidence to support the relationship between welding and PD because of a lack of exposure data and selection bias with the patients. However, welding fumes may contain various neurotoxic substances in addition to manganese such as iron which may increase oxidative stress. Further investigation is warranted.

In: New Research on Parkinson's Disease   ISBN: 978-1-60456-601-7
Editors: T. F. Hahn, J. Werner   © 2008 Nova Science Publishers, Inc.

Chapter I

Therapeutic Potential of Metallothioneins in Parkinson's Disease

*Sushil K. Sharma** and Manuchair Ebadi*

Cyclotron and Positron Imaging Research Laboratory,
Center of Excellence in Neurosciences
University of North Dakota School of Medicine and Health Sciences,
Grand Forks, ND, USA

Abstract

Recently we developed gene manipulated mice to determine the therapeutic potential of metallothioneins (MTs) in Parkinson's disease. Metallothioneins transgenic (MT_{trans}) mice were genetically resistant to 1-methyl, 4-phenyl, 1,2,3,6-tetrahydropyridine (MPTP) parkinsonism as compared to metallthioneins 1 and 2 gene knock out (MT_{dko}) mice. Furthermore MPTP-induced α-synuclein nitration was significantly inhibited in MT_{trans} mice. The striatal coenzyme Q_{10} was significantly reduced upon chronic intoxication of MPTP in MT_{dko} mice as compared to MT_{trans} mice. This was confirmed by the observation that $MT-1_{sense}$ oligonucleotides transfected human dopaminergic (SK-N-SH) neurons were resistant where as $MT1_{antisense}$ oligonucleotide-transfected neurons were susceptible to MPP^+ apoptosis. A potent peroxynitrite ion generator, 3-morpholinosydnonimine (SIN-1)-induced oxidative and nitrative stress and apoptosis were also attenuated in $MT-1_{sense}$ oligonucleotides transfected SK-N-SH neurons. As such MT_{dko} mice did not exhibit typical Parkinsonism however they were highly susceptible to MPTP, 6-hydroxy dopamine, salsolinol, and rotenone neurotoxicity. We developed a rare colony of α-synuclein-metallothioneins triple knock out (α-Syn-MT_{tko}) mice by crossbreeding α-synuclein knock out male mice with MT_{dko} females. The litter size of α-Syn-MT_{tko} mice was significantly reduced and these genotypes exhibited increased head size, reduced body weight, and reduced life span. The striatal coenzyme

* Correspondence: Sushil K. Sharma, Ph. D; D.M.R.I.T. Director, Cyclotron and Positron Imaging Research Laboratory, Center of Excellence in Neurosciences, University of North Dakota School of Medicine and Health Sciences, Grand Forks, ND, U.S.A., Tel (701) 777-2031; Fax (701) 777-4158, Email skumar@medicine.nodak.edu

Qs could not be detected by conventional procedures. Therefore we developed a sensitive method of coenzyme Qs determination from these genetically susceptible mice. Furthermore weaver mutant (wv/wv) mice exhibited typical Parkinsonism characterized by severe body tremors and postural irregularities. The striatal coenzyme Q_{10} and MTs were significantly reduced in wv/wv mice and they exhibited progressive nigrostriatal dopaminergic neurodegeneration as seen in Parkinson's disease. The striatal ^{18}F-DOPA uptake was significantly reduced in wv/wv mice. Progressive reduction in the striatal ^{18}F-DOPA uptake was correlated with the depletion in coenzyme Q_{10}. Cross-breeding wv/wv female mice with MT_{trans} male mice produced a rare colony of metallothioneins over-expressing wv/wv (wv/wv-MTs) mice. wv/wv-MTs mice possessed significantly increases striatal dopamine and mitochondrial bioenergetics as determined by microPET neuroimaging with ^{18}F-DOPA and ^{18}FdG respectively. The striatal coenzyme Q_{10} and dopamine synthesis were also significantly augmented in wv/wv-MTs mice, suggesting that MTs provide neuroprotection by acting as potent free radical scavengers, by augmenting brain regional coenzyme $Q_{10,}$ and dopamine synthesis in Parkinson's disease. Since MTs provide neuroprotection by ameliorating the brain regional mitochondrial bioenergetics and dopaminergic neurotransmission, therapeutic interventions augmenting brain regional MTs may provide neuroprotection in Parkinsons's disease.

Abbreviations

Parkinson's Disease:	PD
α-Synuclein	α-Syn
Metallothionein	MT
Metallothionein double knock out	MT_{dko}
Metallothionein Transgenic	MTtrans
α-Syn knock out	$α-Syn_{ko}$
Dopamine Transporter	DAT
Glutamate Transporter	GAT
Dopamine beta Hydroxylase	DBH
3-Morpholino Sydnonimone	SIN-1
1, Methyl 4-phenyl, 1,2,3,6, Tetrahydropyridine	MPTP
1- Methyl, 4-phenyl, Pyridinium ion	MPP^+
Nitric Oxide Synthase	NOS
Tumor Necrosis Factor-α	TNF-α
Interleukin-6	IL-6
Tetrahydroisoquinolines	THIQs
Nitric Oxide	NO
Serial Analysis of Gene Expression	SAGE
Glial Fibrillary Acidic Proteins	GFAP
Dihydroxy phenyl acetaldehyde	DOPAL
Cytochrome-C	Cyt-C
Apoptosis-Inducing Factor	AIF
Metal Responsive Transcriptional Factor	MTF-1
Nuclear Export Signal	NES

Metal Response Elements   MREs

Introduction

Metallothioneins (MTs), a class of low molecular weight, cysteine-rich, ubiquitous intracellular proteins with high affinity for metal binding including zinc, occur in all eukaryotes were first identified in the horse kidneys (Margoshes and Vellee 1957). Rodents possess four isoforms (MT-1 to MT4) (Palmiter et al., 1992, Quaife et al., 1994). Only three isoforms are expressed in the brain namely MT-1+2 (which are also widly expressed and regulated coordinately) and MT3 (also known as growth inhibitory factor). MTs bind zinc and copper and presumably function in metal ion regulation and detoxification in peripheral tissues as well as in CNS. More recent evidence suggests that MTs could be significant antioxidant proteins (Ashner et al 1997; Hidalgo et al 1997, 2001, Penkova 2006 for review). MT-1+2 are dramatically increased in brains of GFAP-IL6 transgenic mice as a physiological adaptation to cope with the CNS injury due to increased cytokine trigger. Crossing GFAP-IL6 mice with MT-1+2 null mice provided a progeny with significantly altered CNS structure as well as function (Giralt et al 2002). These findings provide evidence that MT1+2 proteins are valuable factors against cytokines-induced CNS injury. Furthermore, high throughput gene screening using serial analysis of gene expression (SAGE), has provided evidence that MT-2 is an important neuroprotective gene as it is three fold increased within 2-16 hrs of focal cerebral ischemia (Trendelenburg et al 2002). All these studies provide evidence that MTs are neuroprotective against, metal ion toxicity, oxidative stress, and cytokines injury due to cerebral ischemia or infection. However the precise neuroprotective role of MTs isoforms in CNS in PD remains elusive.

Brain MT isoforms-I and II were first discovered in our laboratory by Itoh et al in 1983, and were shown to be induced only following intracerebraventricuar but not intra-peritoneal administration of zinc (Ebadi et al 1986). In mammals, MT-1, and II are expressed in most organs and their synthesis is regulated by metal ions, glucocorticoids, endotoxins, cytokines, stress, and radiation (for review Kagi and Kojima 1987, Suzuki et al 1993). Uchida et al (1991) identified first MT-III and named a brain inhibitory factor, and subsequently Palmiter et al 1992 characterized in detail and renamed a brain-specific MT-III. MT-III exists in zinc containing neurons, and is thought to play a role in zinc uptake into neurons and transport of zinc within neurons and their synaptic vesicles (Masters et al 1994). MT isoform IV is restricted to pseudostratified squamous epithelial cells (Quaiffe et al 1994). Various MT isoforms have been postulated to participate in the synthesis of metalloenzymes, regulate metal homeostasis, and protect against metal toxicity and oxygen radicals (Zheng et al 1995; Erickson et al 1995, Ebadi et al 1995; Dalton et al 1995; Aschner, 1996; Ebadi 1991). The function of MT in the nucleus is to protect from DNA damage, apoptosis, and regulate gene expression during certain stages of the cell cycle (Cherian and Apostolova 2000). MT may react directly with ONOO⁻ to prevent DNA and lipoprotein damage (Cai et al., 2001).

We postulated that a specific signal transduction mechanism must exist to foster the induction of MT1 and II by numerous and diversified factors, and searched and identified for the first time, MT receptors in U373MG cells using flow cytometric analysis of fluorescinated MT (FMT)1 probe and confocal microscopic techniques, and by employing cysteine, glutathione (GSH), and other cysteine-containing substances, and MT isoforms I-IV, to determine high affinity and specific binding (ElRefaey et al 1997). Recently we have discovered that MPTP-induced nitration of α-Syn is inhibited by MT gene over-expression in MT transgenic (MT_{trans}) mice striatum. Mitochondrial Coenzyme Q_{10} levels remained preserved in MT_{trans} mice striatal tissue as compared to MT double knock out (MT_{dko}) mice, which exhibited significant depletion in coenzyme Q_{10} upon chronic MPTP (30 mg/kg, i.p) treatment of seven days. Furthermore a potent peroxynitrite ($ON00^-$) ion generator SIN-1-induced lipid peroxidation, caspase-3 activation, and apoptosis were also attenuated by MT gene over-expression in SK-N-SH neurons, while down-regulation of MT gene rendered these neurons highly vulnerable to MPP^+ and SIN-1-induced apoptosis (Sharma and Ebadi 2003; Ebadi and Sharma 2003).

Although MTs serve as potent metal ion regulators and are induced by metals, glucorticoids, and inflammatory signals in a coordinated manner, yet their exact functional significance remains elusive. MT-transgenic mice models in particular are useful for the characterization of the mechanisms underlying cytokine-induced pathological conditions in the CNS as well as for identifying potentially important genes for coping with CNS damage. Cytokines are essential mediators of inter-neuronal communication in the CNS astrocytes, microglia, and macrophages (Hopkins and Rothwell 1995; Rothwell and Hopkins 1995, Stichel and Verner-Muller 1998; McIntosch et al 1998). Yet, in various neuropathological conditions the expression of some cytokines is significantly altered (Campbell 1998 for review). Such alterations could contribute to the clinicopathological features of many neurological disorders such as PD and AD. Recent studies have shown that MT-1+2 deficiency in GFAP-IL6XMTKO mice induces clear symptoms of oxidative stress and apoptotic cell death. This is represented by induction of cytokines such as IL-1α, β, IL6, and other host response genes including TNFα, GFAP, ICAM-1, the acute phase protein-EB22/5, and complement C3 protein followed by recruitment and activation of macrophages and T cells through out the CNS, with clear symptoms of neurodegeneration, astrocytosis, microgliosis, angiogenesis, and up-regulation of several unknown inflammatory processes (Penkova et al 2002), suggesting that the MT1+2 proteins are valuable factors against cytokines-induced CNS injury (Giralt et al 2002). By employing serial analysis of gene expression (SAGE) and high throughput screening, it has been demonstrated that MT-2 was the major neuroprotective gene during mouse focal cerebral ischemia (Trendelenburg et al., 2002).

Extensive studies including our own have shown that 1-methyl-4-phenyl-1,2,3,6-tetrahydropyridine (MPTP)-induced oxidative and nitrative stress produces clinical, biochemical, and neuropathologic changes similar of those that are observed in idiopathic PD [Dawson 1998, Dawson et al., 1999; Dehmer et al., 2000; Du et al., 2001, Ebadi et al., 2002]. Among several toxic oxidative species, NO has been proposed as a key element on the basis of the increased density of glial cells expressing iNOS in the substantia nigra (SN) of patients with PD. Thus sustained production of neurotoxic NO by activated microglial cells may cause detrimental consequences to surrounding neurons (Chang and Liu 1999). Recently we have shown that MTs provided neuroprotection against MPTP, 6-OHDA, salsolinol, and rotenone-induced oxidative and nitrative stress and apoptosis in SK-N-SH neurons and MT-gene-manipulated mice striatum (Ebadi and Sharma 2003). MPP^+ and SIN-1-induced lipid peroxidation, caspase-3 activation, and α-Syn nitration were attenuated by MT gene over-expression in cultured DA neurons and in MT_{trans} mice striatum (Sharma et al 2002a). We have estimated brain regional microdistribution of coenzyme Q_{10} with a primary objective to establish its neuroprotective potential in MT gene manipulated mice (Albano et al., 2002). Striatal coenzyme Q_{10} levels remained preserved in chronic MPTP intoxicated MT_{trans} mice striatum (Sharma et al 2002b). Furthermore, an iron chelator, deferoxamine attenuated iron-induced oxidative stress, mitochondrial damage, and nucleocytoplasmic shuttling of α-Syn in SK-N-SH neurons, suggesting the neuroprotective role of ferritin (Sangchot et al., 2002). Ferritin levels also remained preserved in MT_{trans} animals as compared to MT_{dko} and $control_{wt}$ mice. Interestingly, MT_{trans} mice synthesized higher levels of SN neuromelanin as a function of aging and were quite resistant to MPP^+ neurotoxicity (Sharma et al., 2002), whereas SN ferritin and melanin in MT_{dko} mice were heavily loaded with Fe^{3+}, Cu^{2+}, Zn^{2+}, and Ca^{2+} following chronic MPTP intoxication as compared to MT_{trans} and $control_{wt}$ animals. Selegiline provided neuroprotection by preserving brain regional glutathione, mitochondrial complex-1, and MT gene induction (Ebadi et al., 1989, Ebadi et al., 2002a). By employing EM, we have confirmed that MPP^+-induced mitochondrial damage was also attenuated by Selegiline pre-treatment (Sharma et al., 2003). Furthermore, 3-Morpholinosydnonimone (SIN-1, a potent vasorelaxant, soluble guanyl cyclase stimulator, and $ONOO^-$ generator)-induced lipid peroxidation, caspase-3 activation, BCl-2 down-regulation and Bax activation, Cyt-C release, and apoptosis were attenuated in MT overexpressed DA neurons as compared to MT_{dko} or MT-1 gene down-regulated DA neurons (Sharma and Ebadi 2003).

The exact molecular mechanism of attenuated mitochondrial apoptosis, pathophysiological significance of enhanced SN neuromelanin, nucleocytoplasmic shuttling of MTs, MTF-1, and α-Syn in MT over-expressed DA neurons and glial cells in response to MPTP or SIN-1 remains ingmatic, hence further study is needed in this direction. There are several areas which remain to be established for instance (i) the exact cellular, molecular, and genetic basis α-Syn-MT and MT/Ferritin interaction in PD, (ii) pathophysiological significance of MT Gene Promoter, MTF-1, MRE, cytokine (IL-6) activation, neuromelanin and DAT, and (iii) possible treatment strategies of PD and various other neurodegenerative diseases named broadly as α-Synculeinopathies by brain regional MT gene induction. In view of the above, we investigated and futher explored the exact molecular mechanism of neuroprotection, afforded by brain regional MT gene expression and induction employing the experiments as described in this report.

Recently we have developed colonies of α-synuclein MTs triple knock out mice and MTs overexpressing weaver mutant (wv/wv-MTs) mice to further explore the therapeutic potential of MTs in PD by performing microPET neuroimaing using ^{18}F-dG and ^{18}F-DOPA as sensitive and specific biomarkers of brain regional bioenergetics and dopaminergic neurotransmission, which is significantly impaired in PD. Brain regional coenzyme Q_{10} in α-Synuclein MTs triple knock out mice could not be detected by conventional methods hence we developed a sensitive procedure of its estimation from rare biological samples (Sharma and Ebadi 2004).

We have discovered that the distribution kinetics of ^{18}F-DOPA is significantly impaired in wv/wv mice. The striatal ^{18}F-DOPA uptake is significantly reduced and is delocalized in the kidneys of wv/wv mice (Sharma and Ebadi 2005). The reduction in the striatal ^{18}F-DOPA uptake was proportional to down-regulation of MTs and the rate limiting enzyme involved in oxidative phosphorylation, ubiquinone-NADH-oxidoreductase (complex-1) associated with progressive dopaminergic neurodegeneration (Sharma et al., 2006). MTs over-expressing wv/wv mice exhibited significantly improved striatal ^{18}F-DOPA uptake and coenzyme Q_{10}, suggesting the neuroprotective role of MTs.

This study was performed to explore the exact pathophysiological significance of MT-induced neuromelanin synthesis and elucidate contribution of MT in mitochondrial coenzyme Q_{10} and iron/ Ferritin hoemostasis during acute and chronic MPTP neurotoxicity. We utilized well known neurotoxins, 6-hydoxy dopamine, MPTP and peroxynitire ion generator, SIN-1 to produce parkinsonism in genetically manipulated [(i) control $_{(wt),}$ MT$_{trans}$, MT$_{dko}$, α-Syn knock out, and α-Syn-transgenic mice in vivo, and cultured dopaminergic cell line (SK-N-SH) in vitro to establish the genetic basis of PD and its effective treatment via MTs gene induction. The primary objective of this study was to establish the neuroprotective role of MTs in PD.

Materials and Methods

Preparation of Gene-Manipulated Mice: Two breeder pairs from each experimental genotypes [Ten males and 10 females] (Control$_{wt}$, MT$_{trans}$, MT$_{dko}$, α-Syn$_{ko}$, and α-Syn$_{trans}$) were purchased from Jackson's Laboratories (Minneapolis, Minnesota, USA). First breeder pair from each genopyte was used for breeding a colony of atleast 25 animals in each group. Twenty-five animals were used as basal controls, 25 were treated chronically with MPTP (30 mg/kg, i.p.), and 25 with SIN-1 (10 mg/kg. i.p.) for 7 days. This required atleast 75 animals. The progeny was monitored and genotyped using tail or ear pinna DNA and PCR, as described earlier. The transgenics, having at least 2.5 times enhanced expression of the gene of interest as compared to wild type controls were used for the present study. For further experiments a pure colony of transgenics was prepared by cross-breading the transgenic male and transgenic females. The second breeder pair was utilized to generate striatal fetal stem cells as described below.

Preparation of Fetal Stem Cells: Experimental protocols were approved by local Animal Care Committee and were maintained according to the guidelines of NIH. Pregnant female mice (Strain C57/BJ6) weighing 35-40 g on the 13th day of gestation were purchased from Jackson's Labs (Minneapolis, MN, USA). Breeding of other genotypes were done as described earlier. On 18th day of gestation developing embryos were removed from the womb by cesarean section under strictly sterilized conditions; washed thrice in Dulbecco's PBS (pH 4.5, 0.15M), and anesthetized over dry ice before decapitation. Different brain regions were isolated using sterio-binocular dissecting microscope. Fetal brain regions (hippocampus, substantia nigra, striatum, and cerebellum) were dissected and placed in 0.1% Trypsin (GIBCO, BRL Life Technologies) in Ca-Mg free Hank's Balanced Salt solution (KBSS) buffered to pH 7.3 with 10 mM HEPES, incubated for 15 min at 37^{0}C and washed thrice with HBSS. They were re-suspended in approximately 1 ml of HBSS and dissociated by passage through series of Pasteur pipettes with flame-narrowed tips. The cells were pipetted into 35 mm tissue culture dishes (Falcon) at a density app 1.5 to 2×10^4 cells/cm^2. The dish was pre-coated with poly-lysine hydrobrimide Mol weight $3\text{-}7 \times 10^4$ (Sigma Chem Co. St. Loius MO, USA). (Solutions of only 0.01% polylysine in borate buffer were used). The cultured medium contains equal volumes of Ham's F-12 and DMEM supplemented with an additional 120 mg/100 ml of glucose, 5 µg/ml of bovine insulin, 100 µg /ml of human Transferrin, 20 nM Progesterone, 100 µM Puteriscine, and 20 nM Selenium dioxide (all from Sigma). The culture was maintained in humidified incubator with 5% CO_2 at 36^0C, after 4-6 days the division of non-neuronal cells was halted by addition of 15 µg/ml of fluorodeoxyuridine and 35 µg/ml of uridine. These cultures were maintained for 6-8 weeks. The cells were maintained initially for 30 min in supplemented minimum essential medium [MEM+Earle's Salts (1:1) composition:(i) glutamine 2 mM, glucose 600 mg/100 ml, penicillin 20 units/ml, sterptomycin 20 µg/ml], followed by conditioned medium for 4 hrs (Composition: MEM 80%, fetal calf serum 10%, heat inactivated horse serum 10%), followed by synthetic medium (Synthetic medium containing supplemented Minimum Essential Medium and Ham's F-12 medium). This medium was used for long term survival of the fetal stem cells in culture, [Composition: bovine Insulin 5 µg/ml (Sigma), human transferrin 100 µg/ml, progesterone 20 nM, puteriscine 20 nM, selinium dioxide 30 nM]. Hippocampal and cerebellar cells were used as non-DA controls.

Cell Culture: SKN-SH neurons were used to prepare RhO$_{mgko}$ neurons (a cellular model of aging) by maintaining them for 4-6 weeks in Dulbecco's Modified Eagle's medium (DMEM), supplemented with 5µg/ml of ethidium bromide. (This treatment specifically down-regulates mitochondrial genome without affecting the nuclear genome). Although RhO$_{mgko}$ cells have compromised intra-mitochondrial bioenergetics (as in aging subjects), they possess proliferative potential and exhibit physiological activities similar to control$_{wt}$ neurons. Basal α-Syn expression is increased in RhO$_{mgko}$ neurons. The detailed procedure to prepare RhO$_{mgko}$ neurons is described by Trimmer et al (2001), Ghosh et al (1999), fall and Bennet (1999), and Puri and Coleman (1997).

Cell Transfection: Cell transfection studies were conducted in 60 mm dishes possessing adherent DA neurons in a subconfluent stage. Usually we use the cells between 4-5th passage. 1 µg of antisense oligonucleotide to α-syn: 5'-CCT-TTT-CAT-GAA-CAC-ATC-CAT-GGC-3', Reverse Sense: 5'-GCC-ATG-GAT-GTG-TTC-ATG-AAA-GG-3'; Scrambled: 5'-TAG-CTC-GCT-ACG-TAA-TCA-CCA-CT-3')., MT-1 antisense: CAC-AGC-ACG-TGC-ACT-TGT-CCG-CCG-CCG-CTT-TGC-AGA-CAC-AGC-C, MT-1 Forward: GTT-CGT-CTC-ACT-GGT-GTG-AGC, MT-1 Reverse: AAA-AGA-AAT-CGA-GGA-AAT-GGC (GIBCO/BRL Life Technologies, U.S.A), mixed with 8 µl of enhancer and 25 µl of Effectine trasnfection reagent as per manufacturer's recommendations. The transfected cells were authenticated using radioimmunoprecipitation, immunoblotting, and RT-PCR with specific primer sets of genes. For stable transfection, the cells were grown to subconfluent stage using 6 well plastic dishes by employing sense primer sequences of the coding region of the gene using pEGFP-N1 vector, and electroporation for cell transfection (Bio-Rad Gene Pulser–II) as per manufacturer's recomendations. We have used pEGFP-N1 vectors sense and sense oligonucleotides or restriction enzyme cut plasmids and inserts of interest to transfect cells with genes of specific interest. Cell transfection studies were conducted in control$_{wt}$, RhO$_{mgko}$, and fetal rat striatal stem cells, using 60 mm dishes possessing adeherent SK-N-SH neurons in a subconfluent stage. Gene Bank Accession No # U55762 ClonTeck Catalog No # 6085, encodes a variant of the Aequorea Victoria green fluorescent protein (GFP) has been optimized for brighter fluorescence and higher expression in mammalian cells. PEGFP-N1 vector allows genes cloned into the multiple cloning sites (MCS) upstream of the EGFP coding sequences to be expressed as fusions to the N-terminus of EGFP. The unmodified vector expresses EGFP in mammalian cells. The plasmid size is 4.7 Kb. It has following multiple cloning sites: Nhe 1, ECO47 III, Xho I, Ecl/136 II, Sacl, Hind III, ECOR I, Pst I, Sal I, Acc I, Asp 718 I, Kpn I, Sac II, Bsp 120 I, Apa I, Xma I, Sma I, BamH I, Age I, and exhibits antibiotic resistance to Kanamycin (30 ug/ml) for propagation in E.Coli, Host strain DH5α. Bio-Rad Gene Pulser-II was used for electroporation (750 V pulse for 25 mSec) using sterilized metallic cuvettes. Stable transfectants were enriched by G-418 (250 μg/ml) and limiting dilution techniques, sub-cultured to obtain large number of EGFP-positive cells to study the influence of MPP^+ or SIN-1 on gene expression.

Multiple Fluorochrome Comet Assay: $Control_{wt}$ and aging (RhO_{mgko}) SK-N-SH neurons were grown overnight in Falcon T25 flasks and the monolayer was washed thrice with PBS (pH 7.4) following treatment overnight with MPP^+, or SIN-1 (10 μM) each. 10^5 cells were suspended in 100 μl of LMP Agarose on an agarose coated microscopic slide. A cover slip was applied to imbed the cellular monolayer in the agarose and removed when agarose was solidified. Then a second layer of LMP Agarose was applied. To release individual nuclei, embedded cells were lysed by incubating the slides overnight in 5 ml Buffer [Composition: 2.5M NaCl, 100 mM EDTA, 10 mM Tris-HCl (pH 10), 1% N-Laurylsarcosine, 1% Triton-X-100, 10% DMSO] and incubated for 5 min in elctrophoresis solution [composition: NaOH = 300 mM, EDTA = 1 mM, pH 12.5]. (Relaxed and broken DNA fragments migrate towards the Anode). The gel was neutralized by washing in 0.4M Tris-HCl (pH 7.5), and restained in 20 ug/ml EtBr for 30 seconds, DNA was inspected at 400X magnification with fluorescence microscopy at 590 nm. DNA Damage was estimated by measuring fluorescence ratio [Head Fluorescence/Tail Fluorescence]). Digitized images of ETBr–stained structures were captured with a CCD camera attatched to fluorescence microscope and converted into false color images and fluorescence intensity distribution was measured by Comet II software (Perceptive Instruments). To determine the extent of mitochondrial DNA damage, which is associated with DNA oxidation to 8-hydroxy, 2 deoxy guanosine (8-OH, 2dG), we treated the cellular monolayer with 1:3000 dilution of antibody to 8-OH, 2dG for 1 hr at room temp, following washing with PBS (pH 7.4), the cellular monolayer was treated with secondary antibody (FITC-conjugated-IgG) for 2 hrs and washed thrice in PBS. (The Comet tails exhibit green fluorescence when mitochondrial DNA damage occurs and red when nuclear DNA damage occurs). Merging of red fluorescence with green fluorescence provided an over all estimate of damage produced in the mitochondrial as well as nuclear DNA.

α-Syn Index (Newly Introduced): α-Syn Index is a ratio of nitrated α-syn vs native α-syn. α-Syn Index was determined by double radioimmunprecipitation method. Following overnight exposure to MPP+ or SIN-1, along with 1 μCi/ml of ^{35}S-methionine, the cells were lysed in the lysis buffer, protein A agarose (100 μl) was added along with the working dilution (1:300) of α-syn antibody. The samples were kept on a rotary shaker at 4^0C for 48 hrs. The immunprecipitate was dissolved in 200 μl of lysis buffer. 100 μl of aliquot was counted to determine total α-Syn immunoreactivity. 100 μl of the supernatant was subjected to second immunoprecipitation employing 1:500 dilution of nitrotyrosine antibody. 100 µl of protein A agarose was added and the samples were kept for 24 hrs at 4^0C on a rotary shaker, centrifuged at 14,000 rpm for 20 min at 4^0C. The immunoprecipitate was dissolved in 100 µl of lysis buffer and counted above background in TriCarb Beckman-Coulter β- Scintillation counter. A qualitative estimation of syn-index in DA neurons in response to MPTP (10 µM) was also made using real time Digital Fluorescence Imaging employing *Spotlite* Digital Camera and *ImagePro* computer software by double immunostaining with anti-α-Syn as well as nitrotyrosine antibodies using subtration and merging fluorescence images (Leeds Instruments Co. Minnesota, MN.USA). Target accentuation and background inhibition protocols were employed to estimate native (non-nitrosylated) vs nitrated α-Syn.

Mitochondrial-Related Apoptosis. The cells were washed thrice by resuspending the pellet in modified Tyrode buffer 150 mM NaCl, 5mM HEPES, 0.55 mM NaH_2PO_4, 7 mM $NaHCO_3$, 2.7 mM KCl, 0.5mM $MgCl_2$, 5.6 mM glucose, 1 mM EDTA (di-K), pH 7.4 pelleted by centrifugation at 1000Xg for 15 min. Subsequent steps were performed at 4^0C. The pellet was suspended in ice-cold buffer (250 mM, sucrose, 1 mM, EDTA, 10 mM Tris, pH 7.4) and transferred to glass homogenizer for cell disruption. The homogenate was centrifuged at 1000g for 15 min and nuclear pellet removed. The supernatant contained mainly mitochondrial activity (represented 85% citrate synthase activity after addition of Triton-X-100). The pooled mitochondria were pelleted by centrifugation at 8650g for 10 min, suspended in 600 µl of ice cold buffer to a protein concentration of 3mg/ml, synapse frozen in liquid nitrogen, and placed at -70^0C for storage before assay within 2 weeks. Mitochondrial complex-1 activity and protein carbonylation were estimated spectrophotometrically.

Lipid Peroxidation: Lipid peroxidation was studied as described previously (Buege and Aust 1998). The cells were grown in 12-well plates for 72 hrs. A fresh medium was added to examine the effect of increasing concentrations of MPP^+ or SIN-1 overnight as described in the text, harvested and suspended in Dulbecco's PBS (pH 7.4), sonicated at low wattage for 30 seconds, 1ml of thiobarbituric acid reagent (Sigma Chemicals Co, St Louis, MO) [composition: 15% Trichloroacetic acid: 0.375% Thiobarbituric acid, and 0.25N hydrochloric acid] were added. The samples were heated for 20 min at 95^0C and cooled in running ice-cold water, centrifuged at 10,000 rpm for 10 min. The O.D was measured at 535 nm using a microtiter plate reader.

Detection of Mitochondria-Related Apoptosis: The cells were grown on either cover slips or in eight chambered microscopic slides for 48 hrs to sub-confluent stage, and exposed to either MPP^+ (100 µM) or SIN-1 (10 µM) overnight, washed thrice in D-PBS thrice and incubated at 37^0C for 30 min to stain with the 5nM mitochondrial marker, JC-1 (Molecular Probes, Eugene, Oregon), for 30 seconds in 10 ng/ml of either DAPI and/or ethidium bromide, washed thrice with Dulbecco's PBS, mounted on microscopic slides using aqua mount supplemented with a photo-bleach inhibitor, and observed under digital fluorescence microscope (Leeds Instruments, CO, Minneapolis, MN) set at three (Blue, Green, and Red) spectral wavelengths. The images were merged to estimate mitochondrial vs nuclear apoptosis simultaneously. To estimate α-syn-Ferritin interaction in response to MPP^+ or SIN-1, double immunofluorescence microscopic procedures were employed using 1:300 and 1:500 primary antibodies to α-syn and ferritin respectively for 1 hr after fixation of cellular monolayer with 10% acetone for 15 min. The cells were washed thrice with D-PBS and secondary antibodies FITC-conjugated IgG, and Cy-3-conjugated IgG (dilution 1:500, and 1:1000 respectively) were used for 1 hr. The fluorescence images were captured using *SpotLite* digital camera and *Image-Pro* computer software. MitoLightTM Apoptosis Detection Kit (Chemicon) was used to detect apoptosis in the DA (SK-N-SH) neurons and genetically-engineered mice in response to chronic MPTP (30 mg/kg, i.p. for 7 days). Human Cyt-C ELISA kit was used to measure Cyt-C released from mitochondria into cytoplasm with a detection sensitivity of < 0.31 ng/ml. IHC apoptosis detection kit was utilized to quantitate apoptosis. APO-BRDU-IHCTM is dual-color staining kit for labeling DNA strand breaks found in apoptotic cells. These strand breaks produce numerous 3'-hydroxyl ends which can be labeled with bromolated nucleotides. A biotinylated BrdU antibody then binds to these labeled ends. Following incubation with strepavidin, the labeled DNA strand breaks are visualized using $DAB/H_2O_2/urea$. This kit can also be used for staining of paraffin embedded tissue sections, cryostat sections, and cell preparations fixed on slides.

Radioimmunoprecipitation: The cells were exposed to log concentrations of MPP^+ or SIN-1, and the suspensions were incubated for 45 min in Falcon T25 flasks containing $1\mu Ci/ml$ ^{35}S-methionine at 37^0C in 5% CO_2 incubator, centrifuged at 12,00 rpm for 6 min and the supernatant was discarded. 10 µl of cell lysate was used to determine protein concentration in each cell suspension using Bio-Rad micro titer protein assay and BSA as standard. The rest of the lysate were treated with respective monoclonal antibody to α-Syn (1:500 dilution). 100 µl/ml of protein-A agarose were added and samples were incubated on a shaker for 18 hrs at 4^0C. The samples were centrifuged at 13,000 rpm at 4^0C in eppendorf centrifuge for 20 min. The radioimmunoprecipitate was reconstituted in 100 µl of PBS-TDS buffer. 25 µl of the immunoprecipitate was dissolved in scintillation fluid and counted above background in a Beckman-Coulter TriCarb β scintillation counter. The rest of the lysate was used for immunoblotting.

Immunoblotting: For immunoblotting 15 µg protein from cell lysates was loaded in 10% polyacrylamide gel. Slab gel electrophoresis was performed in a buffer containing Tris:Glycine:SDS buffer at 4^0C using Bio-Rad electrophoresis power supply at 200 V for 1 hr. The gels were electroblotted on to PVDF membranes and incubated in 5% nonfat milk overnight at 4^0C, probed with respective antibodies for 1 hr (α-Syn: 1:500) at room temperature. Following washing thrice in 1% nonfat milk in PBS treated with 1:3000 secondary antibody (Horse radish peroxidase-labelled antimouse IgG) for 1 hr. The blots were washed thrice in PBS containing 0.1% Triton X-100 for 15 min and exposed to ECL chemiluminescence enhancement reagent as per instructions of the manufacturers and exposed to Kodak X-Ray X-OMAT film for 5-10 min. The autoradiograms were analysed using Bio-Rad GS-800 Imaging densitometer. The expression of nitrosylated (32 kDa band) bands was quantitatively estimated using Sigma plot version 4.02 software. The expression of α-Syn, in response to $MPP^{+,}$ and SIN-1 in different experimental genotypes was quantified UVP Gel documentation system equipped with Labworks software.

Immunofluorescence Microscopy: Brain regional expression of α-Syn and MTs (1,2), and Ferritin was estimated employing digital fluorescence imaging microscopy. The animals were perfused with 10% buffered formaldehyde. 5-8 µm thick brain sections were cut using Hacker Brite microcryostat set at -20^0C. The sections were placed on microscopic slides coated with 1% bovine serum albumin and brought to water by progressive hydration. Nonspecific binding was blocked by treating the sections with 3% BSA solution for 1 hr and exposed to α-Syn (dilution 1:5000), MT-1 (dilution 1:3000), and ferritin (dilution 1:8000) primary antibodies for 20 min and washed thrice in PBS, pH 7.4, treated with FITC and cy3 labeled anti-mouse IgG secondary antibodies (dilution 1:30,000) for 2 hrs. The slides were washed thrice in PBS (pH 7.4) for 15 min and mounted in aquamount supplemented with a photo bleach inhibitor. The tissue sections were examined, using *SpotLite* digital camera and analyzed using *ImagePro* software. The images were merged to determine the exact functional interaction of MT-1 with α-Syn and ferritin.

Neuromelanin Estimation: Melanin was estimated as described by Zecca et al (2002). Cell pellet (1 mg) was suspended in 1 ml of phosphate buffer (50 mM). The tubes were shaken, centrifuged at 9000Xg for 30 min and the supernatant discarded. The pellet was incubated with shaking for 2 hrs at 37^0C with 1 ml of Tris buffer (50 mM, pH 7.4) solution containing sodium dodecyl sulphate (5mg/ml) and 200 µg/ml proteinase K (Sigma St Louis, MO USA). The fine suspension of the pigment was centrifuged at 9000g for 30 min. The pellet was washed with 0.5 ml of NaCl solution (9 mg/ml) and 0.5 ml of water and then centrifuged as described above. The Melanin residue was dissolved in 1 ml of 1M NaOH at 80^0C for 1 hr. The obtained solution was centrifuged and the supernatant was transferred to quartz cuvette; its absorbance was measured at 350 nm. Standard curves were run by dissolving known amounts (1, 5, 10, 20 30 and 50 µg) of melanin in 1m l of 1M NaOH at 80^0C for 1hr. The detection limit of this assay is 30±5 ng/mg protein. Metal ions (Fe^{3+}, Cu^{2+}, Zn^{2+}, and Ca^{2+}) analysis of melanin was done by Atomic absorption spectrometry as describe earlier (Sharma and Ebadi , 2003).

[18]F-dG synthesis. [18]FdG was synthesized by SN-2 nucleophilic substitution reaction in a single reaction vessel configuration with trap and release column using supervisory control and documentation analysis (SCADA) node and view node software of the Siemens-CTI, 11 MeV Negative Ion, RDS-111 Cyclotron. The detailed procedure of the cyclotron operation and [18]F⁻ production is described in our recent publications (Sharma and Ebadi 2005; Sharma et al., 2006). The [18]F⁻ ions were trapped in kryptofix (K-222) [composition: 100 mg of K-222; 30 mg of K_2CO_3 in 9 ml of anhydrous acetonitrile]. K_2CO_3 (2.07g in 30 ml of water) was used for the activation of QMA column and for the separation of [18]O water from ^{18}F water. The trapped ^{18}F ions were released into the reaction vessel for aziotropic distillation with CH_3CN. The precursor, 1,3,4,6 tetra-O-acetyl, 2-O-trifluromethanesulphonyl, β-D-mannopyranose (Mannose Triflate) was subjected to SN-2 nucleophilic substitution reaction with [18]F⁻ ions to obtain tetra acetyl ^{18}F-dG. The tetra acetyl [18]FdG was hydrolyzed with 1N HCl to obtain crude [18]FdG, which was passed through AG-50 to remove K-222, AG-11 to remove unreacted HCl, through alumina (Al_2O_3) column to remove free [18]F⁻ ions, and through C-18 column to remove traces of tetra acetyl ^{18}F-dG intermediates. Ten ml of Milli-Q water was added in the reaction vessel and passed through the columns to recover [18]FdG. The final product was passed through Millipore 0.22-µm-syringe tip filter to remove pyrogens and other impurities. Routine quality control procedures were performed before administration of [18]FdG in animals.

^{18}F-DOPA Synthesis. ^{18}F-DOPA was synthesized by regioselective electrophilic substitution reaction using GINA Star synthesis module as described in our recent

publications (Sharma and Ebadi 2005; Sharma et al., 2006). Briefly; ^{18}F-DOPA was synthesized essentially in two synthesis steps (i) electrophilic substitution and (ii) fluorodestannlyzation. The reagent vessels were filled with chemicals in the following sequence: Vessel 1: 3.5 ml of precursor (30-mg triboc, trimethyl stanalyl L-dihydroxyl phenyl alanine in Freon), Vessel 2: 48% of 1.8 ml hydrobromic acid (HBr), Vessel 3: 1.2 ml buffer [composition: $(NH_4)_2HPO_4$ (1M)+$(NH_4H_2PO_4$ (1M) (50/50)], and Vessel 4: 1.1 ml of 25% NH_4OH. The Dewar flask was filled with liquid nitrogen to trap fluorine from Freon in the reaction vessel. Cold runs of F-DOPA were performed in the synthesis module to monitor the position of the ^{18}F-DOPA before running the cyclotron beam. The eluant was monitored for UV absorbance (282 nm) and radioactivity simultaneously.

MicroPET Imaging. Neuroimaging with ^{18}FdG and ^{18}F-DOPA was performed because these radioliopharmaceuticals are used frequently in clinical practice. Recently we have also used these radiopharmaceuticals in wv/wv mice and MTs gene manipulated mice to determine brain regional mitochondrial bioenergetics and dopaminerergic neurotransmission (Sharma et al., 2006). The scanning was performed by microPET (R-4) imaging system equipped with microPET Manager for the data acquisition in list mode and ASIPro for preparing the sinograms and image reconstruction. The microPET scanner was calibrated using plastic phantoms (150 mmX15 mm with 7 mm central hole along with ^{68}Ge Line Source). Random radioactivity correction, electronic dead time correction, normalization correction, attenuation correction, scatter correction, and injection dead time corrections was made before image reconstruction. To establish a functional relationship between DA-ergic neurotransmission and mitochondrial oxidative phosphorylation, ^{18}F-DOPA imaging was performed on the first day and ^{18}FdG imaging of the same animal on the second day at same settings. No residual activity is detected from the previous experiment after 24 hrs. The animals were anesthetized with 350-mg/kg i.p. tribromoethane and 250 µCi/0.1 ml of radioactivity was injected through the caudal vein. The list mode data was fast Fourier transformed (FFT) to generate sinograms. The sinograms were used to generate histograms, which were back-projected to reconstruct final images using ASIPro software. Ordered subset expectation maximization (OSEM) statistics was applied to quantitatively estimate voxel by voxel brain regional radioactivity and establish a functional relationship between mitochondrial bioenergetic and dopaminergic neurotransmission.

Quantitative Analysis: A positron emitting ^{68}Ge source of 500-µCi was used to quantitatively estimate ^{18}FdG or ^{18}F-DOPA uptake in the region of interest (ROI: striatum). ^{68}Ge source scanning was performed with a spatial resolution of 1.2 mm, temporal resolution 12.5 nSec, slice thickness 800-µm, and electronic resolution 10-nSec. 127 slices were prepared in the longitudinal plan and 62 slices in the transverse plan to estimate radioactivity in nCi/CC using ASIPro software. The factor was determined by taking a ratio of calculated vs the actual radioactivity. This factor was used to determine *Mean and Standard Deviation* of radioactivity from the image slices as described in our recent publication (Sharma and Ebadi 2005; Sharma et al 2006; Ebadi and Sharma 2006).

Statistical Analysis: Repeated measures analysis of variance (Repeated-ANOVA) was employed for the statistical evaluation of the experimental data using Sigma-Stat (version 2.03). Values of $p < 0.05$ was considered significant.

Observations and Results

Although there could be several genetic, environmental, and dietary factors, which might play a role in the etiopathogenesis of PD, world wide survey has indicated that the incidence of PD is high among population of European decent as compared to African Americans, Chinese and Indians (Lang and Lozano 1998). We have discovered that MT_{trans} mice had significantly high levels of melanin in their skin, hair and substantia nigra as compared to $control_{wt}$, α-syn knock out, and MT_{dko} mice (Sharma etal 2004). In particular, melanin levels were significantly reduced in MT_{dko} as well as α-syn knockout mice (Figure 1). Furthermore MT_{dko} mice exhibited significantly reduced threshold to MPTP-induced Parkinsonism. Chronic treatment of MPTP (30 mg/kg, i.p) induced severe tremors in MT_{dko} as compared to $control_{wt}$ and MT_{trans} mice as illustrated in Figure 2. We also established that MT gene over-expression suppresses Lewy Body synthesis by inhibiting α-Syn nitration (Sharma and Ebadi 2003).

A   **B**

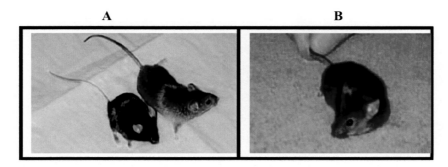

Figure 1. **A** Photographs illustrating that MT gene over-expression enhances melanin, while knocking out this gene suppresses melanin production in the skin, hair, and substantia nigra. Left Panel Black: MT_{trans}, Grey: MT_{dko}. **B:** Right Panel Grey: α-synko. MT_{dko} mice exhibit lethargic behavior, obesity, and reduced threshold to MPTP-Induced parkinsonism as compared to MT_{trans} mice. MT_{trans} mice exhibited increased vigilance state and genetic resistance to MPTP neurotoxicity. Photographs were taken using Olympus camera set at autofocus.

MT_{trans}   MT_{dko}

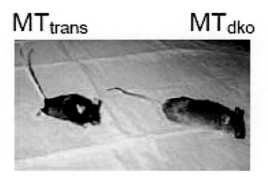

Figure 2. Left: MT_{trans} mice were lean, agile, and possessed dark silky smooth coat (left), while MT_{dko} mice were obese, lethargic and exhibited dull gray coat (right). Chronic treatment of MPTP (30 mg/kg, i.p.) for 7 days induced immobilization and muscular rigidity in MT_{dko} mice, while MT_{trans} mice could still walk with their stiff legs and erect tail, suggesting genetic resistance of MT_{trans} mice to experimental Parkinsonism.

α-Syn-MT$_{tko}$ Mice were prepared by crossbreeding α-synuclein knock out males with MT$_{dko}$ female mice. The progeny was genotyped with tail DNA analysis employing PCR and immunoblotting. Absence of three genes (MT1, MT2, and α-Syn) confirmed that these genetically engineered animals remain alive. α-Syn-MT$_{tko}$ mice possessed brown coat, while control$_{wt}$ litter-mates black coat. α-Syn-MT$_{tko}$ mice exhibited stiff tail, reduced body movements, and lethargic behavior. They were obese as compared to control$_{wt}$ and MT$_{trans}$ mice. Hair, skin, and SN-melanin were significantly reduced in α-Syn-MT$_{tko}$ mice as compared to control$_{wt}$ and MT$_{trans}$ mice. Mitochondrial coenzyme Q$_9$, and Q$_{10}$ were also significantly (p <0.05, ANOVA) reduced in α-Syn-MT$_{tko}$ mice striatum.

α-Syn-Ferritin Interaction in Mice Striatum

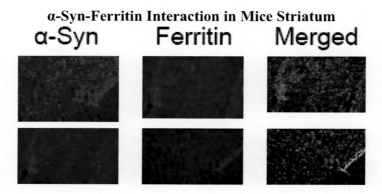

Figure 3. Upper panels: MT$_{trans}$, Lower panels: MT$_{dko}$ mice striatum. Immunofluorescence microscopic examination of striatal α-Syn and Ferritin immunoreacitivity, illustrating increased α-Syn and reduced Ferritin expression in MT$_{dko}$ as compared to MT$_{trans}$ mice striatum.

α-Syn-MT-1 Interaction: Cerebellar Cortex

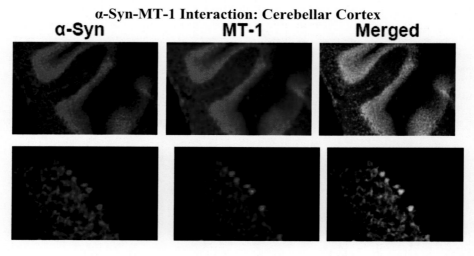

Figure 4. Upper panels: Cerebellar cortex at low magnification (X100), Lower panels: Cerebellar cortex at higher magnification (X400). Purkinje cells are highly rich in MT-1 immunoreactivity. Granular neurons are rich in α-Syn.

Multiple fluorochrome comet assay was developed to determine 8-OH, 2dG synthesis and DNA fragmentation simultaneously in response to Parkinsnian neurotoxins. By performing multiple fluorochrome comet assays, we have demonstrated that transfection of SK-N-SH neurons with MT-1$_{sense}$ oligonucleotides suppressed MPP$^+$-apoptosis and remained restricted to mitochondrial damage (Figure 4, middle panel) [Green fluorescence due to 8-OH, 2dG], while with antisense oligonucleotides to MT-1 enhanced apoptosis and it was extended to nuclear DNA damage (as illustrated by ethidium bromide (red) fluorescent comet tails (Figure 4, lower panel).

MTs Neuroprotection

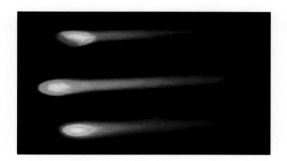

Figure 5. Multiple fluorochrome comet tail assay illustrating resistance of MT-1$_{sense}$-transfected as compared to MT-1$_{antisense}$ oligonucleotide-transfected SK-N-SH neurons in response to overnight exposure to MPP$^+$ (10µM). Upper panel: Control$_{wt}$, Middle panel:MT-1$_{sense}$, Lower panel: MT-1$_{Antisense.}$

MT$_{trans}$ striatal fetal stem cells exhibited genetic resistance to SIN-1-induced apoptosis, characterized by plasma membrane perforations, nuclear DNA fragmentation and condensation as illustrated in Figure 6.

MT$_{trans}$ Fetal Mice striatal stem cells

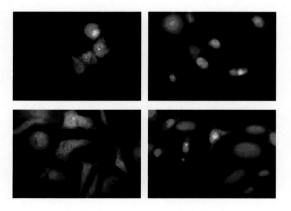

Figure 6. MT$_{trans}$ fetal mice striatal stem cells were resistant to MPP$^+$ (10 µM) apoptosis as compared to MT$_{dko}$ fetal stem cells. MPP$^+$ (10 µM) neurotoxicity in MT$_{dko}$ mice was represented by both apoptosis as well as necrosis. Digital fluorescence images were captured using *SpotLite* Digital camera and *ImagePro* computer software.

Molecular Mechanisms of MT-Induced Neuroprotection

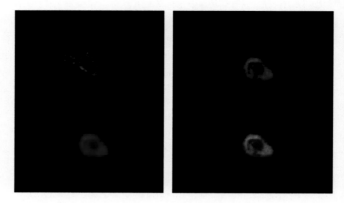

Figure 7. Molecular translocation of MT-1 towards the perinuclear and endonuclear regions during MPP$^+$ (10 μM)-induced apoptosis in mouse striatal fetal stem cells. Digital fluorescence images were captured by *SpotLite* digital camera and analyzed using *ImagePro* computer software. Target accentuation and background inhibition computer software was employed to improve the quality of fluorescence images. Green: FITC-conjugated MT-1 antibody, Red: JC-1. A: Control: Metallothionein, B: Mitochondria, C: Metallothionein, D: Metallothionein+Mitochondria.

Overnight treatment of 6-OH-DA induced peri-nuclear aggregation of α-Syn in control$_{wt}$ as well as MT$_{trans}$ striatal fetal stem cells. MT$_{trans}$ striatal fetal stem cells exhibited significantly suppressed peri-nuclear accumulation of α-Syn as illustrated in Figure 8.

Induction and Translocation of MT-1 by 6-OH-DA

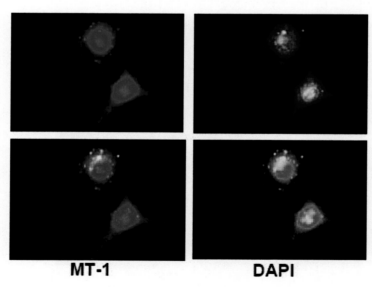

MT-1   **DAPI**

Figure 8. Digital fluorescence imaging microscopy of 6-OH-DA (1μM)-induced apoptosis in SK-N-SH neurons. Dopamine oxidation product, 6-OH-DA-induced apoptosis and translocated MT-1 in the perinuclear and endonuclear regions within 24 hrs in the DA neurons, suggesting the neuroprotective role of MT-1 in PD. (Fluorescence images were captured with SpotLite Digital Camera equipped with ImagePro software.

MT depletion in aging RhO$_{mgko}$ neurons triggers not only mitochondrial but also nuclear apoptosis via enhanced production of DNA oxidation product, 8-OH 2dG. α-Syn over-expressed aging RhO$_{mgko}$ neurons exhibited enhanced DNA damage in response to overnight exposure to MPP$^+$.

6-OHDA-Induced Caspase-3 Activation and Mitochondrial Apoptosis
Basal   6-OH-DA (100 µM)

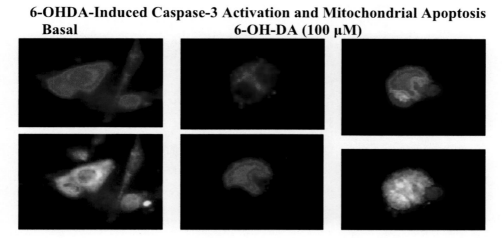

Figure 9. Digital Fluorescence Imaging Microscopy of dopaminergic neurons in response to overnight exposure to 6-OH-DA demonstrating perinuclear and endonuclear accumulation of activated Caspase-3 (Green), and aggregation of mitochondria (Red). (Caspase-3 is localized predominantly in the aggregating Mitochondria) Green: FITC-Conjugated Anti-caspase-3, Red: JC-1, Blue: DAPI.

MPP+-induced α-Syn-positive aggregates in Fetal Stem Cells

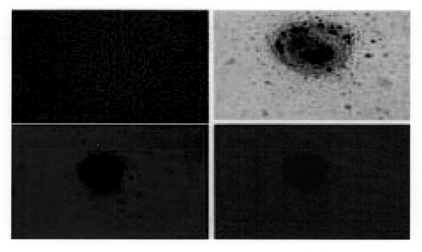

Figure 10. Formation of α-Syn-positive aggregates in response to chronic low doses of MPP$^+$ (100 nM) for 6-8 weeks to striatal fetal stem cells. Upper left panel: control, Upper right panel: phase contrast microscopic picture of α-Syn-positive aggregates surrounded by neuromelanin. Lower left panel; α-Syn-immunoreactivity; Lower right panel: Nitrated α-Syn immunoreactivity. MT$_{trans}$ striatal fetal stem cells were quite resistant to MPP$^+$ neurotoxicity and exhibited α-Syn –positive aggregates.

FeSO$_4$-Induces Mitochondrial damage and α-Syn Aggregation

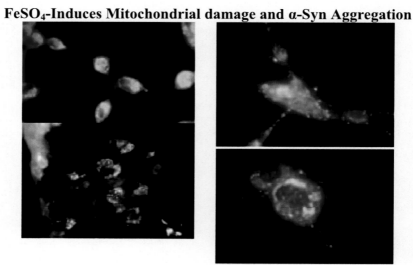

Figure 11. Digital Fluorescence Imaging Microscopy illustrating α-Syn and mitochondrial aggregation in the perinuclear region in response to overnight exposure to FeSO$_4$. Fluorescence images were digitized by SpotLite digital camera and analyzed using ImagePro computer software. Green: FITC-Anti-α-Syn, Red: JC-1. Upper left panel: Basal, Lower left panel: FeSO$_4$:100 nM, Upper right panel: FeSO$_4$: 100 μM; FeSO$_4$: 1000 μM.

MTs Inhibit α-Syn Nitration *(A Lewy Body Rudiment)*
Basal   6-(OH)DA

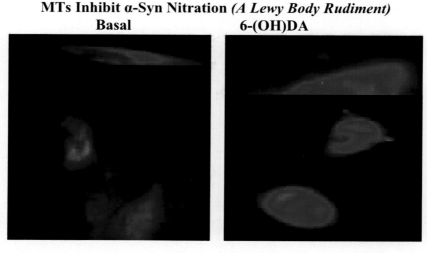

Figure 12. Immunofluorescence of nitrated alpha-Syn in control$_{wt}$ and MT$_{trans}$ fetal stem cells in response to 6-OHDA (10 μM) treatment overnight. 6-OHDA exposure induced induction as well as perinuclear aggregation of nitrated α-Syn particularly in contol$_{wt}$ cells. Nitration of α-Syn iresponse to 6-OHDA is significantly suppressed in MT$_{trans}$ fetal stem cells, suggesting the neuroprotective action of MT gene overexpression in PD. Cells were immunostained using FITC-congugated nitrated α-Syn recognizing primary antibody. Fluorescence images were captured by SpotLite digital camera and analyzed using ImagePro Computer software.

Melanin-Induced Neuroprotection

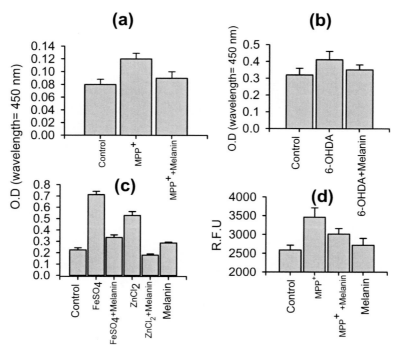

O.D. = Optical Density R.F.U= Relative Fluorescence Intensity Units.
MPP+ and 6-OHDA = 10 μM Melanin = 10 μM $FeSO_4$ and $ZnCl_2$ = 100 μM.

Figure 13. Lipid peroxidation and caspase-3 activation were studied in DA (SK-N-SH) neurons following overnight exposure to MPP$^+$ (10 μM), 6-OHDA (10 μM), $FeSO_4$ (100 μM), and $ZnCl_2$ (100 μM). Lipid peroxidation was determined colorimerically using thiobarbituric acid reagent, while capase-3 activation was estimated spectrofluorometrically employing a fluorogenic caspase-3 substrate, AC-DEVD-AMC, and inhibitor AC-DEVD-CHO. Melanin suppressed MPP$^+$, 6-OHDA, $FeSO_4$, and $ZnCl_2$-induced increase in lipid peroxidation and caspase-3 activation in DA (SK-N-SH) neurons.

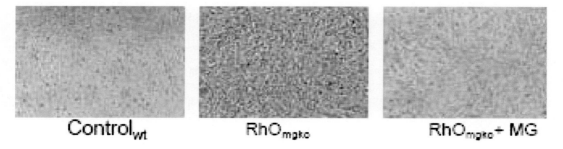

Figure 14. A: Phase contrast microscopic picture of control$_{wt}$ SK-N-SH) neurons; B: Aging mitochondrial genome knock out (RhO$_{mgko}$) neurons; C: Aging mitochondrial genome knock out (RhO$_{mgko}$) neurons transfected with mitochondrial genome encoding complex-1 activity.

Selective down-regulation of the mitochondrial genome was done by growing the neurons in Dulbecco's modified Eagle's medium, supplemented with high glucose, glutamine, 3.7g/l $NaHCO_3$ and 5 µg/ml ethidium bromide for 6-8 weeks. This treatment selectively down-regulates the mitochondrial genome without affecting the nuclear genome. Aging RhO_{mgko} neurons exhibit typical granular appearance, reduced proliferative potential, exaggerated neurotoxicity in response to Parkinsonian agents and compromised recovery in response to antioxidants. Partial recovery was observed in aging RhO_{mgko} neurons, transfected with mitochondrial genome encoding complex-1 activity. This was confirmed by estimating SIN-1-induced lipid peroxidation, caspase-3 activation, protein carbonylation, complex-1 activity, and α-Syn nitration. Phase contrast images of the neurons were captured with SpotLite Digital camera and analyzed by ImagePro computer software.

We have measured mitochondrial membrane potential ($\Delta\Psi$) in $control_{wt}$ and aging mitochondrial genome knock out RhO_{mgko} neurons employing dual fluorochrome analysis. Mitochondrial $\Delta\Psi$ was significantly reduced in RhO_{mgko} as compared to $control_{wt}$ neurons as assessed by Desipher. A digital fluorescence microscopic picture illustrating $\Delta\Psi$ is presented in Figure 9.

α-Syn expression was significantly induced upon exposure of SK-N-SH neurons to MPP^+ overnight in control as well as aging RhO_{mgko} neurons. α-Syn was translocated in the perinuclear region in control and endocnuclear region in the RhO_{mgko} neuron upon MPP^+ exposure. Pretreatment with Selegiline suppressed these changes.

| 1. Ferrtin | 2 Ferritin+α-Syn | 3:α-Syn | 4:LB | 5:Degeneration |

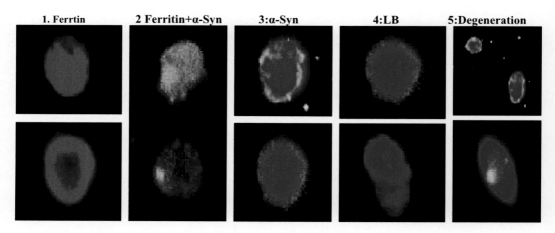

Figure 15. Based on double immunofluorescence microscopic examination of ferritin and α-Syn immunmoreactivity in SK-N-SH neurons in response to increasing concentrations (10-1000 µM) FeSO4, we have arbitrarily divided five different phases of neurodegenration. 1: Ferritin-dominant phase 2: Ferritin+ α-Syn-dominant phase, 3: α-Syn-dominant phase, 4: LB phase, and 5: Neurodegenerative phase.

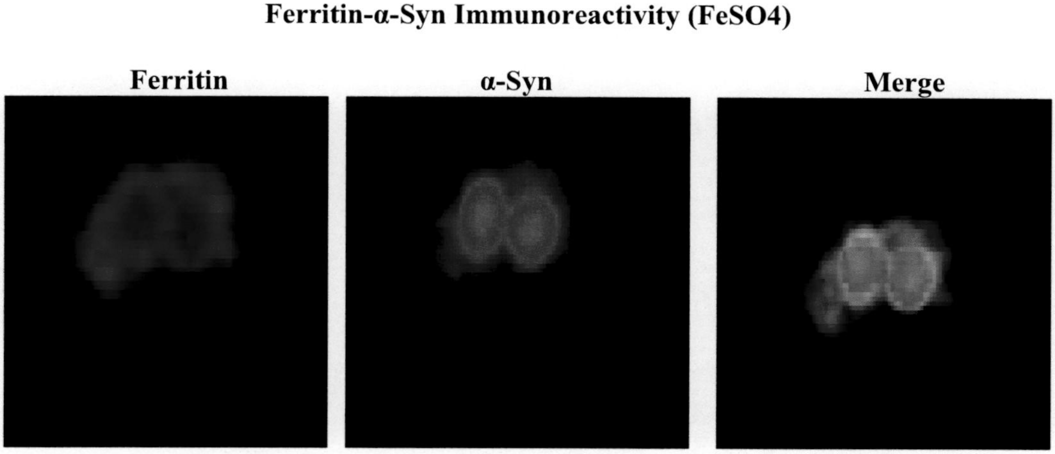

Ferritin-α-Syn Immunoreactivity (FeSO4)

Ferritin	α-Syn	Merge

Figure 16. FeSO₄-induced lipid peroxidation induced structural degradation of plasma membranes in SK-N-SH neurons (FeSO₄ = 250 µM; overnight treatment).

α-Syn was translocated in the nuclear region, while Ferritin remained restricted in the degraded plasma membrane. Ferritin is large molecular weight protein (440 kDa), while MT-1 and α-Syn are low molecular weight proteins (6-7kDA and 14 kDa respectively). During oxidative stress, ferritin remains restricted to cytoplasmic compartment, while MT-1 and α-Syn are translocated in the perinuclear and endonuclear regions in order to afford neuroprotection. Free radical-induced lipid peroxidation-induce plasma membrane perforations and release of ferritin in the extracellular space.

MTs Augment Striatal ^{18}F-DOPA and ^{18}FdG uptake in wv/wv mice

Crossbreeding of wv/wv female mice with MT_{trans} male mice provided colonies of wv/wv-MTs mice with significantly improved ^{18}F-DOPA and ^{18}FdG uptake as illustrated below. Chronic METH (2.5 mg/kg i.p for 1 month) reduced striatal dopamine and body weight whereas 4 months withdrawal induced obesity in C57BL6J mice. METH withdrawal obesity and reduction in the striatal dopamine were attenuated in wv/wv-MTs mice suggesting the neuroprotective role of MTs in drug addiction.

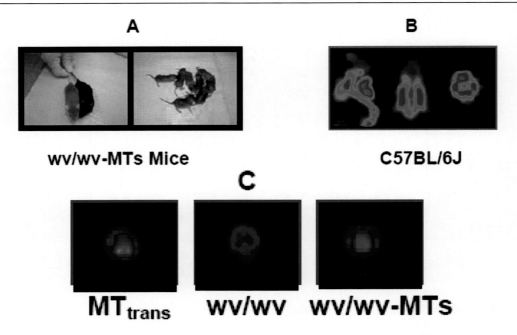

Figure 17. A: Left: Parents; Brown wv/wv female; Black: MT$_{trans}$ Male; Right: Progeny of wv/wv-MTs mice. B: ^{18}FdG microPET imaging of C57Bl/6J mouse in transverse, coronal, and sagittal planes. Right panel: ^{18}FdG is localized primarily in the CNS, adipose tissue, lungs, and in the myocardium. C: ^{18}FdG uptake is reduced in wv/wv mouse brain as compared to MT$_{trans}$ mouse. wv/wv-MTs mouse exhibits increased ^{18}FdG uptake as compared to wv/wv mouse as illustrated in the right panel, indicating that MTs augment DA-ergic neurotransmission. The microPET imaging was performed as described in our recent publications (Sharma et al., 2006).

Discussion

We have studied the role of oxidative and nitrative stresss in the etiopathogenesis of PD using in-vitro SK-N-SH neurons and genetically-engineered mice over-expressing either MTs or under-expressing α-Syn as well as MT. To correlate and confirm in-vitro observations, we have employed in-vivo approach utilizing MT$_{trans}$, MT$_{dko}$, and α-syn knock out mice. We have determined the extent of neurotoxicity of various Parkinsonian agents, (including MPP$^+$, MPTP, and 6-OHDA) and have evaluated the neuroprotective potential MTs in these animals as well as in cultured and fetal stem cells derived from the mesenchymal regions of these genetically-engineered animals. MT gene over-expression enhanced melanin biosynthesis in the dopaminergic neurons. We have estimated melanin in the SK-N-SH neurons in reponse to Zn^{2+} and Fe^{2+} ions which enhance MT gene expression. Our studies have established for the first time, that MT gene over-expression (i) inhibits α-Syn nitration (ii) and augments melanin biosynthesis in order to afford neuroprotection in the dopaminergic neurons. MT$_{trans}$ mice had shiny dark coat, while MT$_{dko}$ and α-syn$_{ko}$ mice were gray in color with significantly reduced melanin content in their hair, skin, and substantia nigra as compared to control$_{wt}$ and MT$_{trans}$ mice. These observations are interpreted to suggest that MT-induced neuroprotection in the MT_{trans} mice and dopaminergic neurons are mediated through melanin synthesis, which is significantly reduced in PD patients.

We have now demonstrated that melanin content in the skin, hair as well as in the SN might have certain important yet unexplored role to perform in the genetic predisposition to Parkinsonism among aging population of various origins. MT promoter is known to enhance α-MSH gene which triggers cAMP-dependent tyrosine kinase gene, involved in the physiological activation and phophorylation of tyrosinase, which synthesizes melanin from tyrosine (Taguchi et al 1998, Ao et al 1998, Borovansky J. (1994). Iwamoto et al 2001, Iwamoto et al 2001, Kupper et al 1990, Larue and Mintz 1990). It has been reported that melanin suppresses lipid peroxidation induced by ferrous ions (Korytowski et al., 1995), and is even more potent scavenger of O_2^- radicals compared to SOD and GSH and participates in the cellular protection against oxidative stress (Corsaro et al., 1995). Microinjections of striatal fetal stem cells in the degenerated substantia nigra of PD patients developed melanin synthesis as a function of aging (Check 2002). Melanin possesses strong chelating ability for iron and an affinity for lipids, pesticides, and MPP^+. Neuronal accumulation of melanin during aging and the link between its synthesis and high cytosolic concentration of catecholes suggests its protective role, which could be attenuated in conditions of toxin overload (Zecca et al., 2001). Furthermore, neuromelanin is the major iron storage site in the SN neurons of normal aging subjects (Zecca et al., 2001). Melanin content is reduced in the SN of PD patients suggesting its neuroprotective role (Zecca et al., 2002). Recent studies have demonstrated that melanin significantly decreases the amount of 3 nitrotyrosine formed by peroxynitrite ions and inhibited peroxynitrite-induced formation of linoleic acid hydroperoxides, both in the absence and presence of bicarbonate, suggesting that it can act as a natural scavenger of $ONOO^-$ ions (Stepien et al., 2000). We have discovered that melanin is significantly increased in MTtrans mice nigrostriatal system hence one of the possible molecular mechanisms of neuroprotection of MTs could be through augmented melanin synthesis.

In fetal stem cells derived from control$_{wt}$ type mice, α-syn-positive aggregates were synthesized within 6 weeks of exposure to low concentrations of MPP^+. The α-Syn-positive aggregates were surrounded by melanin, suggesting that melanin synthesis might inhibit Lewy body formation in PD as reported by Betarbet et al (2001). Melanin also forms a storehouse for various metal ions involved in the progression of PD, such as Fe and Zn. These ions are increased in the SN of Parkinson's patients. Excessive iron and zinc could also enhance α-Syn aggregation, which could eventually participate in Lewy body synthesis. Melanin also suppressed SIN-1 induced mitochondrial damage in the dopaminergic neurons as confirmed by E.M. Examination. By employing double radioimmunprecipitation, we have established that SIN-1-induced increase in Syn index *(Syn Index SI = Nitrated α-Syn/Native α-Syn)*, is suppressed in the presence of melanin, suggesting that MT gene over-expression suppresses α-Syn nitration by enhanced melanin biosynthesis in the nigrostriatal DA neurons.

We have now demonstrated that MT is translocated in the peri-nuclear and endo-nuclear regions in response to SIN-1. SIN-1-induced oxidation of dopamine to 6-OH-DA caused apoptosis in the SK-N-SH neurons. Furthermore, overnight exposure of 6-OH-DA caused molecular induction and translocation of MTF-1 as well as MT-1 in SK-N-SH neurons, as assessed by immunofluorescence microscopy, suggesting its neuroprotective role through zinc-mediated transcriptional regulation of antiapoptotic genes.

It seems that DAT remains genetically stable in MTs-over-expressed DA neurons and vise versa and MTs protect DA-ergic neurons by attenuating oxidative and nitrative stress to DAT. This hypothesis is based on recent studies which have shown that DAT is highly sensitive to redox imbalance and is blocked by ONOO⁻ attack. Peroxynitrite ions bind with dopamine to produce dopamine-quinones, which bind specifically with the DAT to block its activity (Park et al., 2002). Blockade of DAT inhibits DBH and TH activities in the DA neurons, hence antioxidants such as MT could have neuroprotective role through scavenging action of free radicals. Furthermore, MPP⁺-induced DA neurotoxicity occurs through an interaction between mutant α-Syn and the DAT (Lehmensick et al., 2002). In view of the above, it will be important to establish the contribution of MTs genes in the modulation of DAT activity in response to MPP⁺ and SIN-1 exposure to establish the neuroprotective potential of MT induction. DAT activity can be estimated in vitro using ^{3}H-Dopamine uptake and β-scintillation spectrometry in vitro, and invivo by employing ^{18}F-DOPA uptake and high-resolution micro-PET neuroimaging as we have reported (Sharma et al., 2006).

The exact pathophysiological significance of MTs-induced attenuation of nitration, and induction of α-Syn phosphorylation in response to MPTP-induced NOS activation and cytokine (IL-6)-induced CNS injury remains elusive. We have discovered that MT protects neurons by suppressing α-Syn nitration and enhancing its tyrosine phosphorylation. Furthermore MT induction suppresses MPTP-induced NOS and cytokine (IL-6) activation, involved in the etiopathogenesis of PD. α-Syn nitration in control$_{wt}$, MT$_{trans}$, and MT$_{dko}$ mice striatum and SN was determined by double radioimmunprecipitation, immunoblotting, and digital fluorescence imaging microscopy using multiple fluorochrome analysis. Quantitative analysis of α-Syn nitration was made by estimating α-Syn indices. This study was based on the hypothesis that MTs scavenge peroxynitrite ions involved α-Syn nitration and IL-6 induction. The rationale of this study was based on the findings that oxidatively-modified α-Syn is more prone to aggregation than native protein (Souza et al., 2000). Elevated α-Syn expression may itself induce oxidative and nitrative stress in PD (Hsu et al., 2000). Chronic low-grade complex-1 inhibition by rotenone also induced accumulation and aggregation of α-Syn and ubiquitin, progressive damage, and caspase-dependent apoptosis (Sherer et al., 2002).

Usually α-Syn is involved in the synthesis, storage, and release of dopamine (Perz et al., 2002), however point mutation at A30P and A53T can induce low grade DA neurotoxicity resulting in terminal degeneration and ultimately cell death (Lotharius et al., 2002). We have reported that MPTP-induced nitration of α-Syn is attenuated by MT gene over-expression in MT$_{trans}$ mice striatum and in DA neurons while down-regulation of MT-1, 2 genes in MT$_{dko}$ mice induced MPP⁺-induced α-Syn nitration (Sharma and Ebadi 2003). Mutant mice lacking the iNOS gene were comparatively more resistant to MPTP neurotoxicity, suggesting that iNOS is important in the MPTP neurotoxic process and indicates that inhibitors of iNOS may provide protective role in the treatment of PD (Dawson et al., 1998). NO, reacts with superoxides to form peroxynitrite, which plays a major role in the pathophysiology of stroke, PD, Huntington's disease and amyotrophic lateral sclerosis (Beckman et al., 1993; Brown et al., 1995; Beckman and Kopenol 1996; Bredt, 1999). Transfection of SK-N-SH neurons with either MT-1 or MT2 genes suppressed SIN-1-induced lipid peroxidation, caspase-3 activation, and apoptosis Furthermore, SIN-1 induced lipid peroxidation induced dopamine oxidation to DOPAL, which induced spontaneous apoptosis when administered in the MT_{dko} striatal fetal stem cells and particularly in aging RhO_{mgko} neurons possessing significantly reduced MT1, 2 levels. Furthermore, fetal stem cells from MT_{trans} mice were resistant to DOPAL-induced apoptosis, suggesting their clinical potential in neuron replacement therapy of PD (Sharma and Ebadi 2003; Ebadi et al., 2005).

We hypothesisized that MTF-1 is induced and translocated in the endonuclear region to influence MT transcription and several candidate genes are induced/repressed simultaneously during oxidative and/or nitrative stress of PD to establish SIN-1 and MPTP-induced activation and nucleocytoplasmic translocation of MTF-1 in MT gene manipulated dopaminergic neurons and its functional association with mitochondrial and nucleus-related apoptotosis. This study was designed to explore the molecular mechanism by which MPTP and SIN-1 activate metal responsive transcriptional factor (MTF-1) and its participation in the modulation of MT gene transcription. Nucleo-cytoplasmic shuttling of MTF-1 and MTs in $control_{wt}$, MT_{dko}, and MT_{trans} mice strital tissue and fetal stem cells under basal, and following acute/or chronic MPTP or SIN-1 intoxication were investigated employing immunoblotting, RT-PCR, and multiple fluorochrome digital fluorescence imaging microscopy. SIN-1-induced lipid peroxidation was measured using thiobarbituric acid reagent and caspase-3 activation assay was peroformed spectrofluorometrically, mitochondrial ultrastructural morphology was examined under electron microscopy, and apoptosis was estimated employing triple fluorochrome analysis, and multiple fluorochrome comet assays. Differential analysis of various genes involved in apoptosis and anti-apoptosis was conducted employing RT-PCR. SIN-1-induced dopamine oxidation to DOPAL and its suppression with MT gene induction were estimated using HPLC-EC. This study was based on recent studies which have shown that Ca^{2+}-dependent metal-Inducible phosphorylation of MTF-1 by protein kinase-C, tyrosine kinase, and casein kinase-II, is essential in the transcriptional activation of MTs during oxidative stress (Radke et al., 1993; Dalton et al., 1996; Saydam et al., 2001; Sydam et al., 2002). This study was designed to further explore the transcriptional regulation of MTs by zinc finger MTF-1. MTF-1 is a key regulator of heavy metal-induced transcription of MTs during metal homeostasis, oxidative and/or nitrative stress, and UV radiation, which is mediated through binding to metal responsive elements (MRE) of consensus TGCRCNC in the target gene promoters. Although MTF-1 has dual nuclear and cytoplasmic localization in response to above stress stimuli, its exact pathophysiological signficance in PD remains unknown. Simialrly, the basic molecular mechanism of MPTP-mediated MTF-1-induced MT-transcriptional activation of NF-κβ and Iκβ requires further elaboration. The amounts of MTF-1-DNA complexes are elevated several fold in zinc-treated cells, and is mediated by several copies of a 15 bp consensus sequence (Metal responsive element, MRE) present in the promoter region of MTs genes. MTF-1 has a consensus leucine-rich nuclear export signal (NES), located just N-terminal to the first zinc finger protein and is highly sensitive to oxidative stress and mediates sub-cellular localization and nucleo-cytoplasmic shuttling of MTs. Under resting conditions, NES is required for cytoplasmic localization of MTF-1. Nuclear localization signal (NLS) of MTF-1, which enters the nucleus not only upon metal load but also upon oxidative stress, heat shock, UV irradiation, low pH, inhibition of protein synthesis by cycloheximide, and serum factors, activate NF-κβ which has been shown to be under redox regulation, controlled by thioredoxin (TRX), and is one of the major endogenous redox-signaling molecules with thiol reducing activity in addition to MTs (Hirota et al., 1999, Das and White 2002).

As determined by microarry membrane hybridization, MPTP altered the expression of atleast 49-51 different genes involved in oxidative stress (oxidative stress-induced proteins A170, Cyt P450, 1A1, and Osp-94), inflammation (cytotoxic cytokines i.e IL-1, Il-6, TNFα), protective cytokines (Il-10), glutamate receptors (NMDA but not AMPA receptors), neurotrophic factors (GDNF, EGF, NOS, and transferrin receptor, cell cycle regulators, signal transduction factors) also induced in parallel to MPTP-oxidative stress and inflammation to converge eventually into a common pathways of neurodegeneration (Mandel et al., 2000). An iron chelator-radical scavenger, R-Apomorphine protected against MPTP-neurotoxicity by preventing the over-expression of above genes involved in apoptosis (Grunblatt et al., 2001). We have now explored the neuroprotective role of MT isoforms in attenuating α-Syn nitration involved in MPTP or SIN-1-induced neurodegenerative Parkinsonism. In view of the above, we investigated MPTP and SIN-1-induced nucleocytoplasmic translocation of MTF-1 and MTs in $control_{wt}$, MT_{dko} and MT_{trans} striatal neurons with a primary objective to.elucidate whether MTs play a role in the regulation of NF-κβ and Iκβ kinases transcription by enhancing their ability to bind DNA. Thus MTs-dependent regulation of the NF-κβ complex may be a novel activation mechanism of redox-sensitive transcription factors, which needs futher explorations. Hence cDNA microarrays will provide in detail high throughput differential screening of candidate and crucial genes involved in MPTP or SIN-1-induced oxidative and nitrative stress and the extent of their attenuation by MT gene induction. In particular it will be of interest to examine parallel interaction of Lewy body molecular markers (α-synuclein, Parkin, and ubiquntin), ferritin, transferrin, with MT isoforms and genes involved in melanin synthesis in SN dopaminergic neurons from different genotypes. This study might provide novel strategies to prevent and cure PD and may further help in new and effective drug designing.

To elucidate the contribution of MT in mitochondrial coenzyme Q_{10} and iron/ Ferritin hoemostasis and iNOS-mediated MTF-1 and NFκβ translocation in the DA neurons during acute and chronic MPTP neurotoxicity, we hypothesized that MT gene induction preserves mitochondrial coenzyme Q_{10} and ferritin levels, and hence α-Syn homeostasis in DA neurons. Mitochondrial coenzyme Q_{10} and ferritin from above described experimental genotypes were estimated employing HPLC with U.V. detector in an isocratic mode. Coenzyme Q_{10} and ferritin levels were estimated from MT-1,2 gene-transfected SK-N-SH neurons to correlate and confirm in-vivo observations. Striatal and SN mitochondrial iron levels from different experimental genotypes were determined using atomic absorption spectrometry. MT, α-Syn and Ferritin levels were estimated using sensitive ELISA and fluorescence immunocytochmistry. MT, α-Syn and Ferritin expressions were estimated at the transcriptional level employing RT-PCR, using specific primer sets. We have reported that glutathione and mitochondrial coenzyme Q_{10} levels are reduced in PD and in MPTP-induced Parkinsonism (Ebadi et al 2001). Brain regional levels of coenzyme Q_{10} remained preserved in the striatal tissue of MT_{trans} mice as compared to $control_{wt}$ and MT_{dko} mice (Sharma et al.,

2002). These experimental findings provided us a lead in further exploring the molecular mechanism of neuroprotection afforded by MTs gene over-expression in PD.

At this moment, it remains unknown, whether MTs gene manipulation could influence ubiquinone levels and hence mitochondrial function. Therefore, we investigated the role of MT gene induction in ferritin metabolism based on our recent report on iron-induced oxidative stress in the SK-N-SH neurons (Sangchot et al 2002). It is known that Ferritin levels are significantly depleted in the striatal and SN regions of PD patients, which would accumulate iron in the DA neurons. Iron participates in the Fenton reaction to generate highly toxic OH radicals, involved in neurodegeneration. Therefore, we hypothesized that MT gene induction would scavenge iron-induced OH radicals generation and thus protect ferritin degradation. Employing dual fluorochrome immunofluorescence microscopy, we have demonstrated that when α-Syn expression is increased, the ferritin expression is reduced and vise versa. These observations encouraged us to investigate further α-Syn-ferritin interaction in SK-N-SH neurons. Recently we have reported that selegline protects the dopaminergic neurons via MT gene induction (Ebadi et al., 1998, Ebadi et al., 2002). In view of the above, we examined the neuroprotective potential of selegline at the mitochondrial level using elecron microscopy. Overnight treatment of complex-1 inhibitor, MPP$^+$ (100 μM) induced mitochondrial damage in SK-N-SH neurons. The mitochondria exhibited swollen appearance, with loss of internal cirstae, and aggregation. Some of them were completely obliterated. Pre-incubation with selegiline attenuated MPP$^+$-induced mitochondrial damage, suggesting that endogenous and/or exogenous induction of MT by drugs such as selegiline could afford neuroprotection against PD (Sharma et al 2003).

To explore the exact pathophysiological significance of MTs-induced neuromelanin synthesis we hypothesized that MT-induced neuroprotection is mediated through preservation of neuromelanin in the dopaminergic neurons. Therefore, SN neuromelanin from above experimental genotypes was isolated as described by Zecca et al (2002) and its neuroprotective effect on FeS0$_4$-induced lipid peroxidation, capase-3 activation, mitochondrial complex-1 activity, and apoptosis was determined by concentration and time-dependent response curves. This was based on the hypothesis that one of the possible mechanisms of neuroprotection afforded by MT could be through enhanced melanin biosynthesis. Since the exact molecular mechanism of neuroprotection afforded by MT remains unknown, we have discovered that MTs inhibit α-Syn nitration and hence its aggregation via enhanced melanin biosynthesis, which acts as a potent free radical scavenger and suppresses SIN-1-induced protein nitrotyrosine synthesis in the DA neurons (Ebadi and Sharma 2006). In view of the above, a detailed study would be required to further explore α-Syn-MT and α-Syn-Melanin interaction in PD. Melanin can be structurally degraded in the lysosomes perhaps due to oxidative and/or nitrative stress during PD. However there is no report confirming this hypothesis. We hypothesize that the enzyme tyrosinase requires substrate specificity, while nitrotyrosine could readily participate in the synthesis of α-Syn, however nitrated α-Syn synthesized by the genetic apparatus would have deleterious consequences, as it might induce aggregation and Lewy body synthesis involved in the etio-pathogenesis of PD. *Hence brain regional MTs induction could provide neuroprotection by preventing α-Syn nitration and by augmenting neuromelanin and ferritin synthesis, both of* which are significantly reduced in PD. Further studies in this direction would go a long way in the clinical management of PD and other neurodegenerative disorders of unknown etiopathogenesis.

References

Ao Y, Park HY, Olaizola-Horn S, Gilchrest BA. (1998) Activation of cAMP-dependent protein kinase is required for optimal alpha-melanocyte-stimulating hormone-induced pigmentation. *Exp. Cell Res.* 244: 117-124.

Albano C, Muralikrishnan D, Ebadi M. (2002) Distribution of Coenzyme Q Homologues in Brain. *Neurochemical Res.* 27: 359-368.

Aschner M. (1996) The functional significance of brain metallothioneins. *FASEB J.* 10: 1129-1136.

Aschner M, Cherian MC, Klassen CD, Palmiter RDm Erickson JC, and Bush AI (1997) Metallothioneins in Brain-The Role in Physiology and Pathology. *Toxicol. Appl. Pharmacol.* 142: 229-242.

Beal, M.F. (1998) Excitotoxicity and nitric oxide in PD pathogenesis. *Ann. Neurol.* 44: S110-114.

Beckman JS, Carson M, Smith CDm Kopnel WH (1993) ALS, SOD, and peroxynitrite. *Nature* 364: 584.

Beckman JS, Koppenol WH (1996) Nitric oxide, superoxide, and peroxynitrite: the good, the bad, the ugly. *Am. J. Physiol.* 271: C1424-C1437.

Betarbet R, Sherer TB, MacKenzie G, Garcia-Osuna M, Panov AV and Greenamyre JT (2000) Chronic systemic pesticide exposure reproduces features of Parkinson's disease. *Nature Neuroscience* 3: 1301-1306.

Bollimuntha S, Singh B, Shavali S, Sharma S, and Ebadi M. (2005) TRPC-1-Mediated Inhibition of MPP+ Toxicity in Human SH-S-Y5Y Neuroblastma Cells. *J. Biol. Chem.* 280: 2132-2140.

Borovansky J. (1994) Zinc in pigmented cells and structures, interactions and possible roles. *Sb Lek* 95: 309-320.

Buege JA, and Aust SD, (1998): Microsomal lipid perpoxidation. *Methods Mol. Bio.* 108: 302-310.

Bredt, D.S. (1999) Endogenous nitric oxide synthesis: biological functions and pathophysiology. *Free. Radic. Res.* 31: 577-96.

Cai, L., Klein, J.B. and Kang, Y.J. (2001) MT inhibits peroxynitrite-induced DNA and lipoprotein damage. *J. Biol. Chem.* 275: 38957-38960.

Campbell, IL. (1998) Transgenic mice and cytokine actions in the brain: Bridging the gap between structural and functional neuropathology. *Brain Res. Rev.* 26: 327-336.

Chang, J.Y. and Liu, L.Z. (1999) Manganese potentiates nitric oxide production by microglia. Brain. *Res. Mol. Brain. Res.* 68: 22-28.

Check, E. Parkinson's patients show positive response to implants. Nature 2002, 18:416:666.

Cherian MG, and Apostolova MD (2000) Nuclear localization of Metallothionein during Cell Proliferation and Differentiation. *Cell Mol. Biol.* 46: 347-356.

Corsaro C, Scalia M, Blanco AR, Aiello I, Sichel G. (1995) Melanin in physiological conditions protect against lipoperoxidation . A study on albino and pigmented Xenopus. *Pigment Cell Res*. 8: 279-282.

Dalton T, Pazdernik TL, Wagner J, Samson F, and Andrews GK (1995) Temporalspatial patterns of expression of metallothionein-1 and II and other stress-related genes in rat brain after kainic acid-induced seizures. *Neurochemistry Int*. 27: 59-71.

Dalton TP, Li Q, Bittel D, Liang L, Andrews GK (1996) Oxidative stress activates metal-responsive factor-1 binding activity. *J. Biol Chem.* 271: 26233-26241.

Das KC and White CW. (2002) Redox system of the cell: possible links and implications. *PNAS* 99: 9617-9618.

Dawson, V.L. and Dawson, T.M. (1998) Nitric oxide in neurodegeneration. *Prog. Brain. Res.* 118:215-229.

Dehmer, T., Lindenau, J., Haid, S., Dichgans, J. and Schulz, J.B. (2002) Deficiency of inducible nitric oxide synthase protects against MPTP toxicity in vivo. *J. Neurochem.* 74: 2213-2216.

Du, Y., Ma, Z., Lin, S., Dodel, R.C., Gao, F., Bales, K.R., Triarhou, L.C., Chernet, E., Perry, K.W., Nelson, D.L., Luecke, S., Phebus, L.A., Bymaster, F.P. and Paul, S.M. (2001) Minocycline prevents nigrostriatal DA neurodegeneration in the MPTP model of PD. *Proc. Natl. Acad. Sci. USA*. 98:14669-14674.

Duggan DJ, Bittner M, Chen Y, Meltzer P, and Trent JM (1999) Expression profiling using cDNA microarrays. *Nature Genetics* (Suppl) 21: 10-14.

Ebadi M, Sharma SK, Shavali S, Sangchot P, and Brekke L. (2002) The Multiple Actions of Selegiline. *Proc. West. Pharmacol. Soc.* 45: 1-3.

Ebadi M. and Sharma S. (2006) Metallothiionein Isoforms Attenuate Peroxynitrite-Induced Oxidative Stress in Parkinson's Disease. *Journal Exp. Biol. and Medicine*. 231: 1576-1583.

Ebadi M and Sharma S (2006) Vitamin E and Coenzyme Q10 in Parkinson's disease. *The Encylopedia of Vitamin E* (eds. V.R. Preedy and R.R. Watson) CAB International. U.K.

Sharma S. and Ebadi M. (2005) Distribution Kinetics of ^{18}F-DOPA in Weaver Mutant Mice. *Molecular Brain Res*. 139: 23-30.

Ebadi M., Sharma S, Ghafourifar P, Brown-Borg H, and Refaey H.El (2005) Peroxynitrite in the Pathogenesis of Parkinson's disease and the Neuroprotective Role of Metallothioneins. *Method in Enzymol*. 396: 276-298.

Ebadi M, Wanpen S, Shavali S, and Sharma S. (2005) Coenzyme Q_{10} Stabilizes Mitochondria in Parkinson's Disease. *Molecular Interventions in Life-Styl-Related Diseases*. Ed. Hiramatsu. pp 127-153.

Ebadi M, Brown-Borg H, Garrett S, Singh B, Shavali S, Sharma S. (2005) Metallothionein-Mediated Neuroprotection in Genetically-Engineered Mice Models of Parkinson's Disease and Aging. *Molecular. Brain Res*. 134: 67-75.

Ebadi M, Sharma S.K, Wanpen S, Amornpan A (2004) Coenzyme Q_{10} inhibits mitochondrial complex-1 down-regulation and nuclear factor-kappa B activation. *J.Cell. Mol. Med.* 8: 213-222.

Ebadi, M., and Sharma S. (2003) Peroxynitrite and Mitochondrial Dysfunction in the Pathogenesis of Parkinson's disease. *Antioxidants and Redox Signaling* 5: 319-335.

Ebadi M., and Sharma, S. (2003) Mitochondrial damage in Parkinson's disease and its Protection by Coenzyme Q$_{10}$. *Proceedings of the International Symposium on Free Radicals and Health*. Sakata City, Yamagata Prefecture, Japan..

Ebadi M, Sharma S, Shavali S, EI Rafaey (2002) Neuroprotective Actions of Selegiline. *J. Neurosci. Res*. 67: 285-289.

Ebadi M, Sharma SK, Muralikrishnan D, Shavali S, Eken J, Sangchot P, Chetsawang B, Brekke L. (2002) Metallothionein provides Ubiquinone-Mediated Neuroprotection in Parkinson's disease. *Proc. West. Pharmacol. Soc*. 45: 1-3.

Ebadi M, Govitropong P, Sharma SK, Muralikrishnan D, Shavali S, Pellet L, Schafer R, Albano C, Eken J (2001) Ubiquinone (Coenzyme Q10) and Mitochondria in Oxidative Stress of Parkinson's disease. *Biol. Signals and Receptors* 10: 224-253.

Ebadi M. (1986) Characterization of metallothionein-like protein in rat brain. *Biol. Trace Elem. Res*. 11: 277-284.

Ebadi M (1991) Metallothionein and other zinc-binding proteins in brain. *Meth. Enzymol*. 205: 363-387.

Ebadi M, Srinivasan S, Baxi M, (1996): Oxidative stress and antioxidant therapy in Parkinson's disease. *Progr. Neurobiol*. 48: 1–19.

Ebadi M, Govitrapong P, Sharma S, Muralikrishnan D, Shavali S, Pellett L, Schafer R, Albano C, Eken, J (2001): Ubiquinone (CoenzymeQ10) and mitochondria in oxidative stress of Parkinson's disease. *Biol. Signals Recept*. 10: 224–253.

Ebadi M, Hiramatsu M, (2000): Glutathione and metallothionein in oxidative stress of Parkinson's disease; in Poli G, Cadenas E, (eds): *Free Radicals in Brain Pathophysiology*. New York, Marcel Dekker, Inc, pp 427–465.

Ebadi, M., Pfeiffer, R.F., Murrin, L.C. and Shiraga, H. (1991) MT and oxidation reactions in PD. *Proc. West. Pharmacol. Soc*. 34:285-290.

Ebadi M, Iversen PL, Hao R, Cerutis DR, Rojas P, Happe HK, Murrin LC, and Pfeiffer RF (1995) Expression and regulation of brain metallothionein isoforms. *J. Neurochem*. 66: 2121-2127.

Ebadi, M., Leuschen, M.P., el Refaey, H., Hamada, F.M. and Rojas, P. (1996) The antioxidant properties of zinc and MT. *Neurochem. Int*. 29: 159-166.

Ebadi, M., Hiramatsu, M., Burke, W.J., Folks, D.G. and el-Sayed, M.A. (1998) MT isoforms provide neuroprotection against 6-hydroxyDA-generated hydroxyl radicals and superoxide anions. *Proc. West. Pharmacol. Soc*. 41:155-158..

Ebadi M. (1998) Glutathione and MT in Neurodegeneration-Neuroprotection of PD. *Neuroendocrinology Letters* 18 No2/3. 111-122.

Ebadi, M, Hiramtsu M, Ramana Kumari MV, Hao R, and Pfeiffer RF (1998) Metallothionein in oxidative stress of Parkinson's disease. In Metallothionein IV (CD Klassen ed) *Advances in Life Sciences*.

EIRefaey H, Ebadi M, Kusznski CA, Sweeney J, Hamada FM, and Hamed A. (1997) Identification of metallothionein receptors in human astrocytes. *Neurosci. Lett*. 231:131-134.

Erickson JC, Masters BA, Kelly EJ, Brinster R, and Palmiter RD (1995) Expression of human metallothionein-II in transgenic mice. *Neurochem. Int*. 27: 35-41.

Gerlach, M., Desser, H.,Youdim, M.B. and Riederer, P. (1996) New horizons in molecular mechanisms underlying PD and in our understanding of the neuroprotective effects of Selegiline. *J. Neural. Transm. Suppl.* 48: 7-21.

Gerlach, M., Blum-Degen, D., Lan, J. and Riederer, P. (1999) Nitric oxide in the pathogenesis of PD. *Adv. Neurol.* 80:239-245.

Gershon D (2002) Microarrays technology: A array of opportunities. *Nature* 416: 885-891.

Giralt M, Penkova M, Hernandez J, Molinero A, Carrasco J, Lago N, Camats J, Campbell IL, Hidalgo J. (2002) Metallothionein-1+2 deficiency Increases Brain Pathology in Transgenic Mice with Astrocyte-Targeted Expression of Interleukin 6. *Neurobiology of Disease.* 9: 319-338.

Grunblatt E, mandel S, Maor G, Youdim MB (2001) Gene expression analysis in N-methyl-4-phenyl-1,2,3,6-tetrahydropyridine mice model of Parkinson's disease using cDNA microarray: effect of R-apomorphine. *J. Neurochem.* 78: 1-12.

Grunewald, T. and Beal, M.F. (1999) NOS knockouts and neuroprotection. *Nat. Med.* 5: 1354-1355.

Gunn TM, Inui T, Kitada K, Ito S, Wakamatsu K, He L, Bouley DM, Serikawa T, and barsh G.S. (2001) Molecular and p[henotypic Analysis of Attractin Mutant Mice. *Genetics* 158:1683-1695.

Hantraye, P., Brouillet, E., Ferrante, R., Palfi, S., Dolan, R., Matthews, R.T. and Beal, M.F. (1996) Inhibition of neuronal nitric oxide synthase prevents MPTP-induced parkinsonism in baboons. *Nat. Med.* 2: 1017-21.

Hidalgo J., Castellano B., and Campbell, IL (1997) Regulation of Brain Metallothionein. *Curr. Top. Neurochem.* 1:1-26.

Hidalgo J, Aschner M, Zatta P, and Vasak M. (2001) Roles of the Metallothionein family of proteins in the central nervous system. *Brain. Res. Bull.* 55: 133-145.

Hirota K, Murata M, Sachi Y, Nakamura H, Takeuchi J, Mori K., and Yodoi J (1999) Distinct roles of Thioredoxin in the cytoplasm and in the nucleus. *J. Biol Chem.* 274: 27891-27897.

Hirsch, E.C. and Hunot, S. (2002) Nitric oxide, glial cells and neuronal degeneration in parkinsonism. *Trends. Pharmacol. Sci.* 21, 163-165.

Hopkin, S, and Rothwell, N. (1995) Cytokines in the nervous system. I: Expression and recognition. *Trends Neurosci.* 18: 83-88.

Hsu LJ, Sagara Y, Arroyo A, Rockenstein E, Sisk A, Mallory M, Wong J, Takenouchi T, Hashimoto M, Masliah E (2000) α-Synuclein promotes mitochondrial deficit and oxidative stress. *Am. J. Pathol.* 157: 401-410.

Hunot, S., Dugas, N., Faucheux, B., Hartmann, A., Tardieu, M., Debre, P., Agid, Y., Dugas, B. and Hirsch, E.C. (1999) FcepsilonRII/CD23 is expressed in PD and induces, in vitro, production of nitric oxide and tumor necrosis factor-alpha in glial cells. *J. Neurosci.* 19: 344-347.

Hunot, S., Boissiere, F., Faucheux, B., Brugg, B., Mouatt-Prigent, A., Agid, Y. and Hirsch, E.C. (1996) Nitric oxide synthase and neuronal vulnerability in PD. *Neuroscience.* 72: 355-63.

Hunot, S., Dugas, N., Faucheux, B., Hartmann, A., Tardieu, M., Debre, P., Agid, Y., Dugas, B. and Hirsch, E.C. (1999) FcepsilonRII/CD23 is expressed in PD and induces, in vitro, production of nitric oxide and tumor necrosis factor-alpha in glial cells. *J. Neurosci.* 19: 3440-3447.

Imam, S.Z., el-Yazal, J., Newport, G.D., Itzhak, Y., Cadet, J.L., Slikker, W., Jr. and Ali, S.F. (2002) Methamphetamine-induced DA neurotoxicity: role of peroxynitrite and neuroprotective role of antioxidants and peroxynitrite decomposition catalysts. *Ann. N. Y. Acad. Sci..* 939:366-380.

Iravani, M.M., Kashefi, K., Mander, P., Rose, S. and Jenner, P. (2002) Involvement of inducible nitric oxide synthase in inflammation-induced DA neurodegeneration. *Neuroscience.* 110: 49-58.

Ischiropoulos, H., Duran, D. and Horwitz, J. (1995) Peroxynitrite-mediated inhibition of DOPA synthesis in PC12 cells. *J. Neurochem.* 65: 2366-2372.

Itoh M, Ebadi M, and Swanson S (1983) The presence of zinc binding proteins in brain. *J. Neurochem.* 41: 823-829.

Itzhak, Y. and Ali, S.F. (1996) The neuronal nitric oxide synthase inhibitor, 7-nitroindazole, protects against methamphetamine-induced neurotoxicity in vivo. *J. Neurochem.* 67: 1770-3.

Jellinger KA, (1999): The role of iron in neurodegeneration: Prospects for pharmacotherapy of Parkinson's disease. *Drugs and Aging* 14: 115–140.

Iwamoto T, Takahashi M, Ohbayashi M, Nakashima I. (1992) The ret oncogene cann induce melanogenesis and melanocyte development in Wv/E=Wv mice. *Exp. Cell Res.* 200:410-415.

Iwamoto T, Takahashi M, Ito M, Hamatani K, Ohbayashi M, Wajjwalku W, Isobe K, Nakashima I (2001) Abberrant melanogenesis and melanocytic tumor developmentin transgenic mcie that carry a MT/ret fusion gene. *EMBO J.* Nov 10:3167-3175.

Kaji JHR, and Kojima Y. (1987) Chemistry and Biocvhemistry of Metallothionein. *Experientia* (Suppl) 52: 25-62.

Kiss, J.P. (2002) Role of nitric oxide in the regulation of monoaminergic neurotransmission. *Brain. Res. Bull.* 52: 459-66.

Klongpanichapak S., Govitrapong P., Sharma S., and Ebadi M. (2006) Attenuation of Cocaine and Methamphetamine Neurotoxicity in SK-N-SH Neurons by Coenzyme Q_{10}. *Neurochemical Res.* 31: 303-311.

Knott, C., Stern, G. and Wilkin, G.P. (2001) Inflammatory regulators in PD: iNOS, lipocortin-1, and cyclooxygenases-1 and -2. *Mol. Cell. Neurosci.* 16: 724-39.

Kooncumchoo P., Sharma S., Govitrapong P., and Ebadi M. (2006) Coenzyme Q_{10} Provides Neuroprotection in Iron-Induced Apoptosis in Dopaminergic Neurons. *Molecular neuroscience* 28:125-142.

Korytowski W, Sarna T, Zar Ba M. (1995) Antioxidant action of neuromelanin: the mechanism of inhibitory effect on lipid peroxidation. *Arch. Biochem. Biophys.* 319:142-148.

Kristal, B.S., Conway, A.D., Brown, A.M., Jain, J.C., Ulluci, P.A., Li, S.W. and Burke, W.J. (2001) Selective DA vulnerability: 3,4-dihydroxyphenylacetaldehyde targets mitochondria. *Free. Radic. Biol. Med.* 30: 924-931.

Kupper U, Linden M, Cao KZ, Lerch K. (1990) Expression of tyrosinase in vegetative cultures of Neurospora crassa transfromedd with a MT promoter/protyurosinase fusion gene. *Curr. Genet.* 18:331-335.

Lacy, M.E. (1984) Phonon-electron coupling as a possible transducing mechanism in bioelectronic processes involving neuromelanin. *J. Theor. Biol.* 111: 201-4.

Lamensdorf, I., Eisenhofer, G., Harvey-White, J., Hayakawa, Y., Kirk, K. and Kopin, I.J. (2001a) Metabolic stress in PC12 cells induces the formation of the endogenous DA neurotoxin, 3,4-dihydroxyphenylacetaldehyde. *J. Neurosci. Res.* 60: 552-558.

Lamensdorf, I., Eisenhofer, G., Harvey-White, J., Nechustan, A., Kirk, K. and Kopin, I.J. (2001b) 3,4-Dihydroxyphenylacetaldehyde potentiates the toxic effects of metabolic stress in PC12 cells. *Brain. Res.* 868:191-201.

Lang AE, Lozano AM. *Medical Progress: Parkinson disease. Part 1 and 2 N. E. J. M.* (1998):339:1130-1143"1044-1053.

Langston, J.W. (1988) Neuromelanin-containing neurons are selectively vulnerable in parkinsonism. *Trends. Pharmacol.* Sci. 9: 347-8.

Langston, J.W. (1989) Mechanisms underlying neuronal degeneration in Parkinson's disease: an experimental and theoretical treatise. *Mov. Disord.* 4 Suppl 1: S15-25.

Larsson, B.S. (1993) Interaction between chemicals and melanin. *Pigment. Cell. Res.* 6: 127-33.

Larue L, Mintz B. (1990) Pigmented cell lines of mouse albino melanocytes containing a tyrosinase cDNA with an inducible promoter. *Somat. Cell Mol. Genet.* 16: 361-368.

LaVoie, M.J. and Hastings, T.G. (1999) Peroxynitrite- and nitrite-induced oxidation of DA: implications for nitric oxide in DA cell loss. *J. Neurochem.* 73: 2546-2554.

Lehmensick V, Tan EM, Schwarz J, Storch A. (2002) Expression of mutant alpha-synuclein enhances dopamine transporter-mediated MPP$^+$ toxicity in vitro. *Neuroreport* 13: 1279-1283.

Levi, A.C., De Mattei, M., Ravazzani, R., Fariello, G.R. and Corvetti, G. (1987) The action of MPTP on Macaca fascicularis nigral neurons. *Boll. Soc. Ital. Biol. Sper.* 63: 365-8.

Lee, H.S., Park, C.W. and Kim, Y.S. (2002) MPP(+) increases the vulnerability to oxidative stress rather than directly mediating oxidative damage in human neuroblastoma cells. *Exp. Neurol.* 165: 164-171.

Liberatore, G.T., Jackson-Lewis, V., Vukosavic, S., Mandir, A.S., Vila, M., McAuliffe, W.G., Dawson, V.L., Dawson, T.M. and Przedborski, S. (1999) Inducible nitric oxide synthase stimulates DA neurodegeneration in the MPTP model of Parkinson disease [see comments]. *Nat. Med.* 5: 1403-1409.

Lindquist, N.G. (1972) Accumulation in vitro of 35S-chlorpromazine in the neuromelanin of human substantia nigra and locus coeruleus. *Arch. Int. Pharmacodyn. Ther.* 200: 190-5.

Lindquist, N.G. (1972) Accumulation in vitro of 35S-chlorpromazine in the neuromelanin of human substantia nigra and locus coeruleus. *Arch. Int. Pharmacodyn. Ther.* 200: 190-195.

Lindquist, N.G., Larsson, B.S. and Lyden-Sokolowski, A. (1987) Neuromelanin and its possible protective and destructive properties. *Pigment. Cell. Res.* 1: 133-136.

LeVine RL, Garland D., Oliver CN, Amici A., Climent I, Lenz AG, Ahn S, Shaltiel S., Stadtman ER. (1990): Determination of carbonyl content in oxidatively modified proteins. *Methods Enzymol.* 186: 464-478.

Li, S.W., Lin, T., Minteer, S. and Burke, W.J. (2001) 3,4-Dihydroxyphenylacetaldehyde and hydrogen peroxide generate a hydroxyl radical: possible role in PD pathogenesis. *Brain. Res. Mol. Brain. Res.* 93: 1-7.

Liberatore, G.T., Jackson-Lewis, V., Vukosavic, S., Mandir, A.S., Vila, M., McAuliffe, W.G., Dawson, V.L., Dawson, T.M. and Przedborski, S. (1999) Inducible nitric oxide synthase stimulates DA neurodegeneration in the MPTP model of Parkinson disease. Nat. Med. 5: 1403-1409.

Lotharius J, O'Malley KL (2000) The parkinsonism-inducing drug 1-methyl, 4-phenyl pyridinium triggers intracellular dopamine oxidation: a novel mechanism of toxicity. *J. Biol Chem.* 275: 38581-38588.

Lotharius J, Barg S, Wiekop P, Lundburg C, Raymon HK, Brundin P. (2002) Effect of mutant alpha-synuclein on dopamine homeostasis in a new human mesencephalic cell line. *J. Biol Chem.* (Publication ahead of print).

Lyden, A., Larsson, B.S. and Lindquist, N.G. (1984) Melanin affinity of manganese. *Acta. Pharmacol. Toxicol. (Copenh).* 55: 133-138.

Ma, S.Y., Ciliax, B.J., Stebbins, G., Jaffar, S., Joyce, J.N., Cochran, E.J., Kordower, J.H., Mash, D.C., Levey, A.I. and Mufson, E.J. (1999) Dopamine transporter-immunoreactive neurons decrease with age in the human substantia nigra. *J. Comp. Neurol.* 409: 25-37.

Mandel S, Grunblatt E, and Youdim M. (2000) cDNA microarray to study gene expression of dopaminergic neurodegeneration and neuroprotection in MPTP and 6-hydroxydopamine models: implications for idiopathic Parkinson's disease. *J. Neural transm. Suppl* 60: 117-124.

Mann, D.M., Yates, P.O. and Barton, C.M. (1977) Neuromelanin and RNA in cells of substantia nigra. *J. Neuropathol. Exp. Neurol.* 36: 379-83.

Mann, D.M. and Yates, P.O. (1983) Possible role of neuromelanin in the pathogenesis of Parkinson's disease. *Mech. Ageing. Dev.* 21: 193-203.

Mann, D.M. (1983) The locus coeruleus and its possible role in ageing and degenerative disease of the human central nervous system. *Mech. Ageing. Dev.* 23: 73-94.

Manaye, K.F., McIntire, D.D., Mann, D.M. and German, D.C. (1995) Locus coeruleus cell loss in the aging human brain: a non-random process. *J. Comp. Neurol.* 358: 79-87.

Margoshes, M. and Vellee, BL. (1957) A cadmium protein from equine kidney cortex. *J. Am. Cehm. Soc.* 79: 4813-4814.

Masters BA, Kelly EJ, Quaife CJ, brinster RL, and Palmiter RD (1994a) Targeted disruption of metallothionein-1 and –II genes increases sensitivity to cadmium. *Proc. Natl. Acad. Sci. USA* 91: 584-588.

Masters BA, Quaife CJ, Erickson JC, Kelly EJ, Froelick GJ, Zambroicz BP, Brinster RL, and Palmiter RD (1994b) Metallothionein is expressed in neurons that sequester zinc in synaptic vesicles. *J. Neurosci.* 14: 5844-5857.

Mattammal, M.B., Haring, J.H., Chung, H.D., Raghu, G. and Strong, R. (1995) An endogenous DA neurotoxin: implication for PD. *Neurodegeneration.* 4: 271-281.

Maruyama, W., Takahashi, T. and Naoi, M. (1998) (-)-Deprenyl protects human DA neuroblastoma SH-SY5Y cells from apoptosis induced by peroxynitrite and nitric oxide. *J. Neurochem.* 70: 2510-5.

McBride AG, Borutaite' V, and Brown GC. Superoxide dismutase and hydrogen peroxide cause rapid nitric oxide breakdown, peroxynitrite production and subquent cell death. *Biochimica et Biophysica Acta* 1454:(1999) 275-288.

McIntosh, T., Juhler, M., and Wieloch, T. (1998) Novel pharamcologic strategies in the treatment of experimental traumatic brain injury. *J. Neurotrauma* 15: 731-769.

McNeill, T.H., Koek, L.L. and Haycock, J.W. (1984) The nigrostriatal system and aging. *Peptides.* 5 Suppl 1: 263-268..

Melamed, E., Soffer, D., Rosenthal, J., Pikarsky, E. and Reches, A. (1987) Effect of intrastriatal and intranigral administration of synthetic neuromelanin on the DA neurotoxicity of MPTP in rodents. *Neurosci. Lett.* 83: 41-46.

Meglio, L. and Oteiza, P.I. (1999) Aluminum enhances melanin-induced lipid peroxidation. *Neurochem. Res.* 24: 1001-8.

Miller, M.A., Kolb, P.E., Leverenz, J.B., Peskind, E.R. and Raskind, M.A. (1999) Preservation of noradrenergic neurons in the locus ceruleus that coexpress galanin mRNA in Alzheimer's disease. *J. Neurochem.* 73: 2028-36.

Naoi, M., Maruyama, W., Yagi, K. and Youdim, M. (2002) Anti-apoptotic function of L- (-) deprenyl (Selegiline) and related compounds. *Neurobiology. (Bp).* 8: 69-80.

Nappi, A.J. and Vass, E. (2002) The effects of nitric oxide on the oxidations of l-dopa and dopamine mediated by tyrosinase and peroxidase. *J. Biol. Chem. 2001.* 276: 11214-22.

Nelson SK, McCord JM, (1998): Iron, oxygen radicals, and disease (1998): *Adv. Mol. Cell Biol.* 25: 157–183.

Obata, T. and Yamanaka, Y. (2001) Nitric oxide enhances MPP (+)-induced hydroxyl radical generation via depolarization activated nitric oxide synthase in rat striatum. *Brain. Res.* 902: 223-228..

Odh, G., Carstam, R., Paulson, J., Wittbjer, A., Rosengren, E. and Rorsman, H. (1994) Neuromelanin of the human substantia nigra: a mixed-type melanin. *J. Neurochem.* 62: 2030-2036.

Offen, D., Ziv, I., Barzilai, A., Gorodin, S., Glater, E., Hochman, A. and Melamed, E. (1997) Dopamine-melanin induces apoptosis in PC12 cells; possible implications for the etiology of Parkinson's disease. *Neurochem. Int.* 31: 207-216.

Offen, D., Gorodin, S., Melamed, E., Hanania, J. and Malik, Z. (1999) Dopamine-melanin is actively phagocytized by PC12 cells and cerebellar granular cells: possible implications for the etiology of Parkinson's disease. *Neurosci. Lett.* 260: 101-104.

Ohm, T.G., Busch, C. and Bohl, J. (1997) Unbiased estimation of neuronal numbers in the human nucleus coeruleus during aging. *Neurobiol. Aging.* 18: 393-339.

Palmiter, RD., Finley SD, Whitmore TE, and Durnam DM (1992) MT-III, a brain-specific member of the metallothionein gene family. *Proc. Natl Acad. Sci. USA.* 89: 6333-6337.

Park, B.E., Netsky, M.G. and Betsill, W.L., Jr. (1975) Pathogenesis of pigment and spheroid formation in Hallervorden-Spatz syndrome and related disorders. *Neurology.* 25: 1172-8.

Park SU, Ferrer JV, Javitch JA, Kuhn DM. (2002) Peroxynitrite inactivates the human dopamine transporter by modification of cysteine 342: potential mechanism of neurotoxicity in dopamine neurons. *J. Neurosci.* 22: 4399-4405.

Penkowa M (2006) Metallothioneins are multipurpose neuroprotectants during brain pathology. *FEBS Journal* 273: 1857-1870.

Perz RG, Waymire JC, Lin E, Liu JJ, Guo F, Zigmond MJ. (2002) A role for alpha-synuclein in the regulation of dopamine biosynthesis. *J. Neurosci.* 22: 3090-3099.

Porebska-Budny, M., Sakina, N.L., Stepien, K.B., Dontsov, A.E. and Wilczok, T. (1992) Antioxidative activity of synthetic melanins. Cardiolipin liposome model. *Biochim. Biophys. Acta.* 1116: 11-16.

Prota, G. and d'Ischia, M. (1993) Neuromelanin: a key to Parkinson's disease. *Pigment. Cell. Res.* 6: 333-5.

Przedborski, S., Jackson-Lewis, V., Yokoyama, R., Shibata, T., Dawson, V.L. and Dawson, T.M. (1996) Role of neuronal nitric oxide in 1-methyl-4-phenyl-1, 2,3,6-tetrahydropyridine (MPTP)-induced DA neurotoxicity. *Proc. Natl. Acad. Sci. USA.* 93: 4565-71.

Quaife CJ, Findley SD, Erickson JC, Forelick GJ, Kelly EJ, Zambrowicz BP, and Palmiter RD (1994) Induction of a new metallothionein isoform (MT-IV) occurs during differentiation of stratified squamous epithelia. *Biochemistry* 33: 7250-7259.

Qureshi, G.A., Baig, S., Bednar, I., Sodersten, P., Forsberg, G. and Siden, A. (1995) Increased cerebrospinal fluid concentration of nitrite in PD. *Neuroreport.* 6: 1642-4.

Radi R, Rodriguez M, Castro L, Telleri R. (1994) Inhibition of mitochondrial transport by peroxynitrite. *Arch. Biochem. Biophys.* 308: 89-95.

Radtke F, Heuchel R, Georgiev O, Hergerberg M, Gariglio, Dembic Z, and Schafner W. (1993) Cloned transcription factor MTF-1 activates the mouse metallothionein 1 promoter. *The EMBO J.* 12: 1355-1362.

Reddy BR, Kloner RA, Przyklenk K, (1989): Early treatment with deferoxamine limits myocardial ischemic/reperfusion injury. Free Radical Biology and Medicine. 7: 45–52.

Rothwell, N, and Hopkins, SJ (1995) Cytokines in the nervous system. II: Actions and Mechanisms of Actions. *Trend Neurol. Sci.* 18:130-136.

Reyes, M.G., Faraldi, F., Chandran, R., Verano, A. and Levi, A.C. (1996) Histopathology of the substantia nigra in Alzheimer's disease. *Panminerva. Med.* 38: 8-14.

Riobo, N.A., Schopfer, F.J., Boveris, A.D., Cadenas, E. and Poderoso, J.J. (2002) The reaction of nitric oxide with 6-hydroxyDA: implications for PD. *Free. Radic. Biol. Med.* 32: 115-121.

Rojas, P., Cerutis, D.R., Happe, H.K., Murrin, L.C., Hao, R., Pfeiffer, R.F. and Ebadi, M. (1996) 6-HydroxyDA-mediated induction of rat brain MT I mRNA. *Neurotoxicology.* 17: 323-334.

Rojas, P., Hidalgo, J., Ebadi, M. and Rios, C. (2001a) Changes of MT I + II proteins in the brain after 1-methyl-4-phenylpyridinium administration in mice. *Prog. Neuropsychopharmacol. Biol. Psychiatry.* . 24: 143-154.

Rojas, P., Rojas-Castaneda, J., Vigueras, R.M., Habeebu, S.S., Rojas, C., Rios, C. and Ebadi, M. (2001b) MPTP decreases MT-I mRNA in mouse striatum. *Neurochem. Res.* 25: 503-509.

Samii A, Markopolou K, Wszolck ZK, Sossi V, Dobko T, Mak E, Calne DB, and Stoessl AJ (1999) PET studies of parkinsonism associated with mutation in the alpha-synuclein gene. *Neurology* 53: 2097-2102.

Salazar, M., Sokoloski, T.D. and Patil, P.N. (1978) Binding of DA drugs by the neuromelanin of the substantia nigra, synthetic melanins and melanin granules. *Fed. Proc.* 37: 2403-7.

Sanghera, M.K., Zamora, J.L. and German, D.C. (1995) Calbindin-D28k-containing neurons in the human hypothalamus: relationship to DA neurons. *Neurodegeneration.* 4: 375-81.

Sangchot P, Sharma SK, Chatsawang B, Govitropong P, and Ebadi, M. Deferaxamine Attenuates Iron-Induced Oxidative Stress and Restores Mitochondrial Functions in SK-N-SH Cells in Culture. *Developmental Neuroscience.* (2002) In Press.

Saydam N, Georgiev O, Nakano MY, Gerber UF, and Schaffner W (2001) Nucleo-cytoplasmic trafficking of metal-regulatory transcription factor-1 is regulated by diverse stress signals. *J. Biol Chem.* 276: 25487-25495.

Saydam N, Adams TK, Steiner F, Schaffner W. (2002) Regulation of metallothionein transcription by the metal-responsive transcription factor MTF-1 *J. Biol. Chem.* 277: 20438-20445.

Schneider, J.A., Bienias, J.L., Gilley, D.W., Kvarnberg, D.E., Mufson, E.J. and Bennett, D.A. (2002) Improved detection of substantia nigra pathology in Alzheimer's disease. *J. Histochem. Cytochem.* 50: 99-106.

Schraermeyer, U. (1996) The intracellular origin of the melanosome in pigment cells: a review of ultrastructural data. *Histol. Histopathol.* 11: 445-62.

Schulz, J.B., Matthews, R.T., Muqit, M.M., Browne, S.E. and Beal, M.F. (1995) Inhibition of neuronal nitric oxide synthase by 7-nitroindazole protects against MPTP-induced neurotoxicity in mice. *J. Neurochem.* 64: 936-9.

Schulz, J.B., Matthews, R.T., Klockgether, T., Dichgans, J. and Beal, M.F. (1997) The role of mitochondrial dysfunction and neuronal nitric oxide in animal models of neurodegenerative diseases. *Mol. Cell. Biochem.* 174: 193-7.

Sharma S., Refaey H.EI., and Ebadi M. (2006a) Complex-1 Activity and ^{18}F-DOPA Uptake in Genetically-Engineered Mouse Model of Parkinson's Disease and the Neuroprotective Role of Coenzyme Q_{10}. *Brain Res. Bullet.* 70:22-32.

Sharma S., Gregory K. and Ebadi M (2006b) Radiation Safety and Quality Control in the Cyclotron Laboratory. *Radiation Protection Dosimetry* 118: 431-439.

Sharma S. and Ebadi M. (2005) Neuroprotection by Metallothionein in Parkinson's Disease. *In Progress in Parkinson's Disease Research.* Nova Science Publishers, Inc N.Y. (in press).

Sharma S. and Ebadi M. (2004) An Improved Method for Analyzing Coenzyme Q Homologues and Multiple Detection of Rare Biological Samples. *J. Neuroscience Methods* 137:1-8.

Sharma S., Kheradpezhou M., Shavali S., EI Refaey H., Eken J., Hagen C., and Ebadi M. (2004a) Neuroprotective Actions of Coenzyme Q_{10} in Parkinson's Disease. *Methods in Enzymology*. Vol. 382, 488-509.

Sharma S. and Ebadi M (2004b) *Neuroprotective Role of Metallothioneins in Parkinson's Disease.* Nova Science Publishers.

Sharma S, Carlson E, and Ebadi M (2003) The Neuroprotective Actions of Selegiline in Inhibiting 1-Methyl, 4-Phenyl, Pyridinium Ion (MPP⁺)-Induced Apoptosis in Dopaminergic Neurons. *J. Neurocytology* 32, 329-343.

Sharma, S.K., and Ebadi, M. (2003) Metallothionein Attenuates 3-Morpoholinosydnonimone (SIN-1)-Induced Oxidative and Nitrative Stress in Dopaminergic Neurons. *Antioxidants and Redox Signaling.* 5: 251-264.

Sharma SK, Shavali S., Rafaey H.E.I and Ebadi, M (2002a) Inhibition of α-Syn nitration and perinuclear aggregation by antioxidants in MT Transgenic and Aging RhO (mgko) DA neurons. *FASEB Meeting*, New Orleans Abstract.

Sharma SK, Sangchot P, Ebadi M. (2002b) MT Gene manipulation influences striatal mitochondrial ubiquinones and MPTP-induced neurotoxicity in DA neurons. *XIV World Congress of Pharmacology.* San-Francisco (Abstract).

Sharma SK and Ebadi M. (2002) Metallothionein Attenuates 3-Morpholinosydnonimone (SIN-1)-Induced Oxidative and Nitrative Stress in Dopaminergic Neurons. *Antioxidants and Redox Signaling* (Submitted).

Sherer TB, Betarbet R, Stout AK, Lund S, Baptista M, Panov AV, Cookson MR, and Greenamyre T. (2002) An in vitro Model of Parkinson's disease: Lanking Mitochondrial Impairment to Altered α-Synuclein Metabolism and Oxidative Damage. *J. Neurosci.* 22: 7006-7015.

Shima, T., Sarna, T., Swartz, H.M., Stroppolo, A., Gerbasi, R. and Zecca, L. (1997) Binding of iron to neuromelanin of human substantia nigra and synthetic melanin: an electron paramagnetic resonance spectroscopy study. *Free. Radic. Biol. Med.* 23: 110-9.

Sinaceur R, Ribiere C, Abu-Murad C, Nordmann J, Nordmann R, (1983): Reduction in the rate of ethanol elimination in vivo by desferrioxamine and diethylenetrimine penta acetic acid: suggestion for involvement of hydroxyl radicals in ethanol oxidation. *Biochem. Pharm.* 32: 2371–2373.

Smythies, J. (1996) On the functional of neuromelanin. *Proc. R. Soc. Lond. B. Biol. Sci.* 263:487-489.

Souza JM, Giasson BI, Chen Q, Lee VM, Ischiropolous H (2000) Dityrosine cross-linking promotes formation of stable α-Synuclein polymers. Implications of nitrative and oxidative stress in the pathogenesis of neurodegenerative synucleinopathies. *J. Biol. Chem.* 275: 18344-18349.

Stamler JS, Singel DL, Loscalzo J (1992) Biochemistry of nitric oxide and its redox-activated forms. *Science* 258: 1898-1902.

Stepien K, Wilczok A, Zaidel A, Dzierzega-Lecznar A, and Wilczok T. (2000). Peroxynitrite mediated linoleic acid oxidation and tyrosine nitration in the presence of synthetic neuromelanin. *Acta Biochim. Pol.* 47: 931-940.

Stichel, C., and Verner Muller H. (1998) Experimental strategies to promote axonal regeneration after traumatic central nervous system injury. *Prog. Neurobiol.* 56: 119-148.

Sulzer D, Bogulavsky J, Larsen K.E., Behr G, Karatekin E, Kleinman M.H, Turro N, Krantz D, Edwards RH, Greene LA, Zecca L. Neuromelanin biosynthesis is driven by excess cytosolic catecholamines not accumulated by synaptic vesicles. *PNAS* 97: 11869-11874.

Suzuki KT, Imura N, Kimura M. (1993) *Metallothionein III. Biological Roles and Medical Implications,* Basal: Berkhauser Verlag.

Taguchi S, Ogawa T, Endo T, Momose H. (1998) Identification of a structural gene encoding a MT-like domain that includes a putative regulator protein for Sreptomyces protease gene expression. *Biosci. Biotechnol. Biochem.* 62: 2476-2479.

Takahashi M, Iwamoto T, Nakashima I. (1992) Proliferation and neoplastic transformation of pigment cells in MT/ret transgenic mice. *Pigment Cell Res.* Nov 5(5Pt 2) 344-347.

Temlett, J.A., Landsberg, J.P., Watt, F. and Grime, G.W. (1994) Increased iron in the substantia nigra compacta of the MPTP-lesioned hemiparkinsonian African green monkey: evidence from proton microprobe elemental microanalysis. *J. Neurochem.* 62: 134-46.

Tief, K., Schmidt, A. and Beermann, F. (1998) New evidence for presence of tyrosinase in substantia nigra, forebrain and midbrain. *Brain. Res. Mol. Brain. Res.* 53, 307-10.

Torreilles, F., Salman-Tabcheh, S., Guerin, M. and Torreilles, J. (1999) Neurodegenerative disorders: the role of peroxynitrite. *Brain. Res. Brain. Res. Rev.* 30: 153-63.

Trendelenburg G, Prass K, Priller J, Kapinya K, Polley A, Muselmann C, Ruscher K, Kannbley U, Schmitt AO, Castell S, Wiegand F, Meisel A, Rosenthal A, and Dirnag U. (2002) Serial Analysis of Gene Expression Identifies Metallothionein-II as Major Neuroprotective Gene in Mouse Focal Cerebral Ischemia. *J. Neurosci.* 22: 5879-5888.

Uchida Y, Takio K, Titani K, Ihara Y, and Tomonaga M. (1991) The growth inhibitory factor that is deficient in the Alzheimer's disease brain is a 68 aminoa acid metallothionein-like protein. *Neuron* 7: 337-347.

Ward PA, Till GO, Kundel R, Beauchamp C. (1983) Evidence for role of hydorxyl radical in complement and neutrophil-dependent tissue injury. *J. Clin. Invest.* 72: 789-801.

Willis ED (1969) Lipid peroxide formation in microsomes. The role of non-haem iron. *Biochem J.* 113: 325-332.

Wu, E.Y., Chiba, K., Trevor, A.J. and Castagnoli, N., Jr. (1986) Interactions of the 1-methyl-4-phenyl-2,3-dihydropyridinium species with synthetic dopamine-melanin. *Life. Sci.* 39: 1695-700.

Wu, D.C., Jackson-Lewis, V., Vila, M., Tieu, K., Teismann, P., Vadseth, C., Choi, D.K., Ischiropoulos, H. and Przedborski, S. (2002) Blockade of microglial activation is neuroprotective in the 1-methyl-4-phenyl-1, 2,3,6-tetrahydropyridine mouse model of Parkinson disease. *J. Neurosci.* 22:1763-1771.

Yang HY, Speed T (2002) Design issues for cDNA microarray experiments. *Nature* 3: 579-588.

Youdim, M.B., Ben-Shachar, D. and Riederer, P. (1989) Is Parkinson's disease a progressive siderosis of substantia nigra resulting in iron and melanin induced neurodegeneration? *Acta. Neurol. Scand. Suppl.* 126: 47-54.

Youdim, M.B. and Riederer, P. (1993) The role of iron in senescence of DA neurons in Parkinson's disease. *J. Neural. Transm. Suppl.* 40: 57-67.

Youdim, M.B., Ben-Shachar, D. and Riederer, P. (1994) The enigma of neuromelanin in Parkinson's disease substantia nigra. *J. Neural. Transm. Suppl.* 43: 113-122.

Youdim, M.B., Ben-Shachar, D., Eshel, G., Finberg, J.P. and Riederer, P. (1993) The neurotoxicity of iron and nitric oxide. Relevance to the etiology of PD. *Adv. Neurol.* 60: 259-266.

Youdim, M.B., Lavie, L. and Riederer, P. (1994) Oxygen free radicals and neurodegeneration in PD: a role for nitric oxide. *Ann. N. Y. Acad. Sci.* 738: 64-68.

Youdim, M.B. and Lavie, L. (1994) Selective MAO-A and B inhibitors, radical scavengers and nitric oxide synthase inhibitors in PD. *Life. Sci.* 55, 2077-2082.

Zhang, Y., Dawson, V.L. and Dawson, T.M. (2002) Oxidative stress and genetics in the pathogenesis of PD. *Neurobiol. Dis.* 7: 240-250.

Zareba, M., Bober, A., Korytowski, W., Zecca, L. and Sarna, T. (1995) The effect of a synthetic neuromelanin on yield of free hydroxyl radicals generated in model systems. *Biochim. Biophys. Acta.* 1271: 343-348.

Zecca, L., Fariello, R., Riederer, P., Sulzer, D., Gatti, A. and Tampellini, D. (2002b) The absolute concentration of nigral neuromelanin, assayed by a new sensitive method, increases throughout the life and is dramatically decreased in Parkinson's disease. *FEBS. Lett.* 510: 216-20.

Zecca, L., Mecacci, C., Seraglia, R. and Parati, E. (1992) The chemical characterization of melanin contained in substantia nigra of human brain. *Biochim. Biophys. Acta.* 1138: 6-10.

Zecca, L., Pietra, R., Goj, C., Mecacci, C., Radice, D. and Sabbioni, E. (1994) Iron and other metals in neuromelanin, substantia nigra, and putamen of human brain. *J. Neurochem.* 62: 1097-101.

Zecca, L., Costi, P., Mecacci, C., Ito, S., Terreni, M. and Sonnino, S. (2000) Interaction of human substantia nigra neuromelanin with lipids and peptides. *J. Neurochem.* 74: 1758-65.

Zecca, L., Fariello, R., Riederer, P., Sulzer, D., Gatti, A. and Tampellini, D. (2002b) The absolute concentration of nigral neuromelanin, assayed by a new sensitive method, increases throughout the life and is dramatically decreased in Parkinson's disease. *FEBS. Lett.* 510: 216-20.

Zecca, L., Gallorini, M., Schunemann, V., Trautwein, A.X., Gerlach, M., Riederer, P., Vezzoni, P. and Tampellini, D. (2002c) Iron, neuromelanin and ferritin content in the substantia nigra of normal subjects at different ages: consequences for iron storage and neurodegenerative processes. *J. Neurochem.* 76: 1766-73.

Zecca, L., Tampellini, D., Gerlach, M., Riederer, P., Fariello, R.G. and Sulzer, D. (2001) Substantia nigra neuromelanin: structure, synthesis, and molecular behaviour. *Mol. Pathol.* 54: 414-8.

Zecca, L. and Swartz, H.M. (1993) Total and paramagnetic metals in human substantia nigra and its neuromelanin. *J. Neural. Transm. Park. Dis. Dement. Sect.* 5: 203-13.

Zecca L, Tampellini D, Gerlach M, Riederer P, Fariello R.G., Sulzer D. (2001) Substantia nigra neuromelanin: structure, synthesis, and molecular behaviour. *J. Clin. Pathol.* 54: 414-418.

Zecca L, Fariello R, Riederer P, Sulzer D, Gatti A, Tampellini D. (2002) The absolute concentrations of nigral neuromelanin , assayed by a new sensitive method, increases through out life and it dramatically decreased in PD. *FEBS lett.* 510:216-220.

Zhang, P., Damier, P., Hirsch, E.C., Agid, Y., Ceballos-Picot, I., Sinet, P.M., Nicole, A., Laurent, M. and Javoy-Agid, F. (1993) Preferential expression of superoxide dismutase messenger RNA in melanized neurons in human mesencephalon. *Neuroscience.* 55: 167-175.

Zheng H, Berman NEJ, and Klaassen CD (1995) Chemical modulation of metallothionein I and II mRNA in mouse brain. *Neurochem. Int.* 27: 43-58.

Ziv, I., Barzilai, A., Offen, D., Nardi, N. and Melamed, E. (1997) Nigrostriatal neuronal death in Parkinson's disease-a passive or an active genetically-controlled process? *J. Neural. Transm. Suppl.* 49:.69-76.

In: New Research on Parkinson's Disease
Editors: T. F. Hahn, J. Werner

ISBN: 978-1-60456-601-7
© 2008 Nova Science Publishers, Inc.

Chapter II

Therapeutic Perspectives Involving Ferritin Heavy Chain FtH in Parkinson's Disease

Haitham Abdelmoaty[1,3], Quentin Pye[3] and Robert H. Broyles[2,3]
[1]University of Oklahoma, Bioengineering program, Norman, OK, USA
[2]University of Oklahoma Health Sciences Center,
Department of Biochemistry, Oklahoma City, OK, USA
[3]Oklahoma Medical Research Foundation, Oklahoma City, OK, USA

Abstract

Parkinson disease *(PD)* is primarily an age-related progressive neurodegenerative disorder affecting as many as 1,500,000 people in the United States alone. Clinically, PD is characterized by bradykinesia, muscular rigidity, resting tremor, and gait abnormalities with later postural instability [1]. Pathologically, PD results in dopaminergic neuronal cell loss in the substantia nigra pars compacta *(SNpc)*, axonal terminal loss in the caudate/putamen (striatum), oxidative stress *(OS)*, dopamine depletion, increased iron levels, increased lipid peroxidation, and decreased mitochondrial complex I activity [2, 3]. The mechanisms underlying the interplay between the rise in oxidative stress and dopaminergic neuronal cell loss are poorly understood. More critically, very little is known regarding the transcriptional changes that occur in Parkinson's disease and its relation to oxidative stress and dopaminergic cell loss. Epidemiological studies suggest an association with pesticides and other environmental toxins [4]. In particular, the toxin 1-methyl-4-phenyl-1,2,3,6-tetrahydropyridine *(MPTP)* and its active metabolite MPP+, are selectively imported into dopaminergic neurons by the plasma membrane dopamine *(DA)* transporter. Once imported, MPP+ induces parkinsonian-like patterns of degeneration [5]. MPTP effects have been extensively studied in vivo using well developed ferritin heavy chain *(FtH)* transgenic mouse models [6, 7]. Recent studies in FtH deficient mice have shown that iron and the iron storage protein FtH, are two major key players in PD disease mechanisms [8]. Both iron and FtH levels are elevated in PD [7, 9]. As iron becomes required for vital biological reactions like dopamine production [10], FtH is degraded through lysosomal activities to release its stored iron [11].

Nevertheless, when iron homeostasis is disturbed, excess iron becomes involved in Fenton reactions producing highly reactive oxygen species *(ROS)* [10]. Excess iron can react with hydrogen peroxide H_2O_2 to produce hydroxyl radicals *(·OH)* [12]. Excess ·OH and other ROS species leads to lipid peroxidation, DNA breakage, and bio-molecular degradation that eventually lead to neuronal death [10]. FtH is known to sequester Fe^{+2} thus it plays a protective role against substantia nigra, gloubus pallidus, and striatum cell death [10]. In this view, it is our hypothesis that the therapeutic potentials of FtH in vivo and in combination with embryonic stem *(ES)* cells would yield greater benefits in understanding and treating PD. ES cells have extensive self-renewal capacity and high potential in differentiating to dopaminergic neurons [13-15]. They also have been extensively cultured in-vitro and shown to successfully differentiate into dopaminergic neurons for parkinson's mice models [15]. On another level, glutathione S-transferase p1 *(GSTP1)* has been shown to mediate protection against H_2O_2 induced cell death [16, 17] and affects the clinical manifestation of PD [18]. Also, NF-E2 related factor 2 *(Nrf2)* is known to bind ARE activators like tert-butylhydroquinone *(tBHQ)* and many antioxidant genes with high relevance to PD [19, 20].

Background

We can generally divide disorders of the basal ganglia into two distinct categories: hypokinesias and hyperkinesias [21]. PD is the most common form of hypokinetic disorders [21]. Major symptoms of PD include tremor, akinesia, and muscular rigidity [21]. The circuitry of neurons in the basal ganglia is rather complex. The basal ganglia filters out signals from the cerebral cortex and the brain stem through projection loops [21]. There are input and output pathways in the basal ganglia. The input is made up of excitatory glutamanergic projection neurons while the output pathway is composed of a direct and an indirect channel. For the purpose of this chapter, we will focus on the direct and indirect output pathways that eventually influence voluntary movement. The direct pathway composed of inhibitory γ-aminobutyric acid *(GABA)* neurons originating from the striatum. However, the indirect pathway is composed of different neurotransmitters, such as GABA, glutamate, enkaphalin and substance P. This indirect pathway passes through the gloubus pallidus, the subthalamic nucleus *(STN)*, the gloubus pallidas internal segment *(GPi)* and the substantia nigra reticulate *(SNR)*. There is a delicate balance between these two pathways that is partly maintained by dopamine release from the substantia nigra to the striatum. Normally, dopamine release seems to exert a resultant inhibitory effect through the indirect pathway by stimulating dopamine D2 receptors; whereas, it exerts a resultant excitatory effect through the direct pathway by stimulating the dopamine D1 receptor. The depletion of dopamine disbalances the direct and indirect pathways from the striatum, which causes the thalamus to be overstimulated. As a result, the frontal cortex is less activated which would account for most of the Parkinsonian symptoms [21].

PD is similar to other neurodegenerative diseases where oxidative stress and neuronal cell death takes place. It has been shown that dopamine itself is associated with dopaminergic cell death [22]. Generation of oxidative stress prior to cellular death involves production of hydroxyl radicals through the metabolism of dopamine [21]. As iron becomes required in vital biological reactions like dopamine production [10], its excess would react with H_2O_2 to produce hydroxyl radicals via the Fenton reaction [12]. Cohen et al. addresses the balance between oxidative stress and anti-oxidant levels. When oxidative stressors are high and anti-oxidant defenses are low, a state of oxidative insult arises [23].

Cellular Mechanisms in PD

As chemical imbalance occurs, oxidizing species such as H_2O_2 or oxy-radicals such as superoxide become increased [23]. Oxidative stress leads cellular systems to an oxidized state and the detoxification and removal of H_2O_2 is primarily done through glutathione (*GSH*) peroxidase [23]. This results in the formation of glutathione disulfide (*GSSG*) and water [23] (Eqn 1).

$$H_2O_2 + 2GSH \rightarrow GSSG + 2H_2O \qquad (1)$$

Excess hydrogen peroxide is particularly harmful to the mitochondrial respiration chain in complex I. The turnover of monoamine neurotransmitters by monoamine oxidase *(MAO)* produces H_2O_2 [23, 24]. As the level of H_2O_2 is increased, oxidation of GSH to GSSH progresses pre and post synaptically in the region of dopamine neurons and nerve terminals [23, 24]. GSSG reacts with protein sulfhydryls (Pr-SH) to produce protein glutathione mixed disulfides (PrSSG) and GSH [23, 24] (Eqn 2).

$$GSSG + Pr\text{-}SH \rightarrow PrSSG + GSH \qquad (2)$$

Accumulation of PrSSG causes damage to the mitochondrial respiratory activities [23]. Suppression of MAO by a combination of clorgyline and pargyline completely suppressed PrSSG accumulation and damage to mitochondrial complex I respiration [23]. Defects in complex I respiration has been associated with a major Parkinson's inducing toxin, MPTP [25]. MPP^+, an MPTP neurotoxin metabolite, binds to complex I of the respiratory chain and stop the electron transport chain leading to energy depletion through ATP loss [25].

MPTP requires a two-step bio-transformation to produce MPP^+. Monoamine oxidase B *(MAO-B)* converts MPTP to 1-methyl-4-phenyl-1,2-dihydroxypyridinium ion *(MPDP$^+$)* which is subsequently oxidized to MPP^+ [26, 27] (Eqn 3).

$$MPTP/MAO\text{-}B \rightarrow MPDP^+ \qquad (3)$$

MPP^+ accumulation and inhibition of complex I [28, 29] impairs ATP production in the mitochondria causing energy failure [30]. Energy failure leads to decreased activity of calcium-ATPase and increased intracellular calcium levels [31-33]. High levels of calcium lead to ROS production followed by cellular membrane degeneration, loss of membrane potential, and finally neuronal loss [31-33]. Accumulation of MPP^+ has also been shown to promote excitotoxicity by enhancing glutamate release. This can be done in two ways: 1- Direct excitotoxicity involving glutamate release and activation of NMDA receptors leading to a large influx of calcium and formation of peroxides with a reduced intracellular glutathione synethsis, 2- Indirect excitotoxicity based on impaired mitochondria function enabling basal or lower levels of glutamate to become cytotoxic [34]. MPP^+ also been shown to increase ROS turnover caused by the catabolism of dopamine through MAO-B [25, 35]. MPP^+ increases dopamine release in the extracellular space making it abundant on a local level. Dopamine oxidation via auto-oxidation or by MAO-B produces H_2O_2 that in turn reacts with excess iron to produce highly toxic hydroxyl radicals [25, 35] (Eqn 4).

$$H_2O_2 + Fe^{2+} \rightarrow Fe^{3+} + OH\bullet + OH^- \qquad (4)$$

Iron in Parkinson's Disease

It was shown in PD as early as 1924 by Lehermitte et al. that iron levels are significantly increased in globus pallidas and SN [36]. To explain the high levels of iron in the SN, studies such as Mash et al. indicated that these regions have relatively low levels of the transferrin receptor [37]. Although abnormal iron transport across the blood brain barrier is possible [38], other possibilities have been proposed to explain the high levels of iron found in the SN: 1- There is a possibility that iron was accumulated prior to the formation of the blood brain barrier, 2- It has been demonstrated that translocation of iron in the brain exist where Fe^{3+} from cortical brain regions in young rats accumulates in the globus pallidas and SN [39], 3- And finally a genetic mutation alters iron metabolism in PD [40].

Recently, sources leading to the elevated SN iron and its relation to neuro-degeneration have been elucidated [7, 41]. Growing evidence suggests a strong involvement of iron in the pathology of PD [42]. Iron metabolism is essential for intracellular mechanisms and excess iron is sequestered by FtH [42]. However, the excess iron release by FtH may result in its high intracellular availability to participate in redox Fenton reactions resulting in oxidative damage of proteins, lipids, or DNA [42] (Eqn 4). In this case, the cell has its own defense mechanism to deal with excess iron. Thus, cellular iron transport and FtH levels become up-regulated [42]. FtH up-regulation requires the interplay between Iron Regulatory Proteins *(IRP's)* and Iron Responsive Elements *(IRE's)* [42]. When cells become rich in iron, IRP-1 remains attached to its [4Fe-4S] cluster and is not able to bind mRNAs [43]. When IRP-1 is not attached to its [4Fe-4S] cluster, it is free to bind IRE containing mRNAs at the 5' end and prevents translation of FtH [44]. Meanwhile, IRP-1 binding to IREs at the 3' end would stabilize the expression of mRNAs and promote the translation of molecules such as transferrin receptor *(TfR)* and divalent metal transporter *(DMT-1)* [44, 45]. In addition to iron levels also FtH levels were measured in the SN and found to be significantly increased [41]. A finding that points out the critical interplay between iron and FtH suggesting that iron buffering is indeed a natural key mechanism in the protection against oxidative damage arising from Fenton reactions. For buffering to be accomplished, iron must be present in its trivalent oxidation state. Certainly, according to recent studies intracellular iron is in fact present in the trivalent ferric iron state Fe^{3+} [46].

Glutathione S-Transferases (*GST*) Role in PD

GSTs are prime candidates for their involvement in Parkinson's disease. Essentially, they are a second line of defense when iron chelation and transport are inadequate in sequestering excess iron. GSTs are involved in the detoxification of oxidizing species; namely, H_2O_2 as well as the metabolism of pesticides, dopamine, and glutathione [47-49]. Other roles of GSTP1 include the inhibition of c-Jun N-terminal Kinase (JNK)-mediated cell signaling pathways that are regulated endogenously in part by glutathione *S*-transferase P1-1 [50]. Inhibition of JNK suggests that GSTP1-1 is a critical ligand-binding protein with a role in regulating kinase pathways [50]. JNK activation is identified as a cellular response to environmental toxins, cytokines, and interleukins [51].

GSTs, as cytosolic isoenzymes have dimeric structures that serve a role in phase II metabolism and xenobiotics [50]. Essentially, their detoxification role against oxidative stress is accomplished by conjugating GSH to electrophilic species which have the potential to produce reactive oxygen species [49]. To test for GSTP1's elevation in PD, genotype association with polymerase chain reaction *(PCR)* showed an excess of Ile104Val GSTP1 heterozygotes between control and PD cases [48]. Ile104Val is one of the known GSTP1 morphs.

As in any biological system, the complexity of the PD mechanism manifests itself at different levels of molecular involvement. As an example, excess H_2O_2 has the potential to increase PrSSG levels indirectly when glutathione initially becomes involved in its detoxification (Eqn 1, 2). Nonetheless, when iron becomes abundant, excess H_2O_2 can further contribute to highly reactive species production; namely, hydroxyl radicals that are injurious to cells (Eqn 4) [7, 52]. This suggests neuronal protection through iron chelators such as FtH is of high importance and relevance to PD treatment.

Ferritin Heavy Chain (FtH) Relevance and Importance to PD

FtH is the natural iron recycler and chelator. It can store up to 4500 iron atoms [53]. It then releases iron in a controlled manner when needed. This release mechanism is predominantly through FtH's own degradation. Iron is needed in a variety of biological mechanisms such as oxygen transfer, electron transfer, nitrogen fixation, and DNA synthesis [53]. Structurally, Ferritin is 12.0 nm in diameter formed from a spherical protein coat known as apoferritin. It is composed of 24 subunits measuring about 20 kDa in mass with an iron-protein interface [53]. There are two forms of the Ferritin molecule; Ferritin heavy chain (FtH) (21 kDa) and light chain (FtL) (19 kDa). The ratio of FtH/FtL varies within different tissues [54]. Brain tissues have higher ratios of heavy chain expression relative to other tissues [55, 56]. FtH possesses a ferroxidase activity that is required for iron uptake [54]. The ferroxidase activity regulates cellular availability of iron giving resistance to oxidative damage by preventing Fenton reactions [56].

Ferritin stability plays a critical role in providing iron to the cell in a controlled manner. As biological mechanisms require iron, FtH degradation proceeds to release iron. Degradation half-lives have been measured in rat liver and found to vary from 25 to 50 hours [57]. Iron release due to FtH degradation displays rather complex kinetics. Studies have shown that such kinetics are governed by PH, buffer ions, and the age of protein coat or iron coat [58]. In addition, a reductase activity is required to convert Fe^{3+} to Fe^{2+}; however, the mechanisms underlying iron reduction remains unknown.

Differential degradation of FtH is the main mechanism for releasing iron into the intracellular space [59]. Proteasomal activities are thought to be involved in the intracellular degradation of FtH. The 20S proteasome is responsible for abnormal FtH turnover. Treatment of human melanoma SK-Mel-28 cells with the proteasomal degradation inhibitor resulted in the accumulation of ^{59}Fe-ferritin suggesting that proteasomal pathways alter ferritin metabolism. Hence, it is reasonable to assume that it influences iron metabolism and its release. The actual release of iron from FtH molecules is still under investigation. However, recent studies indicated that lysosomal protease inhibition slows ferritin iron release in three different cell types [60]. Interestingly, such lysosomal activity has been shown to diminish with age [60]. Knowing the storage capacity of FtH (4500 atoms) [52], age-related diminished lysosomal activity is expected to negatively affect iron uptake when protective chelation is needed. It is noteworthy to keep in mind that PD progression is also age-related [61].

FtH as a natural chelator has a clear advantage over other known chemical chelators like clioquinol (CQ). Inducing the expression of FtH in transgenic cells did not yield any of the harmful side effects found with chemical chelators. The side effects of chemical synthetic chelation compounds forced companies such as Prana Biotechnology to abandon its CQ clinical trial, pull its product from the market, and discontinue any further production. To elucidate FtH's natural and beneficial therapeutic effects, a study involving the suppression of FtH by siRNA, triggered cells to become less resistant to oxidative stress [55]. Studies by Andersen et al. and others have shown that FtH expression protects against MPTP toxicity and provides the same protection as CQ without the harmful side effects [7, 8].

Clearly, the interplay between FtH, neuronal communication dysfunctions in the SN, and basal ganglia are important to understand. More fundamental is the understanding of gene regulation, DNA changes, and their relation to oxidative stress and neuronal death. It has been shown that the depletion of dopamine affects the overall neuronal communication pattern in the basal ganglia and SN [2, 3]. However, the question is not as simple as knowing the relation between dysfunctions in the basal ganglia, neuronal communication, and other established features of the disease such as oxidative stress. The underlying question is much more profound and should consider precisely the timing of events through investigating the most basic stage of involvement at the DNA level. FtH has been shown to be a natural iron chelator and to influence transcription at the DNA level with a major role in gene regulation through its repression to the β-globin gene in sickle cell disease [62].

Gene Regulation Mechanisms Involving FtH

Our laboratory has extensive experience in working with the iron binding hemoglobin molecule [62]. In 2001, such work led to the introduction of FtH as a major repressor to the β globin gene [62]. Broyles et al. published data showing that FtH would bind to a highly conserved CAGTGC motif on the β globin gene promoter region between −153 and −148 bp from the cap site [62]. Binding of FtH represses the β globin gene as shown by the expression of the chloramphenical acetyltransferase (CAT) reporter plasmid [62]. This discovery revealed FtH to be a trans-acting protein [62]. At this point, FtH multilevel involvement begins to be revealed and its importance as a critical player in iron related mechanisms becomes more evident.

Two studies have identified the genetic sequence of GSTP1 in human and rat [63, 64]. We utilized this information by performing a thorough scan of both sequence in the GenBank database. As a result, we confirmed the presence of a highly conserved CAGTGC motif in the human and rat GST promoter region. Curiously, we found an ARE protein binding sequence also present (GTGACTCAGC). ARE's are well known for promoting many genes with chemoprotective roles [62]. Our search in the GenBank database led us to two GST genes that include the FtH and ARE binding sequences at various locations on the promoter as well as the coding sequence. The first gene is *a Homo sapiens* glutathione S-transferase pi (GSTP1) with ID: NM 000852 from the national center for biotechnology information NCBI database. The second gene is a *Rattus norvegicus* glutathione S-transferase (GST) NCBI ID: L29427.

The detoxification role of FtH through the removal of iron and the prevention of hydroxyl radical production [55] is essentially similar to that of GSTP1. Fenton reaction requires H_2O_2 to react with iron to produce free radicals (Eqn 4). Either the removal of iron by FtH or the detoxification of H_2O_2 by GSTP1 would prevent toxic radical production. From this junction of events, FtH and GSTP1 roles appear to be "two faces" of a single coin. However, their overall protective role in gene regulation may take a very different turn with PD progression. With the presence of the FtH binding sequence in the GSTP1 promoter and what is known about the role of this sequence, we strongly expect that the elevation of FtH would influence the expression GSTP1.

If our future experimental data indicate that in fact FtH binds ARE genes and influences GSTP1, then for the first time that aspects of genetic regulation involving Ferritin in Parkinson's will be clearly understood. To date, Parkinson's mechanisms on the DNA level are ambiguous at best.

Nrf2 Gene Regulation Mechanisms in PD

Nuclear related factor 2 (Nrf2) is well known for its transcriptional regulation role at the DNA level [19, 20, 65-67]. In neuronal cells, Nrf2 is found in the cytoplasm with a molecular mass of about 67 KDa in humans, rats and mice [20]. Human Nrf2 is made up of 605 amino acids with a strong interspecies homology [20]. The Keap1-Nrf2 complex reacts with inducers/stressors in the cytoplasm causing the release of Nrf2 prior to ARE activation [20].

In PD, there is a considerable amount of evidence indicating that Nrf2 binds ARE sequences (RTGACnnnGC) on the promoter region and coordinates activation of a series of endogenous cytoprotective genes that encode for both antioxidant- and anti-inflammatory proteins [19, 20, 65, 66].

There are two main lines of evidence that lead us to hypothesize that Nrf2 is expected to bind GSTP1 and positively influence its transcription: 1- Nrf2 has been shown to bind a specific ARE sequence (RTGACnnnGC) and give rise to antioxidant genes such as Hmox-1, NADPH and glutathione [68-76], and that 2- Stabilization and/or activation of Nrf2 by ARE inducer tert-butylhdroquinone (tBHQ) protects against H_2O_2 induced cell death [20, 74-78].

FtH Expression in Mice Models

Given the importance of FtH in its significant involvement in neurodegenerative disorders and in particular Parkinson's, the need for a FtH transgenic mouse model became inevitable. Among others, a ferritin transgenic mouse was created by Kaur et al. [7] via injection of an 8.3 kb Hind III DNA fragment containing 4.8 kb of 5' upstream sequences from the rat TH gene [79], a 2.6 kb of human genomic ferritin DNA containing 4 coding exon regions [80], a 3' SV40 splice and a polyadenlylation transgenic sequence. This DNA fragment was injected into fertilized B6D2 mouse embryos to make the p-TH transgenic mouse [7]. Initially, FtH played a neuro-protective role in these mice following MPTP treatment; however, prolonged upregulation of FtH after 12 months of age have shown an adverse result with a measured progressive neuro-degeneration [6]. Thus, the experimental procedure is set up to test these mice at early (2-4 month) as well as later stages (8-12 month) of age.

An alternative method for studying the effect of high levels of FtH is through injections of FtH inducers into mice or through diet supplementation [81, 82]. Treatment with retinoic acid (RA), an endogenous molecule and the acidified form of Vitamin A [83, 84], has shown a 4 fold increase in FtH levels [82]. Astroglia derived RA has also been identified as a key factor in glia-induced neurogensis [85]. RA is lipophilic with a molecular weight of 300 g/mol (Daltons) [84, 86]. Substances with a molecular weight lower than 500 g/mol (500 daltons) generally can cross the blood-brain barrier [87]. RA is acquired from diet through retinyl esters present in animal meat or β-carotene present in plants [84]. It is well established that RA is an FtH inducer in the brain [82]. Thus, RA will serve as a standard we will use to compare to out test compound abscisic acid (ABA).

Administration of ABA formulated mouse diet has been tested before in other disease models like type II diabetes (T2D) [81] but not in Parkinson's. Several studies have focused on ABA involvement in the mammalian brain [81, 88]. ABA, a naturally occurring phytochemical hormone with structural similarities to thiazolidinediones (TZDs), has been shown to increase ferritin levels [89, 90]. TZDs are generally known to cross the blood brain barrier, in particular pioglitazone [91]. TZD pioglitazone has been administered orally to autism patients, autism is a complex neuro-developmental disorder. Administration of pioglitazone to patients showed a statistically significant clinical improvement [92]. Abscisic acid ($C_{15}H_{20}O_4$) has a molecular weight of 264.32 g/mol. ABA has been found in the central nervous system of pigs and rats [88]. Its conjugates esters and glucosides found in plants has also been identified and detected in the brain [88]. Pidoplichko et al. showed that trans,trans-ABA, not an ABA isomer used by plants, has a role in increasing the fast component of NMDA-gated currents in isolated rat hippocampal neurons [93]. However, the link to the exact mechanism underlying ABA engagement in FtH up-regulation and its NMDA role is yet to be elucidated.

Embryonic Stem Cells Therapeutic Potentials in PD

Embryonic stem cell ES differentiation into neurons has been studied for many decades. Early studies demonstrated embryonic stem cells (ESC-BLC 6) exhibiting morphological characteristics that are specific to neurons [94]. In-vivo and in-vitro studies have shown that dopaminergic stem cells can in fact be derived from embryonic stem cells [13, 14, 95]. Earlier in-vitro studies indicated that mouse embryonic stem cells exposed to retinoic acid expressed multiple phenotypes that are normally specific to neurons [95]. Recent In vitro co-culture of stromal feeder cells and human ES cells (line H1, H9, HES-3, and monkey line R366) were shown to induce differentiation into DA neural cells [14]. The study showed a successful differentiation of up to 79% of all differentiated neurons expressing tyrosine hydroxylase TH, the rate-limiting enzyme in DA synthesis [14]. Meanwhile, in vivo studies focused mostly on the transplantation of ES and its therapeutic potentials [96-100]. Earlier, In vivo transplantation of ES has encountered many challenges [101] ranging from the ability to generate a highly purified and homogenous population of dopamine neurons and the ability of ES cells to completely survive, restore, and re-innervate in the striatum to more basic challenges such as contamination of differentiated cells with undifferentiated ones [101]. Recently, many of these challenges been surpassed with improved ES transplantation results and enhanced cell preparation protocols that show clear evidence of a dopamine neuronal phenotype [102-104].

ES differentiation to dopamine neurons has been successfully demonstrated by Lee at al [102] and later was successfully replicated by Kim et al [98]. ES differentiation was confined to 5 stages with clear genetic expression of specific makers in each differentiation stage. Among others, these markers include the homebox genes *OTX1* and *OTX2* [102]. Characterization of the different stages have shown that *OTX2* is expressed in the undifferentiated stage 1 and is present at low levels in stage 2 and 3 [102]. In stage 3, *OTX1* is expressed at high levels. Other genes such as *Pax2, Pax5, Wn1, En1, Nurr1* became also elevated in stages 3 and 4 [102]. Stage 3 and 4 is also know for its high expression of nestin [102]. At stage 5, TuJ1$^+$ antibody with its neuron specific β-III tubulin was directed toward and bound to many cells that possess clear neuronal morphology [102]. Immunocytochemistry with TH monoclonal antibody directed toward these β-III tubulin (TuJ1) bound neurons showed a significant increase in TH$^+$ neurons [102]. This increase was due to an improved modification to the cell culture protocol by excluding HEPES from the cell medium during stages 4 and 5 [102]. Dissociation of EB cells (stage 2) into single cells in culture yielded astonishing results with a 3.5 fold increase in nestin-positive cells in stage 3 [102].

Summary

Parkinson disease is primarily an age-related progressive neurodegenerative disorder affecting as many as 1,500,000 people in the United States alone. To date, very little is known regarding the transcriptional changes that occur in Parkinson's disease and its relation to oxidative stress and dopaminergic cell loss. Particularly, the genetic regulatory roles of the iron storage protein ferritin-H and the ARE binding protein Nrf2 with respect to significantly relevant antioxidant genes such as GSTP1.

The use of a transgenic mouse model and ES cell cultures in testing their PD therapeutic potential offers benefits that are critical on a multi-dimensional level. In additional to their therapeutic potentials, our studies offer the opportunity to answer pure scientific questions regarding PD mechanisms. Different methods of FtH induction is expected to shed light on further FtH mechanisms with regard to MPTP induced parkinsonism. Eventually this will lead to understanding parkinson's disease mechanism as a whole.

To further reveal genetic regulation mechanisms in PD, future investigations would be necessary. The next step is to set forth new aims that would look further into the interplay between FtH, Nrf2, and GSTP1 with a focus on the multi-layered mechanistic details leading to dopaminergic cell death. Upon proving our hypothesis, another critical question would follow addressing additional FtH and Nrf2 genetic regulation roles and how such roles assemble together to reveal greater framework details in regard to PD. For example, are there other regulators that compete with FtH and Nrf2 for the GSTP1 promoter? Is there a common inducer/inhibitor that influences both FtH and Nrf2 in different ways? Possibly test a new therapeutic candidate and examine its potential is dealing with high iron levels and dopaminergic cell loss.

To date, Parkinson mechanisms on the DNA level are ambiguous at best. With this proposed study we are building a solid foundation for understanding genetic regulation in PD. On the basis of our findings we would open a main gate leading to several avenues that would hopefully converge into the same final destination in fully understanding and treating PD.

References

[1]   Berardelli, A., et al., Pathophysiology of bradykinesia in Parkinson's disease. *Brain*, 2001. 124(Pt 11): p. 2131-46.

[2]   Bernheimer, H., et al., Brain dopamine and the syndromes of Parkinson and Huntington. Clinical, morphological and neurochemical correlations. *J. Neurol. Sci.*, 1973. 20(4): p. 415-55.

[3]   Damier, P., et al., The substantia nigra of the human brain. II. Patterns of loss of dopamine-containing neurons in Parkinson's disease. *Brain*, 1999. 122 (Pt 8): p. 1437-48.

[4]   Gorell, J.M., et al., The risk of Parkinson's disease with exposure to pesticides, farming, well water, and rural living. *Neurology*, 1998. 50(5): p. 1346-50.

[5]   Javitch, J.A., et al., Parkinsonism-inducing neurotoxin, N-methyl-4-phenyl-1,2,3,6 -tetrahydropyridine: uptake of the metabolite N-methyl-4-phenylpyridine by dopamine neurons explains selective toxicity. *Proc. Natl. Acad. Sci. USA*, 1985. 82(7): p. 2173-7.

[6]   Kaur, D., et al., Chronic ferritin expression within murine dopaminergic midbrain neurons results in a progressive age-related neurodegeneration. *Brain Res*, 2006.

[7]   Kaur, D., et al., Genetic or pharmacological iron chelation prevents MPTP-induced neurotoxicity in vivo: a novel therapy for Parkinson's disease. *Neuron*, 2003. 37(6): p. 899-909.

[8]   Ill, A.M., et al., Metabolic analysis of mouse brains that have compromised iron storage. *Metab. Brain Dis.*, 2006. 21(2-3): p. 77-87.

[9]   Zecca, L., et al., Iron, brain ageing and neurodegenerative disorders. *Nat. Rev. Neurosci.*, 2004. 5(11): p. 863-73.

[10] Lee, D.W., J.K. Andersen, and D. Kaur, Iron dysregulation and neurodegeneration: the molecular connection. *Mol. Interv.*, 2006. 6(2): p. 89-97.

[11] Kidane, T.Z., E. Sauble, and M.C. Linder, Release of iron from ferritin requires lysosomal activity. *Am. J. Physiol. Cell Physiol.*, 2006. 291(3): p. C445-55.

[12] Ebadi, M., S.K. Srinivasan, and M.D. Baxi, Oxidative stress and antioxidant therapy in Parkinson's disease. *Prog. Neurobiol.*, 1996. 48(1): p. 1-19.

[13] Andersson, E., et al., Development of the mesencephalic dopaminergic neuron system is compromised in the absence of neurogenin 2. *Development*, 2006. 133(3): p. 507-16.

[14] Perrier, A.L., et al., Derivation of midbrain dopamine neurons from human embryonic stem cells. *Proc. Natl. Acad. Sci. USA*, 2004. 101(34): p. 12543-8.

[15] Barberi, T., et al., Neural subtype specification of fertilization and nuclear transfer embryonic stem cells and application in parkinsonian mice. *Nat. Biotechnol.*, 2003. 21(10): p. 1200-7.

[16] Baez, S., et al., Glutathione transferases catalyse the detoxication of oxidized metabolites (o-quinones) of catecholamines and may serve as an antioxidant system preventing degenerative cellular processes. *Biochem J.*, 1997. 324 (Pt 1): p. 25-8.

[17] Tew, K.D. and Z. Ronai, GST function in drug and stress response. *Drug Resist. Updat*, 1999. 2(3): p. 143-147.

[18] Golbe, L.I., et al., Glutathione S-transferase polymorphisms and onset age in alpha-synuclein A53T mutant Parkinson's disease. *Am. J. Med. Genet B Neuropsychiatr. Genet*, 2007. 144(2): p. 254-8.

[19] Clements, C.M., et al., DJ-1, a cancer- and Parkinson's disease-associated protein, stabilizes the antioxidant transcriptional master regulator Nrf2. *Proc. Natl. Acad. Sci. USA*, 2006. 103(41): p. 15091-6.

[20] Li, J., et al., Stabilization of Nrf2 by tBHQ confers protection against oxidative stress-induced cell death in human neural stem cells. *Toxicol. Sci.*, 2005. 83(2): p. 313-28.

[21] Sian, J., et al., Parkinson's disease: a major hypokinetic basal ganglia disorder. *J. Neural. Transm*, 1999. 106(5-6): p. 443-76.

[22] Cantuti-Castelvetri, I., B. Shukitt-Hale, and J.A. Joseph, Dopamine neurotoxicity: age-dependent behavioral and histological effects. *Neurobiol. Aging*, 2003. 24(5): p. 697-706.

[23] Cohen, G., Oxidative stress, mitochondrial respiration, and Parkinson's disease. *Ann. NY Acad. Sci.*, 2000. 899: p. 112-20.

[24] Cohen, G. and N. Kesler, Monoamine oxidase inhibits mitochondrial respiration. *Ann. NY Acad. Sci.*, 1999. 893: p. 273-8.

[25] Schmidt, N. and B. Ferger, Neurochemical findings in the MPTP model of Parkinson's disease. *J. Neural. Transm.*, 2001. 108(11): p. 1263-82.

[26] Chiba, K., A. Trevor, and N. Castagnoli, Jr., Metabolism of the neurotoxic tertiary amine, MPTP, by brain monoamine oxidase. *Biochem. Biophys. Res. Commun.*, 1984. 120(2): p. 574-8.

[27] Markey, S.P., et al., Intraneuronal generation of a pyridinium metabolite may cause drug-induced parkinsonism. *Nature*, 1984. 311(5985): p. 464-7.

[28] Nicklas, W.J., I. Vyas, and R.E. Heikkila, Inhibition of NADH-linked oxidation in brain mitochondria by 1-methyl-4-phenyl-pyridine, a metabolite of the neurotoxin, 1-methyl-4-phenyl-1,2,5,6-tetrahydropyridine. *Life Sci.*, 1985. 36(26): p. 2503-8.

[29] Ramsay, R.R., et al., Interaction of 1-methyl-4-phenylpyridinium ion (MPP+) and its analogs with the rotenone/piericidin binding site of NADH dehydrogenase. *J. Neurochem.*, 1991. 56(4): p. 1184-90.

[30] Di Monte, D.A., Mitochondrial DNA and Parkinson's disease. *Neurology*, 1991. 41(5 Suppl 2): p. 38-42; discussion 42-3.

[31] German, D.C., et al., Midbrain dopaminergic cell loss in Parkinson's disease and MPTP-induced parkinsonism: sparing of calbindin-D28k-containing cells. *Ann. NY Acad. Sci.*, 1992. 648: p. 42-62.

[32] Kupsch, A., et al., Pretreatment with nimodipine prevents MPTP-induced neurotoxicity at the nigral, but not at the striatal level in mice. *Neuroreport*, 1995. 6(4): p. 621-5.

[33] Kupsch, A., et al., 1-Methyl-4-phenyl-1,2,3,6-tetrahydropyridine-induced neurotoxicity in non-human primates is antagonized by pretreatment with nimodipine at the nigral, but not at the striatal level. *Brain Res.*, 1996. 741(1-2): p. 185-96.

[34] Beal, M.F., et al., Neurochemical and histologic characterization of striatal excitotoxic lesions produced by the mitochondrial toxin 3-nitropropionic acid. *J. Neurosci*, 1993. 13(10): p. 4181-92.

[35] Busciglio, J., et al., Stress, aging, and neurodegenerative disorders. Molecular mechanisms. *Ann. NY Acad. Sci.*, 1998. 851: p. 429-43.

[36] Youdim, M.B., D. Ben-Shachar, and P. Riederer, The possible role of iron in the etiopathology of Parkinson's disease. *Mov. Disord*, 1993. 8(1): p. 1-12.

[37] Mash, D.C., et al., Distribution and number of transferrin receptors in Parkinson's disease and in MPTP-treated mice. *Exp. Neurol.*, 1991. 114(1): p. 73-81.

[38] Kortekaas, R., et al., Blood-brain barrier dysfunction in parkinsonian midbrain in vivo. *Ann. Neurol.*, 2005. 57(2): p. 176-9.

[39] Dwork, A.J., et al., An autoradiographic study of the uptake and distribution of iron by the brain of the young rat. *Brain Res.*, 1990. 518(1-2): p. 31-9.

[40] Dekker, M.C., et al., Mutations in the hemochromatosis gene (HFE), Parkinson's disease and parkinsonism. *Neurosci. Lett.*, 2003. 348(2): p. 117-9.

[41] Zucca, F.A., et al., Neuromelanin and iron in human locus coeruleus and substantia nigra during aging: consequences for neuronal vulnerability. *J. Neural. Transm.*, 2006. 113(6): p. 757-67.

[42] Berg, D. and H. Hochstrasser, Iron metabolism in Parkinsonian syndromes. *Mov. Disord.*, 2006. 21(9): p. 1299-310.

[43] Li, Q., et al., Effects of 12 metal ions on iron regulatory protein 1 (IRP-1) and hypoxia-inducible factor-1 alpha (HIF-1alpha) and HIF-regulated genes. *Toxicol Appl. Pharmacol.*, 2006. 213(3): p. 245-55.

[44] Siddappa, A.J., et al., Iron deficiency alters iron regulatory protein and iron transport protein expression in the perinatal rat brain. *Pediatr. Res.*, 2003. 53(5): p. 800-7.

[45] Huang, E., W.Y. Ong, and J.R. Connor, Distribution of divalent metal transporter-1 in the monkey basal ganglia. *Neuroscience*, 2004. 128(3): p. 487-96.

[46] Chwiej, J., et al., Investigations of differences in iron oxidation state inside single neurons from substantia nigra of Parkinson's disease and control patients using the micro-XANES technique. *J. Biol. Inorg. Chem.*, 2007. 12(2): p. 204-11.

[47] Menegon, A., et al., Parkinson's disease, pesticides, and glutathione transferase polymorphisms. *Lancet*, 1998. 352(9137): p. 1344-6.

[48] Yin, Z., et al., Glutathione S-transferase p elicits protection against H2O2-induced cell death via coordinated regulation of stress kinases. Cancer Res, 2000. 60(15): p. 4053-7.

[49] Kelada, S.N., et al., Glutathione S-transferase M1, T1, and P1 polymorphisms and Parkinson's disease. *Neurosci. Lett.*, 2003. 337(1): p. 5-8.

[50] Wang, T., et al., Glutathione S-transferase P1-1 (GSTP1-1) inhibits c-Jun N-terminal kinase (JNK1) signaling through interaction with the C terminus. *J. Biol. Chem.*, 2001. 276(24): p. 20999-1003.

[51] Ip, Y.T. and R.J. Davis, Signal transduction by the c-Jun N-terminal kinase (JNK)--from inflammation to development. *Curr. Opin. Cell Biol.*, 1998. 10(2): p. 205-19.

[52] Puppo, A. and B. Halliwell, Formation of hydroxyl radicals from hydrogen peroxide in the presence of iron. Is haemoglobin a biological Fenton reagent? *Biochem. J.*, 1988. 249(1): p. 185-90.

[53] Theil, E.C., Ferritin: structure, gene regulation, and cellular function in animals, plants, and microorganisms. *Annu. Rev. Biochem.*, 1987. 56: p. 289-315.

[54] Pinero, D.J., J. Hu, and J.R. Connor, Alterations in the interaction between iron regulatory proteins and their iron responsive element in normal and Alzheimer's diseased brains. *Cell Mol. Biol.* (Noisy-le-grand), 2000. 46(4): p. 761-76.

[55] Connor, J.R., et al., A quantitative analysis of isoferritins in select regions of aged, parkinsonian, and Alzheimer's diseased brains. *J. Neurochem.*, 1995. 65(2): p. 717-24.

[56] Cozzi, A., et al., Overexpression of wild type and mutated human ferritin H-chain in HeLa cells: in vivo role of ferritin ferroxidase activity. *J. Biol. Chem.*, 2000. 275(33): p. 25122-9.

[57] Richter, G.W., Studies of iron overload. Rat liver siderosome ferritin. *Lab. Invest*, 1984. 50(1): p. 26-35.

[58] Ihara, K., et al., Cell-specific properties of red cell and liver ferritin from bullfrog tadpoles probed by phosphorylation in vitro. *J. Biol. Chem.*, 1984. 259(1): p. 278-83.

[59] Goralska, M., et al., Differential degradation of ferritin H- and L-chains: accumulation of L-chain-rich ferritin in lens epithelial cells. *Invest Ophthalmol. Vis. Sci.*, 2005. 46(10): p. 3521-9.

[60] Shang, F., et al., Age-related decline in ubiquitin conjugation in response to oxidative stress in the lens. *Exp. Eye Res.,* 1997. 64(1): p. 21-30.

[61] Le Couteur, D.G., et al., Age-environment and gene-environment interactions in the pathogenesis of Parkinson's disease. *Rev. Environ Health*, 2002. 17(1): p. 51-64.

[62] Broyles, R.H., et al., Specific repression of beta-globin promoter activity by nuclear ferritin. *Proc. Natl. Acad. Sci. USA*, 2001. 98(16): p. 9145-50.

[63] Moscow, J.A., et al., Expression of anionic glutathione-S-transferase and P-glycoprotein genes in human tissues and tumors. *Cancer Res.*, 1989. 49(6): p. 1422-8.

[64] Okuda, A., M. Sakai, and M. Muramatsu, The structure of the rat glutathione S-transferase P gene and related pseudogenes. *J. Biol. Chem.*, 1987. 262(8): p. 3858-63.

[65] van Muiswinkel, F.L. and H.B. Kuiperij, The Nrf2-ARE Signalling pathway: promising drug target to combat oxidative stress in neurodegenerative disorders. *Curr. Drug Targets CNS Neurol. Disord.*, 2005. 4(3): p. 267-81.

[66] Hara, H., M. Ohta, and T. Adachi, Apomorphine protects against 6-hydroxydopamine-induced neuronal cell death through activation of the Nrf2-ARE pathway. *J. Neurosci. Res.*, 2006. 84(4): p. 860-6.

[67] Zhang, D.D., Mechanistic studies of the Nrf2-Keap1 signaling pathway. *Drug Metab. Rev.*, 2006. 38(4): p. 769-89.

[68] Ramos-Gomez, M., et al., Sensitivity to carcinogenesis is increased and chemoprotective efficacy of enzyme inducers is lost in nrf2 transcription factor-deficient mice. *Proc. Natl. Acad. Sci. USA*, 2001. 98(6): p. 3410-5.

[69] Kwak, M.K., et al., Modulation of gene expression by cancer chemopreventive dithiolethiones through the Keap1-Nrf2 pathway. Identification of novel gene clusters for cell survival. *J. Biol. Chem.*, 2003. 278(10): p. 8135-45.

[70] Fahey, J.W., et al., Sulforaphane inhibits extracellular, intracellular, and antibiotic-resistant strains of Helicobacter pylori and prevents benzo[a]pyrene-induced stomach tumors. *Proc. Natl. Acad. Sci. USA*, 2002. 99(11): p. 7610-5.

[71] Cao, T.T., et al., Increased nuclear factor-erythroid 2 p45-related factor 2 activity protects SH-SY5Y cells against oxidative damage. *J. Neurochem.*, 2005. 95(2): p. 406-17.

[72] Nakaso, K., et al., Novel cytoprotective mechanism of anti-parkinsonian drug deprenyl: PI3K and Nrf2-derived induction of antioxidative proteins. *Biochem. Biophys. Res. Commun.*, 2006. 339(3): p. 915-22.

[73] Satoh, T., et al., Activation of the Keap1/Nrf2 pathway for neuroprotection by electrophilic [correction of electrophillic] phase II inducers. *Proc. Natl. Acad. Sci. USA*, 2006. 103(3): p. 768-73.

[74] Shih, A.Y., et al., Coordinate regulation of glutathione biosynthesis and release by Nrf2-expressing glia potently protects neurons from oxidative stress. *J. Neurosci.*, 2003. 23(8): p. 3394-406.

[75] Li, J., M.L. Spletter, and J.A. Johnson, Dissecting tBHQ induced ARE-driven gene expression through long and short oligonucleotide arrays. *Physiol. Genomics*, 2005. 21(1): p. 43-58.

[76] Johnson, D.A., et al., Activation of the antioxidant response element in primary cortical neuronal cultures derived from transgenic reporter mice. *J. Neurochem.*, 2002. 81(6): p. 1233-41.

[77] Kraft, A.D., D.A. Johnson, and J.A. Johnson, Nuclear factor E2-related factor 2-dependent antioxidant response element activation by tert-butylhydroquinone and sulforaphane occurring preferentially in astrocytes conditions neurons against oxidative insult. *J. Neurosci.*, 2004. 24(5): p. 1101-12.

[78] Nguyen, T., et al., Increased protein stability as a mechanism that enhances Nrf2-mediated transcriptional activation of the antioxidant response element. Degradation of Nrf2 by the 26 S proteasome. *J. Biol. Chem.*, 2003. 278(7): p. 4536-41.

[79] Banerjee, S.A., et al., 5' flanking sequences of the rat tyrosine hydroxylase gene target accurate tissue-specific, developmental, and transsynaptic expression in transgenic mice. *J. Neurosci.*, 1992. 12(11): p. 4460-7.

[80] Hentze, M.W., et al., Cloning, characterization, expression, and chromosomal localization of a human ferritin heavy-chain gene. *Proc. Natl. Acad. Sci. USA*, 1986. 83(19): p. 7226-30.

[81] Guri, A.J., et al., Dietary abscisic acid ameliorates glucose tolerance and obesity-related inflammation in db/db mice fed high-fat diets. *Clin. Nutr.*, 2007. 26(1): p. 107-16.

[82] VanLandingham, J.W. and C.W. Levenson, Effect of retinoic acid on ferritin H expression during brain development and neuronal differentiation. *Nutr. Neurosci.*, 2003. 6(1): p. 39-45.

[83] Chen-Roetling, J., L. Benvenisti-Zarom, and R.F. Regan, Cultured astrocytes from heme oxygenase-1 knockout mice are more vulnerable to heme-mediated oxidative injury. *J. Neurosci. Res.*, 2005. 82(6): p. 802-10.

[84] Maden, M. and M. Hind, Retinoic acid, a regeneration-inducing molecule. *Dev. Dyn.*, 2003. 226(2): p. 237-44.

[85] Kornyei, Z., et al., Astroglia-derived retinoic acid is a key factor in glia-induced neurogenesis. Faseb J, 2007.

[86] Crick, F., Diffusion in embryogenesis. *Nature*, 1970. 225(5231): p. 420-2.

[87] Tanobe, K., et al., [Blood-brain barrier and general anesthetics]. *Masui*, 2003. 52(8): p. 840-5.

[88] Le Page-Degivry, M.T., et al., Presence of abscisic acid, a phytohormone, in the mammalian brain. *Proc. Natl. Acad. Sci. USA*, 1986. 83(4): p. 1155-8.

[89] Fobis-Loisy, I., et al., Structure and differential expression of two maize ferritin genes in response to iron and abscisic acid. *Eur. J. Biochem.*, 1995. 231(3): p. 609-19.

[90] Lobreaux, S., T. Hardy, and J.F. Briat, Abscisic acid is involved in the iron-induced synthesis of maize ferritin. *Embo J.*, 1993. 12(2): p. 651-7.

[91] Maeshiba, Y., et al., Disposition of the new antidiabetic agent pioglitazone in rats, dogs, and monkeys. *Arzneimittelforschung*, 1997. 47(1): p. 29-35.

[92] Boris, M., et al., Effect of pioglitazone treatment on behavioral symptoms in autistic children. *J. Neuroinflammation.*, 2007. 4: p. 3.

[93] Pidoplichko, V.I. and K.G. Reymann, Abscisic acid potentiates NMDA-gated currents in hippocampal neurones. *Neuroreport*, 1994. 5(17): p. 2311-6.

[94] Wobus, A.M., R. Grosse, and J. Schoneich, Specific effects of nerve growth factor on the differentiation pattern of mouse embryonic stem cells in vitro. *Biomed. Biochim. Acta*, 1988. 47(12): p. 965-73.

[95] Bain, G., et al., Embryonic stem cells express neuronal properties in vitro. *Dev. Biol.*, 1995. 168(2): p. 342-57.

[96] Lindvall, O. and A. Bjorklund, Cell therapy in Parkinson's disease. *NeuroRx*, 2004. 1(4): p. 382-93.

[97] Wagner, J., et al., Induction of a midbrain dopaminergic phenotype in Nurr1-overexpressing neural stem cells by type 1 astrocytes. *Nat. Biotechnol.*, 1999. 17(7): p. 653-9.

[98] Kim, J.H., et al., Dopamine neurons derived from embryonic stem cells function in an animal model of Parkinson's disease. *Nature,* 2002. 418(6893): p. 50-6.

[99] Takagi, Y., et al., Dopaminergic neurons generated from monkey embryonic stem cells function in a Parkinson primate model. *J. Clin. Invest.*, 2005. 115(1): p. 102-9.

[100] Nikkhah, G., G. Falkenstein, and C. Rosenthal, Restorative plasticity of dopamine neuronal transplants depends on the degree of hemispheric dominance. *J. Neurosci.*, 2001. 21(16): p. 6252-63.

[101] Singec, I., et al., The leading edge of stem cell therapeutics. *Annu. Rev. Med.*, 2007. 58: p. 313-28.

[102] Lee, S.H., et al., Efficient generation of midbrain and hindbrain neurons from mouse embryonic stem cells. *Nat. Biotechnol.*, 2000. 18(6): p. 675-9.

[103] Zhao, M., et al., Evidence for neurogenesis in the adult mammalian substantia nigra. *Proc. Natl. Acad. Sci. USA*, 2003. 100(13): p. 7925-30.

[104] Winkler, C., et al., Transplantation in the rat model of Parkinson's disease: ectopic versus homotopic graft placement. *Prog. Brain Res.*, 2000. 127: p. 233-65.

In: New Research on Parkinson's Disease
Editors: T. F. Hahn, J. Werner

ISBN: 978-1-60456-601-7
© 2008 Nova Science Publishers, Inc.

Chapter III

Race and Ethnicity in Parkinson's Disease: Genetic and Prevalence Data

Masharip Atadzhanov[1] and Gretchen L. Birbeck[2]

[1]University of Zambia, Department of Medicine, Lusaka, Zambia
[2]Michigan State University, International Neurologic and Psychiatric Epidemiology
Program (INPEP), East Lansing, Michigan, USA

Abstract

Parkinson's disease (PD) prevalence various significantly globally and its etiology remains unknown. Both genetic and environmental factors as well as their interactions are believed to be important in the etiology of PD. Published epidemiological studies indicate that the prevalence of PD in Asian and African population is much lower than in the Caucasian population. This suggests that the incidence of PD may vary by race. Migration studies indicate that environmental exposures potentially mediated or modified by ethnicity-related lifestyle exposures may also be important. Efforts to characterize gene-environment interactions have intensified in the last decade. For example, genetic studies show that the MAO B G/A genotype frequency in Asian population differ from frequencies in Caucasians and the prevalence of the LRRK2 G2019S mutation is rare in Asian population. Recently, a common genetic variant (LRRK2 G2385R) has been found to be associated with a two-fold increased risk of sporadic PD in ethnic Chinese populations in Singapore and Taiwan. Epidemiological and genetic studies suggest that race/ethnicity effects should be considered in the context of new genetic breakthroughs and haplotype mapping given the extensive population heterogeneity due to genetic admixture. In this article we review the available data and discuss the possible contributions of race and ethnicity to the epidemiological, clinical and pathological features, and genetics of PD.

Introduction

Parkinson's disease (PD) is one of the most prevalent neurodegenerative diseases in the middle and elder age. The prevalence of the disease varies significantly on a global scale. The disease known as Parkinson's disease was first described by J. Parkinson in 1817. Most of researchers accept that both genetic and environmental factors are important in the etiology of PD. Nevertheless, controversy over the role of genetic and environmental risk factors in the etiology of PD has continued for many years.

The environmental hypothesis in the etiology of PD was strongly suggested ~20 years ago after the report of a parkinsonian syndrome in young adults that were intoxicated by a neurotoxin called MPTP, which selectively destroys nigrostriatal dopaminergic neurons. Several chemical products used in herbicides and pesticides are similar structurally to MPTP. However, no causative environmental chemical agent has been identified in the etiology of PD [1]. However, there are recently identified genes associated with familial and sporadic PD [2-4]. These data support an important role of genetic factors and lead some investigators to the conclusion that there is no evidence that the environment plays a role in the etiology of PD [2-5]. Results of twin studies show that monozygotic (MZ) and dizygotic (DZ) twin concordance rates (CR) are low however, lending support to the role of environmental factors since heritability estimates determine less than 50% indicating that environmental variance is greater than genetic variance [6]. These debates highlight the importance of gene-environment interactions (or incompletely penetrant mutations) and the role of self-propagating stochastic factors that may underlie the disease.

Efforts to investigate gene-environment interactions have only begun recently and the role of each of them is not yet clear. If PD results from a combination of genetic and environmental factors, then an interaction of genetic factors with key environmental exposures should result in a high prevalence of the disease [7]. PD is heterogeneous disease and whether clinical presentation of genetic heritability factors should guide categorization for research purposes and epidemiological studies remains unclear.

Advances in genetics and the Human Genome Project significantly increased attention to the importance of race and ethnic background in biomedical research and clinical practice[8-11]. The sequencing of the human genome and the ongoing international effort to catalog common haplotypes in several populations [12] make this an opportune time to examine the complex relationships between genetics research and the categories of race, ethnicity and ancestry [13]. However, increasing attention to racial and ethnic categories in medicine and biomedical research meet growing controversy and has generated much discussion. Recently, the New England Journal of Medicine [14-17], the International Journal of Epidemiology [10, 18, 19] and other journals [10, 18-22] have published commentaries, articles and editorials, some criticizing and others arguing in favor of the use of race and ethnicity in medical research. We do not wish to enter into these debates, but medical literature categorizing clinical, epidemiologic, and biomedical differences across peoples based upon race and ethnicity with the presumed basis being genetic variability are widespread in various fields of medicine [23-27]. For the foreseeable future, racial and ethnic descriptors will continue to be used in medical and scientific research. Ignoring racial and ethnic differences in medicine and biomedical research will not eliminate them. In the context of current genetic advances, the use of 'racial' categorization is inevitable. Focusing attention on these issues can help to understand causes, expression and prevalence of various diseases and develop strategies for their prophylaxis and treatment.

Although "any two human beings on this Earth are 99.9% identical at the DNA level" [12], the human population is not homogeneous in terms of risk of disease. The 10th of a percent of the genome's 3 billion letters that are different translates into roughly 3 million sequence differences, which dramatically contribute to the causes, expression and prevalence of various diseases. Although differences between human populations have been a focus of scientific investigation since at least the 18th century [28] and ethnicity, race and ancestry have been categorized in biomedical research since the 20th century, categorization of humans in biomedical research still suffers from many shortcomings. This is partly due to the complexities offered by immigration and populations mixing. How can accurate classifications schemes that are simple enough to offer quantitative comparisons be developed that still corresponds to real biological differences rather than culturally defined stereotypes? The absence of detail and inconsistencies that occur as one tries to answer to this question affects the replicability or comparability of results from biomedical research in different countries [8, 29]. Efforts of anthropologists to provide such categories using typological, population, and clinical models were also far from ideal [30].

Much of the persistent controversy over the use of the terms "race' and "ethnicity" may be attributable to the imprecision of their use. The enormous variation in terms used today suggests that the most appropriate approach is to avoid using them as general concepts and in each study should explain how and why they used. At present there is not a single most appropriate classification system for the races of humanity. One problem with using *race* as an identifier is the lack of a clear definition of *race*. The popular concept of five races corresponds well to both geographic regions (Africa, Europe, East Asia, Oceania and the Americas) and bureaucratic definitions (e.g., the US census bureau)[21, 31], which define racial groups on the basis of the primary continent of origin and ethnicity as a self-defined construct that may be based on geographic, social, cultural and religious grounds. On the basis of numerous population genetic surveys, most categorize *Africans* as those with primary ancestry in sub-Saharan Africa; this group includes African Americans and Afro-Caribbean. *Caucasians* include those with ancestry in Europe and West Asia, including the Indian subcontinent and Middle East; North Africans typically also are included in this group as their ancestry derives largely from the Middle East rather than sub-Saharan Africa. *Asians* are those from eastern Asia including China, Indochina, Japan, the Philippines and Siberia. By contrast, *Pacific Islanders* are those with indigenous ancestry from Australia, Papua New Guinea, Melanesia and Micronesia, as well as other Pacific Island groups further east. *Native Americans* are those that have indigenous ancestry in North and South America. Populations that exist at the boundaries of these continental divisions are most difficult to categorize simply. For example, east African groups, such as Ethiopians and Somalis, have great genetic resemblance to Caucasians and are clearly intermediate between sub-Saharan Africans and Caucasians. African Americans frequently have a greater genetic contribution from European rather than African ancestors. Undoubtedly, the categorization of genetic admixed groups, persons with multiple races or ethnic backgrounds poses special challenges [14].

An alternative to the use of racial or ethnic categories in genetics research is to categorize individuals in terms of ancestry. Ancestry may be defined geographically (e.g., Asian, sub-Saharan African, or northern European), geopolitically (e.g., Vietnamese, Zambian, or Norwegian), or culturally (e.g, Brahmin, Lemba, or Apache). The definition of ancestry may recognize a single predominant source or multiple sources [32]. Rebbeck and Sankar [33] attempt to construct concepts of ethnicity, ancestry, or race that can serve research effectively and which recognize and benefit from the complexity inherent to these concepts. They defined four general terms that may be used when comparing groups of individuals: "Minor ethnicity", "Major ethnicity", "Ancestry", and "Race". Unfortunately, such detailed categorization is rarely available in mainstream biomedical or epidemiological studies.

In this study we review articles published since 1970 that provided genetic or epidemiological PD data by race, ethnicity, or 'population group' categories in order to evaluate the possible contribution of race and ethnicity on prevalence, clinical and pathologic features and genetics of PD and try to understand the role of genetic and environmental factors in the etiology and pathogenesis of the disease. Methodological differences and the lack of truly population based data for most regions do limit the comparability of study results and interpretation of data in different racial and ethnic groups. Population-based epidemiological research is limited. Three important limitations deserve consideration when we compare results of epidemiological studies. First, there is an absence of appropriate, validated standardized tools and diagnostic criteria for PD in many countries. Secondly, clinical criteria at best can only lead to a diagnosis of probable PD. A definite diagnosis of PD requires post-mortem confirmation which is rarely available in any of the studies reviewed. And thirdly, since PD is an age-related disease and life expectancy varies widely across regions, age-adjusted rates are needed but often not available. Nevertheless, existing data with all its categorical and methodological limitations may offer some insights into the role of genes and environment in PD etiology. For our purposes, we use common racial classification based on geographical regions: *Africa, Europe, Asia, Oceania/Australia and Americas.*

I. Parkinson's Disease in Africa and African-American Populations

According to the Internet World Statistics [34], 14.2 % of the world population (933, 448, 292) live in the African region, which includes 58 countries. The African population is not homogeneous in terms of race and ethnicity. There are several thousand ethnic groups in Africa, ranging in physical stature from the short Pygmies to the tall Massai, each with its own cultural traditions [35]. The genetic landscape in northern Africa is an east-west pattern of variation pointing to the differentiation between the Berber and Arab population groups of the northwest and the populations of Libya and Egypt. Moreover, Libya and Egypt show the smallest genetic distances from the European populations [36]. The Ethiopian population, which is genetically heterogeneous, sits between Sub-Saharan Africa and western Eurasia. There is evidence of a close relationship between Ethiopian and Yemenite Jews, likely a result of indirect gene flow [37, 38]. Various loci studies reveal lose similarity between the

Berbers and other North African groups, mainly with Moroccan Arabic-speakers, which is in accord with the hypothesis that the current Moroccan population has a strong Berber background [39]. Some genetic differences and similarities have been observed between regions or clusters of regions of the Algerian population, which is explained by a combination of gene flow, ecology and history [40].

We reviewed full text articles, abstracts, and other publications with a focus on the prevalence, clinical and pathological features, and genetics of PD in Africa and African-American (AA) populations.

Prevalence of PD

There is little information on the prevalence of PD on the continent of Africa [41]. Aspects of the epidemiology of PD in individuals of African ancestry, including African Americans have been reviewed in a few articles [41-44]. In these articles study design including primarily hospital-based, community-based, or other special cohorts and were rarely population-based. Table 1 reviewed the diagnostic criteria for PD, survey methods, and results of such studies.

Several epidemiologic studies in the 1970s indicated that idiopathic PD was much less prevalent among Africans and African Americans [44-47](Table 2). Studies conducted in 1980s and 1990s in several African countries confirmed a lower prevalence of PD among African patients (Table 1). However, age-adjustment and sampling methods were problematic in these works. An epidemiological study (Table 2) with more optimal surveying techniques investigated the prevalence of PD in the biracial community of Copiah County, Mississippi, US and found an equal prevalence of PD among African Americans and Caucasians [1][48].

Using the least stringent diagnostic criteria ("possible PD"), the prevalence rate was found to be similar in both groups (338/100,000 and 353/100,000 for African Americans and Caucasians, respectively). Caucasians, however, had a higher age-adjusted prevalence rate if the more stringent criteria (definite PD) were used (196/100,000 and 280/100,000 for African Americans and Caucasians, respectively). To compare the prevalence of PD in the African American populations living under different environmental conditions, authors [49] conducted a door-to-door survey in Copiah County, Mississippi, US, and Ibgo-Ora, Nigeria. After age adjustment, the prevalence rates were dramatically different. The overall prevalence rates were 67/100,000 and 341/100,000 for Igbo-Ora and Copiah County populations, respectively. The age-adjusted prevalence rate in Nigerian Africans was fivefold lower than the prevalence in American Africans. This may reflect the heterogenous mix of Caucasian and African populations in US African Americans. In a study Kaiser Permanente Medical Care recipients in Northern California [50], the age- and gender-adjusted rates were lowest among African Americans (10.2) and highest among Hispanics (16.6). A study of PD in South Carolina showed that African Americans have a lower prevalence than Americans of European origin. Estimated prevalence was 2-29 per 10,000 black South Carolinians

---

[1] The Caucasian race is defined by the Oxford English Dictionary as "relating to a broad division of humankind covering peoples from Europe, Western Asia, Middle East, South Asia and North Africa" or "white-skinned; of European origin" or relating to the region of the Caucasus in SE Europe.

compared to 9-57 per 10,000 white residents [51]. In a recent hospital-based study of a university neurology clinic in Ethiopia, PD was particularly uncommon among all neurological patients [52], but this may reflect the age demographic of the population and/or care-seeking patterns.

Table 1. Prevalence studies of Parkinsonism and Parkinson's disease in Africa [41, 234]

Country	Year (duration)	Popula-tion Size	Crude Prevalence per 100,000	Age-Specific Prevalence	Diagnostic Criteria
Nigeria [235]	1982 (1.5 yrs)	20,000	10	59 (>39 yrs)	WHO protocol plus 3 of 4 cardinal signs
Libya [236]	1985 (2 yrs)	518,745	31.4	285 (>50 yrs)	2 of 4 cardinal signs
Tunisia [237]	1985 (1 mo)[2]	34,874	43	216 (>40 yrs) 296 (>50 yrs)	WHO protocol
Ethiopia [238]	1986 (2 yrs)	60,820	7	---------------	Not provided
Togo [239]	1989	19,241	20	---------------	WHO protocol
Togo [239]	1995	4,182	20	---------------	WHO protocol
Ghana[3][240]	1968 (1 yr)	472	11	---------------	Not provided
Kenya[b][241]	1973 (5 yrs)	750	27	---------------	Not provided
Zimbabwe[b][242]	1969	561	3	---------------	Not provided

Table 2. Prevalence studies of PD in African American populations [44]

Location	Population	Sample size	# cases	Crude prevalence (per 100,000)	Adjusted prevalence
Baltimore[45]	Community clinics	Not provided	1,183 (black) 87 (white)	8.67 (female) 30.66 (male) 121 (female) 128 (male)	---------
New Orleans[46]	Inpatient records	Black 333,280 White 112,878	75 165	22[4] 147	----------
Mississippi[205]	Door-to-door	Black 11,666 White 11,981	12 19	341 352	338 353
New York[207]	Healthcare recipients	Not provided	Not provided	---------	Black 57[c] White 116
California[50]	HMO[5] patients	Black 192,316 White 969,286	16 291	8.3 2.2	---------

---

[2] Three phases: (1) pilot study, screened 908 people; (2) full-scale study screened 34,874; (3) control study screened 1,530 people
[3] PD cases among neurological inpatients.
[4] Statistically significant difference.
[5] HMO=health maintenance organization.

Clinical studies: A few studies have shown a younger age at onset, more often tremulous form of PD, slower progression of the disease, and a differing response to levodopa [52-55] in African patients or patients of African origin compared to the European and Asian patients with PD. Greater disease severity and disability have been observed in African Americans vs. Caucasians in tertiary care centers, likely reflecting differential access to specialty care [56]. Clinical comparison of Tunisian and North American Caucasian patients with familial PD found that non-motor symptoms and cognitive impairment were less common in Tunisia patients[57].

Pathology: The pathological hallmark of PD is the selective and progressive degeneration of dopaminergic (DA) neurons of the substantia nigra pars compacta (SNpc) and the presence of Lewy bodies. Despite extensive research, the exact cause(s) of neuronal death in PD are still unknown [58]. Apoptotic cell death has been implicated as a major mechanism in PD and other neurodegenerative disorders. Pathologically, the number of pigmented neurons and their size decreases with age. Despite the reduced prevalence of PD in Nigerian population relative to the US, no significant difference was found in the number of melanized nigral neurons between the Nigerian and British subjects [59] at autopsy. Muthane et al. suggested that differences in melanized nigral neuronal numbers may not explain differences in the prevalence of PD between white and non-white populations under study.

Genetic studies: Recent research has provided increasing support for the origins of anatomically and genetically "modern" human populations in Africa between 150,000 and 200,000 years ago[60-62]. Analysis of data derived from African and European Americans for twenty two genes spanning a total of 516 kb and the HapMap ENCODE data across 500 kb on chromosome 2p16.3 from three major world populations show strong pairwise linkage disequilibrium (LD) between SNPs selected from populations having African ancestry[63]. These findings also support the African origin of modern humans. Given the evolutionary conservation in other out-of-Africa populations, the haplotype frameworks are likely ancestral haplotype backgrounds upon which more recent mutations have been superimposed[63]. Hence, a lower prevalence of PD in African populations may be due to PD mutation occurring relatively recently.

Studies of genetic variation enhance our understanding of the differential predisposition to diseases in various ethnic populations. For this purpose, a comprehensive haplotype map based on the most abundant form of genetic variation, single nucleotide polymorphisms (SNP), are principal. At the present time, however, our knowledge of the similarities and differences of haplotype structure among different ancestral populations is rather poor.

Mitochondrial DNA (mtDNA) haplotypes have become important tools for tracing maternal ancestry. Common mtDNA haplotypes are shared among multiple ethnic groups. A recent comparison of mtDNA sequences from 1148 African Americans living in the US with a database of African mtDNA sequenced showed that more than 55% of US lineages have a West African ancestor, while fewer than 41% came from Central or South West Africa[64, 65]. Few studies of the genetics of PD in Africa have been reported, most of them have been from North Africa [41]. Tunisian and Zambian patients with familial PD have a younger age at onset and inheritance of PD in these countries are most commonly autosomal dominant with reduced penetrance [41, 53]. A younger age demographic in these populations relative to the US may be a confounder, however. In Zambia, clinic-based studies indicate that men have a higher risk of PD than women [53], but care-seeking behaviors and access issues may have influenced these findings. Linkage of autosomal juvenile PD caused by a mutation in the parkin gene have been confirmed in Algerian and Tunisian families [66-68].

Recently, several pathogenic mutations in the highly conserved leucine-rich repeat kinase2 gene (LRRK2) have been associated with autosomal dominant familial late onset and sporadic PD [69, 70]. LRRK2 is a huge gene encompassing 144 kb and the open reading frame consists of 1449 base pairs in 51 exons. LRRK2 protein consists of 2527 amino acids and it is ubiquitously expressed in the cytoplasm of many orphans [2-4]. To date, 6 missence mutations have been reported [71, 72]. Reports on the common LRRK2 G2019S mutation have generated considerable interest in genetic testing [73-75]. Studies show that patients with autosomal dominant (ADPD), autosomal recessive (ARPD) and sporadic PD may have LRRK2 mutations. Moreover, LRRK2 mutations in late- and early onset PD have been identified [76]. A shared LRRK2 G2019S haplotype in the vast majority of carriers argues against *de novo* occurrence [74]. Based on the widely variable age at onset and various modes of inheritance, the phenotype of PD patients with LRRK2 mutations must be influenced by stochastic, environmental, and other genetic factors [77]. The clinical features of most patients with LRRK2 mutations are similar to those of patients with typical idiopathic PD[57, 76]. Comparisons of homozygous and heterozygous Tunisian carriers of LRRK2 G2019S mutations could not find significant differences in PD characteristics between the two groups, suggesting no gene dosage effect [57].

G2019S LRRK2 mutation have been found in families with PD from Morocco, Algeria and Tunisia [78]. The frequency of the G2019S mutation was significantly greater in North African (7/17, 41%) than European cases (5/174, 2.9%)[78]. Results of other investigations also indicate a high frequency of the G2019S mutation in North African patients with PD [70]. The frequency of the mutation was very high (42%) in Tunisian families with PD [57].

These data suggested that the G1920S mutation constitutes a significant risk factor for PD in this population [70] and may be associated with human migration history. Indeed, patients from Europe and North Africa have the same haplotype [79-81]. A study of six families of North African or European origin carrying G2019S estimated that these individuals shared a common founder ~725 years ago[82]. The high prevalence of this mutation in Ashkenazi Jews and North African Arabs has led to the hypothesis that the mutation originated in the Middle East [83]. Using a maximum-likelihood method, estimations are that the families with haplotype 1 shared a common ancestor 2,250 years ago, whereas those with haplotype 2 appear to share a more recent founder [81].

In Sierra Leone, the nucleotide sequence of the hypervariable 1 (HV1) region of mtDNA in the two major ethnic groups (the Mende and Temne) and two minor ethnic groups (the Loko and Limba)showed that the distribution of studied haplotypes within the Limba sample was significantly different from that of the other ethnic groups. No significant genetic variation was seen between the Mende, Tempe, and Loko. These results suggest that distinguishing genetic differences can be observed among ethnic groups residing in historically close proximity to one another [84]. Mutations in the DJ-1 gene have not identified in African American patients with PD [85]. The PINK-1 mutation has been identified in Tunisian family with autosomal recessive early onset Parkinsonism [86]. A genetic study of 30 South Africans(Xhose), mixed ancestry and Afrikaner patients with PD detected 4 mutations in the PARK2 gene, 2 novel variants in the DJ-1 gene, and one in the LRRK2 G2019S gene[87].

II. Parkinson's Disease in Asian Populations

Definition: The term "Asian" refers to people who live in the continent of Asia, although geologists and physical geographers consider Asia as the major eastern constituent of the continent of Euroasia. Given the scope and diversity of the landmass, it is sometimes not even clear exactly what "Asia" consists of. Some definitions include only the Far East, Southeast Asia and the Indian Subcontinent [88, 89] also called the continent of Tripartite Asia. Using this term, an indigenous Asian is a person born in tripartite Asia who lives in tripartite Asia with ancestry from the original Proto-Asian population [89]. But the term may also refer to other Asian groups [90]. New Asians and Asian ancestry mixes include Eurasian ancestry, Afrasian ancestry, Amerasian ancestry, Mideastasian ancestry and Pacifasian ancestry. Citizens of Asian ancestry living in non-Asian countries are defined as Asian diaspora and include Asian American, Asian British, Asian Canadian, Asian Latin American, Asian African and Asian Australian [89]. Asia is the world's largest and most populous continent containing more than 60% of the world's current human population [91]. Regions of Asia include: Northern Asia, Central Asia, Western Asia, Southern Asia, Eastern Asia, and Southeastern Asia[91]. According to the World's Statistics, Asia include 35 countries [92] and the Middle East includes 14 countries.

Prevalence of PD: The prevalence of PD has been studied in a few Asian countries mainly in the Far East (China, Japan, Taiwan, and South Korea), Southeast Asia (Singapore, Malaysia), The Indian Subcontinent (India, Pakistan) and the Middle East (Israel). See Table 3.

Chinese populations: Early Asian studies reported the lowest prevalence of PD in China (crude prevalence ratios of 14.6-44 per 100,000 see Table 3). Later, a door-to-door community survey in the Hong-Kong Chinese population showed a prevalence of 188 per 100,000[93], which is comparable with other door-to-door surveys in industrialized countries [47, 94] and Taiwan[95], but lower than in the Australian population[93]. The prevalence of PD after 70 years of age in rural China and Taiwan is particularly high (902 and 819.7, respectively) but is still lower than in European populations [94, 96]. A community-based survey in central Singapore among Chinese, Malays, and Indians aged 50 years and above showed that prevalence rates increased significantly with age. Studies of Chinese and Philippinos in the US found a very low prevalence of PD 10.8 per 100,000[50].

Korean population: We found only one published prevalence study in Korea [97]. The calculated prevalence of PD in the South Korean population was 19/100,000, similar to data from China.

Japanese population: The population of Japan is significantly older than that of either China or Korea, and the prevalence of PD in Japan in early studies in the 1980s was higher (81/82 per 100,000) than in China and South Korea [98] [99]. See Table 3 for details. Overall, the incidence of PD was 7.1/10,000 person-years in a cohort of 8,006 Japanese-

American men was generally higher than in Asia and similar to rates observed in Europe suggesting a role for environmental and/or lifestyle exposures [100].

Table 3. Prevalence of PD in Asian countries [47, 94]

Region	Population Size	# cases	Crude Prevalence per 100,000	Prevalence (age-adjusted)
China (6 cities)[243]	63,195	28	44	57
China (29 provinces)[244]	3,869,162	566	15	18
China (Linxian)[245]	16,488	86	522	--------
Hong Kong[93]	1,078	--------	188	--------
South Korea[97]	---------	--------	19[6]	--------
Taiwan (Kinmen)[246]	--------	--------	119	50-60:273 60-70:535 70-80: 565 <80: 1,839
Taiwan (Ilan)[95]	---------	--------	367.9	--------
Japan (Yonago)[98]	125,291	101	81	73
Japan (Izumo) [247]	80,639	66	82	61
Japan (Yonago)[99]	140,911	205	145.5	135
India (Parsi)[101]	14,010	46	328	148
India[248]	---------	--------	60-100	--------
India (Bangalore)[249]	612[7]	109	---------	--------
Saudi Arabia (Thugbah)[250]	22,613	6	27	128
Southern Israel[251]	250,000	156	62	---------
Israel (kibbutz)[103]	73,767	180	244	--------

Indian population: The prevalence of PD in India has been found to be highest among the Parsi population (328 per 100,000) [101]. Of note, the reported prevalence of PD is nearly five times higher amongst Indians compared to the Anglo-Indians [102].

Israel population: In the Israeli Kibbutz population, a cross-sectional prevalence rate was 0.24% for the population of 73,767 people aged over 40 years. Age-adjusted prevalence was 0.94% in the population over 60 years and 0.33% in the population over 40 years [103].

Arab populations: The crude prevalence of PD in Saudi Arabia is similar to China and Korea, whereas age-adjusted prevalence is higher in Arabic relative to other Asian countries. A door-to-door survey in Arabic villages of Wadi Ara (Northern Israel) estimated that the prevalence of PD was similar to that observed in elderly populations in Europe and Northern America [104].

Clinical Studies: Only a few studies in the literature focus on ethnic differences in the clinical characteristics of PD. Most studies indicate there are no difference in the clinical presentation, disease duration and the prevalence of fluctuations, dyskinesias, and depression between different ethnic populations. However, in Korean patients with early-onset PD (EOPD), the most frequent initial symptom is resting tremor, which does not correlate with

---

[6] Calculated prevalence based upon health insurance statistics.

[7] Elderly home-based study.

age at onset. Earlier onset of levodopa-induced dyskinesia and off-dystonia are found in EOPD, especially when onset of symptoms is <30 years [105]. A comparative study of clinical characteristics in three ethnic groups (Chinese, Malays and Indians) in Singapore failed to identify any differences among the three groups [106]. A study comparing Asian Indians and Anglo-Indians showed that in Anglo-Indians tremor is strongly dominant, whereas in the Asian Indians 45.3% experience akinetic-rigid type PD. The rate of PD progression may be more rapid in Yemenite Jews relative to Ashkenazi Jews [107]. In Russia and Uzbekistan, tremor predominates in Russian families, whereas the akinetic-rigid type is more common in patients of Uzbekistan [53]. A high prevalence (20%) of atypical parkinsonism with a late-onset, akinetic-rigid has been reported among parkinsonian patients of Africo-Caribbean and Indian origin attending movement disorder clinics in London Hospitals [55].

Pathology: Autopsy studies of neuronal loss in the SN and clinical studies of parkinsonian signs in elderly populations demonstrate that both loss of pigmented neurons in the SNpc and the presence of Lewy bodies occurs with aging [108, 109]. In the Honolulu-Asia Aging Study, investigations assessing the anatomical correlates of parkinsonian signs in elderly persons without PD showed a significant association of increasing number of Parkinsonian signs present with decreasing neuron density in the SN leading the authors to suggest that low SN neuron density may be the basis for parkinsonian signs in the elderly without PD[110]. However, according one study [59] the absolute number of melanized neurons in the SNpc of people from India was about 40% lower than brains from UK patients. Ultrasonographic studies showed that SN hyperechogenicity is a characteristic finding in PD patients. SN hyperechogenicity has been found in almost 80% of the Japanese PD patients. The SN hyper-echogenicity seen in Chinese patients with PD in Taiwan suggests the possibility of racial and ethnic differences in hyper-SN in Asians and Caucasians [111].

Genetic studies: Asia encompasses a vast region but genetic studies have been able to delineate some distinctions. The genetic profiles of 28 populations sampled in China support the presence of genetic distinctions between southern and northern populations [112]. Analysis of data on 58 DNA markers (mitochondrial [mt], Y-chromosomal, and autosomal) and sequence data of the mtDNA hypervariable sequence I (HVS1} from an ethnically diverse population of India showed that the tribal and the caste populations are highly differentiated and the Tibeto-Burman tribes share considerable genetic commonalities with the Austro-Asiatic tribes. The upper casts have a close genetic affinity to Central Asian populations [113].

Archeological and genetic evidence points to a single successful dispersal event, which impacted culturally modern populations fairly rapidly across southern and southeastern Asia into Australasia with only a secondary and later dispersal into Europe[61]. One of the first waves of out-of-Africa migration came into India, therefore India served as a major corridor for the dispersal of modern humans[114]. Study of mtDNA and Y-chromosome haplo groups reveal asymmetric gene flow in population of Eastern India [115].

To date 6 genes have been identified as causative genes for PD; alpha-synuclein (SNCA), parkin, UCH-L1 (ubiquitin-C terminal hydrolase-L1), DJ, PINK1 (PTEN-induced kinase1), and LRRK2 in familial PD an/or early-onset PD [2-4, 69, 116-118].

In a systematic review of 78 publications on genetic studies in Asian populations (Table 4), most studies were conducted in the Far East (China, Japan, Taiwan, South Korea, Mongolia), Southeast Asia (Singapore, Thailand), the Indian Subcontinent (India) and the Middle East (Israel).

Table 4. Frequency of LRRK2 mutations in Asian populations

Population	Mutation(s)	Frequency % (n)[8]	Familial %	Sporadic %
North African Arabs[82]	G2019S	41 (17)	100	0
North African Arabs[70]	G2019S	39 (59)	17	83
Ashkenazi Jews[83]	G2019S	18.3 (120)	31	69
Ashkenazi Jews[122]	G2019S	1.4 (208)	24.5	75.5
Ashkenazi Jews[76]	G2019S	9.9 (181)	12.7	87.3
Yemenite Jews[124]	G2019S	0 (61)	0	100
Ashkenazi Jews[252]	G2019S	17.6 (153)	0	100
Ashkenazi Jews[253]	G2019S	14.8 (472)		
Non-Ashkenazi Jews[253]	G2019S	2.7 (472)		
Indian [125]	G2019S	0.12 (800)	10	90
Chinese[254]	G2019S	0 (675)	8.6	91
Chinese[126]	G2019S	0 (624)	0	100
Chinese[127]	G2019S	0 (343)	0	100
Chinese[255]	G2019S	0 (141)	0	100
Korean[130]	G2019S	0 (453)	3.8	96.2
Japanese[81]	G2019S	0.34 (586)	5.5	94.5
Russian[256]	G2019S	0.98 (304)	4.6	95.4
Arabic[104]	G2019S	0 (11)	9	91
Indian[125]	R1441C	0 (800)	10	90
Ashkenazi Jews[76]	R1441C	0 (181)	12.7	87.3
Indian[125]	R1441G	0 (800)	10	90
Indian[125]	R1441H	0 (800)	10	90
Chinese[126]	I2020T	0 (624)	0	100
Indian[125]	I2020T	0 (800)	10	90
Ashkenazi Jews[76]	L1114L	0 (181)	12.7	87.3
Ashkenazi Jews[76]	I1122V	0 (181)	12.7	87.3
Ashkenazi Jews[76]	Y1699C	0 (181)	12.7	87.3
Chinese[257]	R1067Q	0.16 (630)	25	75
Japanese[258]	R1067Q	0.34 (590)	0	100
Chinese[127]	G2385R[9]	9 (305)	0	100
Chinese[255]	G2385R	7.3 (989)	0	100
Non-Chinese Asian[129]	G2385R	1.4 (145)	0	100
Chinese[133]	G2385R	10 (608)	0	100

Specific MDR1 (a multidrug transporter) alleles of the 2 SNPs were found to be positively selected among ethnic Chinese, but not in the Caucasian populations. An MDR1

---

[8] n=Number of subjects analyzed
[9] LRRK2 Glu2385Arg variant.

specific haplotypes formed by SNPs e21/2677 and e26/3435 appears to be protective against PD in ethnic Chinese [119]. Apolipoprotein E (APOE) was found to be associated with PD Chinese populations [120, 121]. The most commonly reported six pathogenic or potentially pathogenic mutations were in the LRRK2 gene.

The most common genetic determinant of PD identified to date is the LRRK2 G2019S mutation which occurs variously in different populations being most frequently identified (39%) in North African Arabs [70]. Studies of 90 unrelated G2019S-bearing subjects of European or Middle Eastern-North African (MENA) origin indicate that all shared the same haplotype, consistent with a common founder [70, 80, 82, 83].

Findings on the frequency of the G2019S mutation in Jewish population was was different across countries: the lowest frequency (4.5%) was found in Ashkenazi Jews in Russia [122] and the highest (18.3%) in Ashkenazi Jews in the US [83]. A higher frequency (10.7%) of the beta-glucocerebrosidase (GBA) gene N370S allelewas identified among Jewish ethnicity [123]. The G2019S identified in Europeans, Ashkenazi Jews, and North African Arabs may have arisen from a common Middle Eastern founder [81, 83]. The Yemenite Jews are a distinctive ancient ethnic group from the Ashkenazi Jews and no Yemenite patients have been identified with the G2019S mutation [124].

Overall, the G2019S mutation is rare in Asian populations studied [81, 104, 119, 125-128] and was not detected in Chinese, Korean Indian or Arabic populations [104, 119, 125, 126, 129, 130]. Five other common mutations of the LRRK 2 gene are also absent or extremely rare in studied Asian populations [125, 131-133]. The absence or rarity of these mutations in one ethnic Asian population does not exclude the possibility of other mutations arising independently in the same ethnic population, but the striking absence of the common G2019S mutation in Chinese populations suggests that this mutation resulted from a common European founder [127, 128]. If modern population dispersed across southern and southeastern Asia into Australasia as suggested [61], the common determinant PD mutation occurred later in European population and have contributed significantly to the prevalence of PD among people of European descent.

A recently identified common genetic variant G2385R[127, 128, 133, 134] is associated with a two-fold increased risk of sporadic PD in ethnic Chinese populations and may be the single most important variant in ethnic Chinese and/or Asian PD patients[134]. A new LRRK2 Ile1371Val mutation has been detected in an Indian family [135]. The frequency of the other genes mutations in Asian population is summarized in Table 5.

Alpha-synuclein was the first gene mutation to be found in PD, and the PD world became a synucleinopathy world [2, 4, 116, 136]. SNCA gene haplotype has been implicated in the risk of PD in a Chinese populations [106]. A study of polymorphisms of the a-synuclein gene in a Japanese population found a significant association with PD in 15 of 21 SNPs[137]. However, other studies of SNCA multiplication have indicated that is rare in Asian populations [138, 139].

Mutations in the parkin gene are the predominant cause of juvenile (autosomal recessive juvenal parkinsonism, ARJP) and early onset recessive PD [140]. However, recent reports suggest that parkin associated PD may not necessarily occur exclusively through autosomal recessive inheritance [141]. Mutations in the parkin gene have been identified in several oJapanese families with autosomal recessive juvenile parkinsonism [142]. These mutations were found mainly in EOPD in Asian populations. The frequency of the mutations differs across populations with the highest frequency reported in Chinese (14.3%) populations and the lowest (2.8%) in Korean populations [139].

Table 5. Frequency of the other genes mutations in Asian populations

Population	Gene	Frequency % (n)[10]	Clinical Category	Familial %
Korean[259]	SNCA	0.2 (453)	-----------------	0.2
Korean[139]	SNCA	1.4 (72)	EOPD[11]	16.7
Indian[144]	parkin	7.2 (138)	-----------------	6
South Indian[143]	parkin	0 (102)	EOPD	19.6
Chinese[260]	parkin	12 (230)	EOPD	0
Chinese[138]	parkin	6.4 (62)	EOPD	14.5
Chinese[225]	parkin	12.5 (72)	AR-EOPD[12]	0
Chinese[221]	parkin	14.3 (28)	EOPD	0
Korean[139]	parkin	2.8 (72)	EOPD	16.7
Arabic[104]	parkin	9 (11)	-----------------	9
Korean[139]	UCH-L1	1.4 (72)	AR-EOPD	0
Chinese, Malays, Indian[261]	PINK1	3.7 (80)	EOPD	0
Chinese[111]	PINK1	3.6 (28)	EOPD	0
Chinese[225]	PINK1	4.2 (72)	AR-EOPD	0
Taiwanese[127]	PINK1	0 (73)	EOPD	0
Korean[138]	PINK1	1.6 (62)	EOPD	14.5
Korean[139]	PINK1	5.5 (72)	EOPD	16.7
Asian[148]	PINK1	15 (39)	AR-EOPD	100
Chinese[154]	DJ-1	0 (41)	EOPD	0
Chinese, Malays, Indian[262]	DJ	0 (80)	EOPD	0
Chinese[225]	DJ	0 (72)	AR-EOPD	0
Korean[138]	DJ	0 (62)	EOPD	14.5
Korean[139]	DJ	0 (72)	EOPD	16.7
Chinese Malays, Indian[262]	Nurr 1	0 (64)	YOPD[13]	37.5

The frequency of the parkin mutations also varied in Indian populations. No mutations were found in the South Indian patients with sporadic EOPD [143], whereas in the Eastern Indian population with sporadic PD the frequency of parkin mutations was 7% [144]. A cross comparison of allele frequencies of G-to-A transition in exon 4 (S/N167) in parkin showed that the frequencies were higher in Japanese and Chinese populations [145-147] than in European and North American populations. In contrast, the V/L380 polymorphism was higher in Caucasians than in Japanese [147].

PINK1 mutations are the second most common cause of autosomal recessive PD after parkin [148, 149]. The frequency of PINK1 mutations among Caucasian patients with EOPD and ARPD is about 1% to 7% [150-153]. The frequency of PINK1 in Chinese familial PD

---

[10] Number of patients=n.
[11] EOPD=early onset.
[12] AR=autosomal recessive.
[13] YOPD=young onset.

patients is 2.5% [119] and in sporadic EOPD of different ethnicity (Chinese, Malays, and Indian) it is 3.7% [134]. The prevalence of the gene in Korean patients with EOPD was estimated 1.6 to 5.5% [138, 139]. High frequency (15%) of the PINK1 mutation was found in AR EOPD Japanese families [148]. It is suggested that the PINK1 mutation is more frequent in the Asian population than in whites. Mutations in the DJ-1 gene is associated with autosomal recessive early onset parkinsonism [2], but DJ-1 mutations have not been identified in Chinese, Japanese or Korean patients with EOPD [4, 138, 139, 154]. A study of Chinese, Malays and Indians with YOPD and fPD did not find any pathogenic mutations in the Nurr1 gene [106].

III. Parkinson's Disease in European Populations

Europe is one of seven continents and physically and geologically, Europe is the westernmost peninsula of Eurasia. Europe is the world's second-smallest continent in terms of area. The only continent that is smaller is Australia. In terms of population, it is the third-largest continent (after Asia and Africa) [155] According to the Internet World Statistics [156], 12.3 % of World population (809,624,686) live in Europe, which includes 52 countries.

European populations are also heterogenic and include hundreds of ethnic groups. In the past, common racial categories used included; Nordic, Alpine, Mediterranean, Atlanto-Mediterranean, Dinaric, and East Baltic among other types. However, few individuals have backgrounds that correspond precisely with one of these racial groups.

Prevalence of PD: There are many more studies of PD prevalence in European populations relative to African or Asian populations 157]. We reviewed studies which provided data on the prevalence of idiopathic PD. Country-specific data on the prevalence of PD are summarized in Table 6. Age-specific prevalence rates suggest a higher prevalence of PD in European populations, but with a great deal of variability across countries.

Bulgaria. Bulgaria is a country of Southeastern Europe. According to the 2001 Census Bulgarian population is mainly ethnic Bulgarians (83.9%) with two sizable minorities, Turks 9.4% and Roma (Gypsies) (4.7%). The crude prevalence ratios varied from 156 [158] to 169.8 and increased steadily with age [159, 160]. However, the prevalence of PD in the Gypsies in a region of Sofia was found to be only 16/100,000 [160]. The origin of Gypsies is thought to be North Indian and in Bulgaria they exist as genetic isolates [160].

Denmark. The kingdom of Denmark is situated in Scandinavia and Northern Europe. People of Danish ancestry are ethnic Danes. Most Danes today trace their heritage to Germanic tribes who have inhabited Denmark since prehistoric times. The Danish population is relatively homogenous with about 85% of the population of Denmark composed of ethnic Danes[161]. Nationals of Denmark also include a German minority and non-European immigrants. Denmark historically included former colonies Greenland and the Faroe Islands. Inuit populations inhabit Greenland. The Faroe Islands are characterized by their geographic isolation and ethnically homogeneous Nordic population with their own language [161]. Prevalence studies of PD in Denmark found higher prevalence in the Faroe Islands

(187.6/100,000) [162] and in Greenland (187.5/100,0000) [163] compared to the island of Als (98.3/100,000) [164] and Arhus.

Table 6. Prevalence of PD in European countries

Location	Design	Population size	# Cases	Crude prevalence per 100,000	Age-specific prevalence
Bulgaria [159]	Hospital-based registry	28,614	47	164	50-60: 70.5 60-70:389 70-80: 1,883 >90: 3,930
Bulgaria [159]	Hospital-based registry	91,296	155	170	50-60: 72 60-70: 368 70-80:1,585 >80: 3,286
Bulgaria (Sofia)[158]	Cross-sectional	1,381,295	2,150	156	---------------
Bulgaria (Sofia gypsies)[160]	Door-to-door	6,163	1	16	---------------
Denmark (Arhus) [263]	Cross-sectional	242,151	203	84	---------------
Denmark (Faroe Islands) [162]	Cross- sectional	43,709	82	188	70-74: 2,020
Denmark (Als)[164]	Cross-sectional	56,839	58	98.3	75-79: 838
Denmark (Greenland)[163]	Cross-sectional	--------------	----------	187.5	---------------
Finland (Turku)[264]	Cross- sectional	402,988	282	120	--------------
France (Limousin)[167]	Door-to-door	1,562	5	320	---------------
France[265]	Cross-sectional	3,337,795	971	121	---------------
Northern Germany[169]	Cross-sectional	--------------	1,018	183	--------------
Germany[168]	Door-to-door	982	7	713	---------------
Iceland[171]	Cross-sectional	187,314	304	162	---------------
Italy (Sassari)[266]	Longitudinal	1,473,800	934	65.6	<50: 205 50-60: 342 60-70:311 >70: 83
Italy (Sicily)[267]	Door-to-door	24,496	63	257	--------------
Italy (San Marino)[268]	Cross sectional	22,322	34	152.3	>60: 476 >70:1593 80-84:949
Italy (Ferrara)[269]	Cross-sectional	38,360	73	190.3	>60:326 70-74: 1,137 >74:1,814.5

Table 6. (Continued)

Location	Design	Population size	# Cases	Crude prevalence per 100,000	Age-specific prevalence
Italy (Ferrara)[270]	Longitudinal	176,621	291	164.7	<40-39:43 41-49:103.9 50-59:186.8 60-69:381.5 70-79:624.3 >80:783.2
Italy (Cossato)[271]	Healthcare setting	61,830	104	168	>50:115.3 >60:288.2 >70:835 >80:972.6
Italy (L'Aquila)[272]	Cross- sectional	---------------	682	229.3	--------------
Netherlands (Rotterman)[172]	Healthcare setting	5,510	74	1,300	55-64:300 65-74:1,000 75-84:3,200 85-94:3,300
Northern Norway[174]	Cross-sectional	48,091	59	133	--------------
Poland (Poznan)[175]	Cross-sectional	1,308,277	862	66	---------------
Portugal[176]	Cross-sectional	219,928	291	130	45-54:36 55-64:169 64-74:652 >75: 890
Spain (Navarra)[273]	Healthcare setting	523,563	789-903	161.5	--------------
Spain (Castilla-LaMancha, and Navarra)[274]	Healthcare setting	1,712,529	4096 and 5,218	270.2	---------------
Spain (Lower Aragon)[275]	Cross-sectional	60,724	134	220.6	40-49:16.5 50-59:100 60-69:435.6 70-79:953.3 80-89:973
Spain (Asturias)[276]	Healthcare setting	1,087,885	2,115	199	---------------
Spain (Cantalejo)[277]	Door-to-door	3,503	20	1,280	60-69:630 70-79:1,300
Central Spain[278]	Cross-sectional	5,278	81	1500	65-69:500 70-74:1,600 75-79:1,900
Spain (Bidasoa)[279]	Door-to-door	2,000	18	1,500	65-74:400 75-84:4,700
Spain (Arosa Island)[280]	Cross-sectional	724	16	220	---------------

Table 6. (Continued)

Location	Design	Population size	# Cases	Crude prevalence per 100,000	Age-specific prevalence
Sweden (Goteborg)[281]	Cross- sectional	--------------	----------	261	--------------
Sweden (Ostergotland)[282]	Longitudinal	147,777	170	115	--------------
Turkey [283]	Population-based	1,529	36	235	>65:410
United Kingdom (Northampton)[177]	Cross-sectional	208,499	226	108	50-59:64 60-69:277 70-79:702 >80:1,136
United Kingdom[178]	Cross-sectional	15,616	249	164.2	40-44:12.5 45-49:76 50-59:77.6 60-69:254 70-79:863 80-84:1,792
United Kingdom [284]	Cross-sectional	302,500	383	121	40-49:7 50-59:93.5 60-69:251 70-79:761 80-74:1,400
United Kingdom (London)[180]	Cross-sectional	121,608	156	128	40-49:12 50-59:109 60-69:342 70-79:961 >80:1,265
United Kingdom (North Wales)[179]	Cross-sectional	--------------	112	105	40-49:32 50-59:63 60-69:228 70-79:537 >80:653
European Community (mixed)[173]	Door-to-door	6,969	97	1,400	55-64:300 65-74:1,000 75-84:3,100

Finland. Most inhabitants of Finland (97.6%) are Finnish with a small population (5.6%) of Swedish speakers. The types of mtDNA markers among Finnish people do not differ from those of other European ethnicities. The prevalence of PD in the country is 120/100,000 [165].

France. Many English-language sources define the French people as an ethnic group consisting of primarily a "Celtic and Latin" population with "Teutonic, Slavic, North African, Sub-Saharan African, Indochinese, and Basque minorities"[166]. French ethnicity, being that of a large and diverse nation-state, is relatively complex, and heterogeneous. However,

"French people" as an ethnic group is not used in French official terminology since according to the French constitution "French" is a nationality, and not a specific ethnicity [166]. In a door-to-door study in the Limousin region, the prevalence of PD was estimated to be320/100,000 [167], but the generalizability of these data is questionable.

Germany. Germany is largest economy and second most populous nation of Europe. The Germans are most commonly defined as a Germanic people. The Germanic peoples are linguistic and ethnic branch of Indo-European peoples, originating in Northern Europe. The division of peoples into West Germanic, East Germanic, and North Germanic is a modern linguistic classification. Ethnic Germans form an important minority group in several countries (Poland, Hungary, southern Brazil, Peru, Argentina, etc.)[161]. At present Germany consists of 91.5% ethnic Germans and 8.5% non-ethnic Germans (Turkish, Italian, etc.). In southern Germany, the estimated prevalence of PD is 713/100,0000 [168]compared to 183/100,000 in northern Germany[169].

Iceland. Iceland is a country of northwestern Europe. Icelanders descended primarily from Norseman of Scandinavia and Celts of the British Isles [170]. Due to their considerable history of relative isolation, Icelanders have often been considered highly genetically homogeneous—a mixture of Norse/Celtic descendants (94%) and others of foreign origin (6%). For this reason, along with the extensive genealogical records for much of the population that reach back to the settlement of Iceland, Icelanders have been the focus of considerable genomics research. Studies of mtDNA, blood groups, and isozymes have revealed a highly variable population from a genetic standpoint, comparable to or exceeding the diversity of other Europeans. Results of the mtDNA studies have been consistent with the genealogical records that trace the ancestry of most Icelanders to Scandinavia and the British Isles. Founder effects and the effects of genetic drift are more pronounced for the Icelandic gene pool than other nearby populations, supporting the assumed genetic isolation of the population [170]. The prevalence of PD in Iceland estimated to be162/100,000[171].

Italy. Italy is a country located in Southern Europe with 95.45% of the population considered ethnic Italians. The history of the Italian peoples is ancient and stretches back millennia to Paleolithic times. Not all Italians originated from the original native Italic tribes. The Gauls in the North, the Etruscans in Central Italy and the Greeks in the south preceded the Romans, who in turn "Latinized' the whole country [155]. Northern Italians are more similar to central Europeans, while most Southern Italians are similar to other peoples of Southern Europe, such as the Spaniards and the Greeks [155]. A wide range of the ethnic Italian Diaspora live throughout Western Europe, the Americas and Australia. The crude prevalence ratios of PD vary across Italy.

Netherlands. The Netherlands is the European part of the Kingdom of the Netherlands and the ethnic origins of the citizens are very diverse. The vast majority (80.8%) of the population are ethnic Dutch people with the remainder being primarily Germans, Indonesians, Turks, Indian, and Moroccan. The Netherlands also has a resident population of mixed Dutch and Indonesian descent (Indonesia being a former colony of the Netherlands) [170]. The Dutch predominantly descend from various Germanic tribes, the main specific ancestry are Franks [170]. The Dutch share their genetics with other European people; nevertheless there are some mutations that arose among the Dutch. that can be found in many countries with Dutch Diaspora. The prevalence of PD in Rotterdam studies was 1300-1400/100,000 [172, 173].

Norway. Norway, in Northern Europe, comprises the western part of Scandinavia. The majority of the population is comprised of ethnic Norwegians--a Nordic/North Germanic people with a small minorities of Sami. The largest concentration of Sami people is found in Norway's capital, Oslo. Norway also has a small Finnish community [170]. According to recent genetic analysis, both mtDNA and Y chromosome polymorphisms show a noticeable genetic affinity for Norwegians and central Europeans. The crude prevalence of PD in Norway iss significantly lower (133/100,000) [174] than in Netherlands (1300/100,000)[172].

Poland. Poland, a country of Central Europe, has 96.7% of the population of Polish descent. The exact ethnicity of the Poles is still hotly debated. Poles belong to the Lechitic subgroup of a western Slavic ethnic group [155], but ethnic minorities include Germans, Ukrainians, Lithuanians, and Jews. A wide-ranging Polish Diaspora exists throughout Western and Eastern Europe, the America, and Australia. A study in Poznan [175] found a PD prevalence of 66/100,000.

Portugal. Portugal, located in southwestern Europe on the Iberian Peninsula, is the westernmost country of mainland Europe. Portugal's population has been remarkably homogenous for most of its history. Native Portuguese people are ethnically a combination of pre-Roman Iberians and Celts with some Roman and Germanic mix. Ethnic minorities of the country include Gypsy populations and Muslim population from North Africa as well as Spaniards, Brits, French, and Germans [155]. The prevalence of PD in Portugal is 130/100,000 and increases with age [176].

Spain. Spain, located in Southern Europe, is the largest of three sovereign states that make up the Iberian Peninsula (the others are Portugal and Andorra). Spain has a Castilian ethnic core and three major peripheral ethnic groups: the Catalans, the Galicians, and the Basques. Some regions have strong local identities and dialects, such as the Asturias, Aragon, the Canary Islands and Andalusia [155]. Y-chromosome and mtDNA analysis suggests that modern-day Spaniards largely trace their ancestry to the paleolithic peoples who began arriving on the European continent around 45,000 years ago. Millions of Spanish descendants can be found throughout the Hispanic countries of Latin America in the form of creoles (predominantly Spaniards born in the Americas), mestizos (mixed Spanish/Amerindian), mulatos (mixed Spanish/African) or triracial (Spanish/African/Amerindian). In the United States, the number of Mexican-Americans represents a significant portion of the Spanish descended populations since the over 70% of Mexicans have Spanish ancestry [155]. There are wide variations in the reported prevalence rates of PD in different parts of Spain.

Sweden. Sweden is a Nordic country on the Scandinavian Peninsula in Northern Europe. The population consists primarily of ethnic Swedes. According to genetic analysis, both mtDNA and Y chromosome polymorphisms show a noticeable genetic affinity between Swedes and central Europeans, especially Germans.

United Kingdom. The United Kingdom of Great Britain and Northern Ireland lies to the northwest of mainland Europe with a population of English (83.6%), Scottish (8.6%), Welsh (4.9%), and Northern Irish (2.9%). Almost 8% of the total population of the UK is composed of ethnic minorities including Indians followed by Pakistanis, Caribbeans, Africans and

Bangladeshis. About 15% of the minority ethnic population describes their ethnic group as mixed [155]. The prevalence of PD in the UK is ranges from 108/100,000[177] in Northampton to 164.2/100,000 in a Scottish city [178]. Age-specific prevalence ratios in 60-69 years ranged from 228/100,000 in a rural area of North Wales [179] to 342/100,000 in London [180].

Clinical studies: Although prevalence varies across European studies, clinical characteristics of PD do not. Small differences have been found in the clinical characteristics of PD patients from the three areas of Denmark: Faroe Islands, the island of Als and Greenland. Patients appear to be significantly younger in Greenland with a faster progression than in the other areas [181] and a study of PD in Cantalejo showed that the disease may be less severe in men than women.

Pathology: No studies focusing on pathological features of PD in various European ethnic groups was identified. Several reports suggest that mitochondrial dysfunction may be involved in the expression of PD. Reduced activity of mitochondrial complex I within SN tissue of patients with PD has been found [182] suggesting that a genetic defect in the ubiquitin-proteasomes system may induces selective nigral neuronal death[183].

Genetic studies: Mutations in the LRRK2 gene are common in several PD populations [184]. The frequency of LRRK2 mutations in European populations with PD is summarized in Table 7. In European populations the G2019S mutation is more frequent [73, 133, 185, 186] than in Asian populations, but less frequent than in North African Arabs and Ashkenazi Jews. This mutation accounts for about 2-6% of familial and 0.3-2% of sporadic cases [74, 82, 131, 187, 188]. A higher number of G2019S mutation were found in populations of the Iberian Peninsula [189, 190]. Modern day Iberians (Spaniards and Portuguese) are a South-Western European population, which shares its predominant genetic relationships with both Mediterranean and Atlantic Europe [191]. This mutation in Iberian populations likely originated from a common founder. European Caucasian patients with PD have the same haplotype as patients from North Africa. Hence, the mutation is likely ancient, not *de novo*. Its frequency in different ethnic groups may be associated with the evolution of ethnic groups and human migration history [76].

One can hypothesize that each ethnic group has its own phylogenic history of the development of PD as illustrated by studies of the R1441G mutation in PD among people of Basque descent. The 1441G mutation was found in 2.7-5% of sporadic cases [192] and 8-20% in families originating from the Basque region [71, 192] which has a relatively homogeneous and historically isolated ethnic group [185]. Analysis the chromosomal region surrounding LRRK2 in carriers of the R1441G mutation suggest that the Basque carriers inherited the mutation as part of an ancestral chromosome [193]. This mutation has not been found in other world populations, including Portuguese patients in the Iberian peninsula [190]. In the Basque county's neighboring region of northern Spain, 2.2% of Asturias PD patients have the mutation [194]. The R1441G Asturia carriers shares the same ancestral haplotype as the Basque patient [194]. In PD patients from Catalonia, the R1441G mutation was present in 0.7% [185] suggesting that the presence of the mutation in Catalonia may be associated with migration from the Basque population [185]. Future studies to identify this mutation in PD patients where there has been a strong migration from the Basque region, such as Argentina or Chili would be of value[193]. Other LRRK2 mutations are rare in

studied European populations (See table 7). Recently, a new LRRK2 Ile1371Val mutation
has been detected in Italian families [133, 195].

Table 7. Frequency of LRRK2 mutations in European populations

Population	Mutation(s)	Frequency % (n)[14]	% Familial
Italian[187]	G2019S	1.74 (1,092)	21.6
Italian[285]	G2019S	1.9 (1,072)	23.3
Italian [286]	G2019S	1.2 (98)	88
Italian[73, 133]	G2019S	6.6 (60)	100
Mixed Brazilian[287]	G2019S	0.8 (80)	12.5
Spanish[189]	G2019S	7.6 (105)	15
Spanish[185]	G2019S	4.3 (286)	29.7
Spanish[288]	G2019S	5.6 (18)	100
Spanish[288]	G2019S	1.5 (133)	0
Portuguese[190]	G2019S	8.6 (128)	20
Portuguese[186]	G2019S	16 (31)	100
Portuguese[186]	G2019S	3.7 (107)	0
Portuguese[186]	G2019S	6.6 (138)	22.4
Swedish[188]	G2019S	1.4 (284)	29.5
British[74]	G2019S	1.6 (482)	0.4
British[289]	G2019S	6.8 (44)	100
French[290]	G2019S	1.9 (103)	0
French-Canadian[291]	G2019S	0 (125)	0
Polish[292]	G2019S	0 (174)	12
Russian[256]	G2019S	1 (305)	4.6
Russian[293]	G2019S	0.9 (345)	4
Norwegian[294]	G2019S	2.1 (435)	1.3
Mixed [295]	G2019S	0.7 (806)	0
Greek[296]	G2019S	0.3 (290)	19
Greek[297]	G2019S	0 (134)	33.6
German[298]	G2019S	0 (162)	24
German[299]	G2019S	0.25 (390)	13.5
Mixed[78]	G2019S	2.9 (174)	100
Turkish[300]	G2019S	1.4 (72)	65.3
Spanish (Catalonia)[185]	R1441G	0.07 (286)	29.7
Spanish (Basque)[193]	R1441G	14.6 (41)	100
Spanish (Basque)[71]	R1441G	8 (137)	22
Spanish (Basque)[193]	R1441G	5 (117)	0
Spanish (Basque)[192]	R1441G	2.7 (147)	0
Spanish (Basque)[192]	R1441G	20 (36)	100
Spanish (Asturias)[192]	R1441G	2.7 (225)	22

---

[14] # subjects analyzed=n0 (284)29.5.

Table 7. (Continued)

Population	Mutation(s)	Frequency % (n)[15]	% Familial
Spanish[189]	R1441G	0 (105)	15
Spanish[288]	R1441G	1.5 (133)	0
Portuguese[190]	R1441G	0 (128)	20
Greek[296]	R1441G	0 (290)	19
Italian[80]	R1441G	0 (629)	28
Swedish[188]	28	0 (284)	29.5
Italian[80]	R1441C	0.16 (629)	28
Mediterranean[73]	R1441C	3.4 (60)	100
Spanish[185]	R1441C	0.3 (286)	29.7
Spanish[189]	R1441C	0 (105)	15
Spanish[288]	R1441C	1.5 (133)	0
Portuguese[190]	R1441C	0 (128)	20
German[72]	R1441C	0.5 (346)	12
Swedish[188]	R1441C	0 (284)	29.5
British[289]	R1441C	2.3 (44)	100
Swedish[188]	R1441H	0 (284)	29.5
Portuguese[190]	R1441H	0 (128)	20
Portuguese[186]	R1441H	0.7 (137)	22.4
Spanish[288]	R1441H	1.5 (133)	0
Norwegian[301]	R1514Q	3.3 (338)	0
Spanish[301]	R1514Q	1 (205)	0
Irish[301]	R1514Q	1.6 (186)	0
German[72]	12020T	0.26 (346)	12
German[131]	12020T	0.25 (390)	13.5
Swedish[188]	12020T	0 (284)	29.5
German[72]	Y1699C	0.26 (346)	12
Italian[80]	Y1699C	0 (629)	28
German[72]	11122V	0.26 (346)	12
German[299]	R793M	0.76 (390)	13.5
German[299]	S1228T	0.25 (390)	13.5

Mutations in alfa-synuclein, parkin, UCH-L1, PINK1, DJ-1 and Nurr1 are comparatively rare in European populations with PD [196, 197] (See Table 5). Although mutations in the SNCA gene have been identified mainly in families of European ancestry (Greek, Italian, Spanish, French) [198], overall mutations in this gene are rare in European populations [131].

Mutations in the parkin gene represent a frequent cause of familial early-onset PD and isolated juvenile Parkinsonism [2]. The mutations in this gene are found in approximately 50% of familial and 15-20% of sporadic EOPD cases among European populations [67, 199], which are more frequent than in Asian patients. Frequencies of the PINK1 mutations vary

---

[15] # subjects analyzed=n0 (284)29.5.

across European populations being highest in Italian patients [2] and lowest in British and Irish patients [151]. PINK1 mutations are less frequent in European populations than Asian [148]. DJ-1 mutations are estimated to be present in 1-2% European patients with EOPD [199, 200], but has not been found in studied Asian populations [4, 154].

Of 16 candidate genes investigated with relation to the etiology of sporadic PD, polymorphisms in MAO-B, dopamine D2 receptor (DRD2), and CYP2D6 may be associated with sporadic PD in Caucasian populations in Europe, America and Australia [121]. Recent studies of familial and sporadic PD in European populations showed that the sepiapterin reductase (SPR) gene appears to be associated with both sporadic and familial PD.

Table 8. Frequency of the other genes mutations in European populations

Population	Gene	Frequency % (n)[16]	Category	% Familial
Finnish[302]	SNCA	0 (147)	Not provided	-----------
British[248, 303]	SNCA	0 (58)	Not provided	-----------
European[131]	SNCA	0.05 (1,912)	Not provided	12.3
German[222]	Parkin	54 (24)	Not provided	100
Russian[256]	Parkin	17.2 (128)	YOPD[17]	0
Russian[293]	Parkin	25 (25)	AR-JP[18]	100
Russian[293]	Parkin	5.8 (345)	Not provided	4
European[67]	Parkin	49 (73)	AR, EOPD	100
European[67]	Parkin	18[19] (100)	EOPD	0
European[199]	Parkin	17 (100)	EOPD	37
Portuguese[186]	Parkin	1.4 (138)	Not provided	22.4
Italian[2]	PINK1	8.9 (90)	EOPD	0
Italian[152]	PINK1	7.7 (90)	EOPD	0
Ireland[151]	PINK1	0.3 (290)	EOPD, LOPD	12
Serbian [304]	PINK1	2.7 (75)	EOPD	24
Italian[304]	PINK1	5.9 (17)	EOPD	35
British[248, 303]	PINK1	1.2 (768)	EOPD	0
Netherlands[200]	DJ-1	1 (200)	AR, EOPD	0
European[199]	DJ-1	2 (100)	EOPD	37
European American[302]	DJ-1	0 (292)	EOPD	100

IV. Parkinson's Disease in Americas' Populations

The Americas include continents of North America and South America with associated islands and regions and contain about 14% of the world population. The population of the Americas is made up of the descendants of eight large ethnic groups [155].

---

[16] # patients analyzed=n.
[17] Young onset PD.
[18] Autosomal recessive juvenile parkinsonism.
[19] Isolated cases.

North America is the third-largest continent but only fourth in population. North America is often divided into sub-regions, but there are no universally accepted divisions. Most of northern North America is occupied by Canada, the world's second-largest country by total area. The US has a highly diverse population, being home to at least 31 ethnic groups [155]. The US Office of Management and Budget [201] recognizes six racial categories: American Indian or Alaska Native, Asian, Black or African-American, Native Hawaiian or Other Pacific Islander, white and Hispanic [202]. The 1997 standards retained only two ethnic categories: Hispanic or Latino, and Not Hispanic or Latino with Hispanic defined as: "A person of Cuban, Mexican, Puerto Rican, South or Central American or other Spanish culture or origin, regardless of race". The Office of Management and Budget acknowledges that these categories are "neither anthropologically nor scientifically based, but rather represent a social-political construct designed for collecting data on race and ethnicity of board population groups in the US" [201]. Among racial demographics, whites with European ancestry remained the largest racial group (75.1%) followed by African Americans (12.3%), and Asians (3.6%) [34]. Latinos are the largest (14%) minority population in the US. From a genetic perspective, Latinos are descended from indigenous American, European, and African populations. Because Latinos are known to be an admixed population, they may be an ideal population for "admixture mapping", an approach that can efficiently identify genomic regions that underlie racial differences in disease [14].

South America includes 33.3% Caucasians, 25.6% Mestizo, 17.3% Mulatto, 11.6% Amerindian or Native Peoples, 6% White/Mestizo, and 4.7% is Black. Many Latin Americans are of European descent, mainly of Spanish, Portuguese or Italian heritage. Southeastern and Southern Brazil, Argentina, and Uruguay contain peoples of Caucasian descent. Overall, the population of Latin America is an amalgam of ancestries and ethnic groups. The composition varies from country to country. Most or all Latin American countries have Asian minorities [155].

Prevalence of PD Epidemiologic studies of PD in the Americas have been conducted mainly in the US and Canada. The prevalence of PD in North America is summarized in Table. 9.

The US: The prevalence of PD in the US ranges from 79/100,000 in Baltimore [45, 203] to 331/100,000 in South Carolina [204], which is similar to European populations. The prevalence of the disease was higher in African Americans than in white populations [204, 205]. The prevalence rate increases with age and was highest in individuals aged from 70 to 80 years [206, 207]. The population prevalence of PD in those over aged 60 was particularly high in an Amish community (566/100,000) with increasing prevalence in every decade [208]. Amish communities geographically and social isolated and are united by a common Swiss-German ancestry [155].

Canada Has a PD Prevalence Similar to the US and Europe

Latin America. There are only six published surveys on the prevalence of parkinsonism and PD in Latin America [209-213]. The prevalence was higher (135-656.8/100,000) than in the US (79-331/100,000) or Canada (69-246/100,000 with rhe highest prevalence

(656.8/100,000) found in Buenos Aires, The age specific prevalence was consistently higher for men (824/100,000) than the one for women (526,7/100,000), and it increased with advancing age for both sexes [209].

Table 9. Prevalence PD in the Americas

Region	Study Design	Population size[20]	#cases	Crude prevalence per 100,000	Age-specific prevalence
US (Baltimore)[45]	Community-based	2.070,000	1,630	79	-------------
US (Mississippi)[49]	Door-to-door	23,597 B: 11,666 W:11,931	31 12 19	131 103 159	-------------
US (New York)[207]	Population-based	Not provided	Not provided	178.3	50-60:125.2 60-70:438 70-80:1,353 >80:846.7
US (Nebraska)[305]	PD registry	Not provided	5,062	329.3	---------------
US (Amish) [208]	Population-based	Not provided	Not provided	Not provided	>60:556
US (South Carolina) [204]	Clinic-based	9,336 B:1,289 W:7,907	Not provided	246 B:119 W:331	---------------
Canada (BC)[303]	Medical record review	80,000	55	69	86.2
Canada (Alberta)[165]	Gender-based	Not provided	Not provided	249	---------------
Canada (Saskatchewan) [306]	Community-based	70	4	------------	-------------
Canada (Ontario)[307]	Cross - sectional	Not provided	Not provided	Not provided	373
Uruguay (Montevideo)[213]	Clinic-based	1,975	8	405	---------------
Uruguay [308]	Clinic-based	Not provided	Not provided	136	---------------
Brazil (Bambui) [211]	Population-based	15,000	39	260	--------------
Argentina (Junin) [209]	Cross-sectional	7,765	51	656.8	---------------
Cuba (Havana City)[309]	Door-to-door	17,784	24	135	---------------
Bolivia[210]	Door-to-door	9,955	5	286	>80:443
Columbia[212]	Capture-recapture	Not provided	Not provided	176.4	---------------

---

[20] B=blacks and W=whites

The clinical features of PD: A comparison of Tunisian and North American Caucasian PD families showed that non-motor symptoms (most commonly autonomic dysfunction) are more common in the US populations than in Tunisians [57]. According to reported studies, patients with PD from North and South America are clinically and pathologically indistinguishable from Caucasian patients from the other regions of the world [214, 215].

Genetic studies (predominantly from North America): The frequency of LRRK2 mutations in patients with PD in American studies are summarized in Table 10.

Table 10. The Frequency of LRRK2 mutations in the Americas

Country	Mutation	Frequency % (n)[21]	% Familial
US[310]	G2019S	0.8 (371)	20
US[76]	G2019S	5.6 (504)	11.5
US[311]	G2019S	0.5 (786)	30
US[312]	G2019S	5 (430)	100
US[313]	G2019S	1.3 (1,425)	0
US[110]	G2019S	2 (405)	0
US[75]	G2019S	5 (767)	100
US[314]	G2019S	1.2 (326)	46
US[315]	G2019S	1.3 (347)	Not provided
US[57]	G2019S	2.6 (39)	100
Mixed [295]	G2019S	2.8 (248)	100
Canada[135]	G2019S	1.7 (121)	42
Canada[291]	G2019S	0 (125)	0
US[310]	R1441C	0.26 (371)	20
US[216]	R1441C	0.4 (247)	100
US[312]	R1441C	0.23 (430)	100
US[76]	R1441C	0 (504)	11.5
US[310]	R1441H	0.26 (371)	20
US[312]	R1441H	0 (430)	100
US[312]	R1441G	0 (430)	100
US[312]	R793M	0 (430)	100
US[311]	M1869T	0.12 (786)	30
US[312]	M1869T	0 (430)	100
US[312]	I2012T	0 (430)	100
US[312]	I2020T	0 (430)	100
US[312]	L1114L	0 (430)	100
US[312]	I1371V	0 (430)	100
US[312]	Y1699C	0 (430)	100
US[312]	G2385R	0 (430)	100
Brazil[218]	G2019S	7.7 (13)	100
Brazil (mixed)[73]	G2019S	6.6 (60)	100
Brazil (mixed)[73]	R1441C	3.4 (60)	100

---

[21] # Subjects analyzed=n

In North America, the G2019S mutation is more common than other mutations of LRRK2. The prevalence of the G2019S mutation in North America resembled that found in North European and Asian countries. The mutation of the G2019S in North America also was prevalent in patients with familial PD [57, 216, 217]. European and North American patients with the G2019S share a common ancestral haplotype suggesting a single founder. Among the few studies conducted in South America, there is a high frequency of the G2019S mutation in familial PD [73, 133, 218].

The frequency of other genes mutations besides LRRK2 in American PD populations is summarized in Table 11. Mutations in the SNCA, UCHL1, PINK1, DJ-1 and Nurr 1 occur relatively infrequently in the American population. Parkin is the only other PD gene besides LRRK2 that has an appreciable mutation frequency in American populations. The parkin mutation is higher (21-33%) in American populations [219, 220] compared to Asian (2.8-14.3%) [221] or European populations (1.4-17%) [186, 199]. However, frequency of the mutation in parkin gene in American patients with familial PD was similar (53%) [220] to Europeans (54%) [222].

A recent study [199] of the origin of the parkin mutations supports a common founder for the most frequent parkin mutation (924C>T) as indicated by a rare allele at marker D6S305. Three other mutations were found in individuals of the same geographic/ethnic origin (1072delT and delEx7 in South Tyrol; delEx3-4 in Puerto Rico). The study results show that certain specific mutations are overrepresented in a given population. A novel homozygous missense mutation (Gly504Arg) was identified in one sporadic case from Brazil with juvenile parkinsonism [223].

Table 11. Frequency of the other genes mutations in the Americas

Country	Gene	Frequency % (n)[22]	Clinical Category	% Familial
US[79]	SNCA	0 (286)	------------------	63
US[316]	SNCA	0 (75)		0
US[302]	SNCA	0 (292)		100
US and Canada[219]	Parkin	31 (42)	EOPD[23]	19
US[316]	UCHL1	0 (75)	------------------	0
US[79]	PINK1	0 (215)	EOPD	47.4
US[79]	PINK1	0 (237)	------------------	46
US[316]	PINK1	0 (75)	------------------	0
Brazil[218]	PINK1	2.2 (45)	EOPD	25
US[85]	DJ-1	0 (89)	EOPD	7
US[316]	DJ	0 (75)	------------------	0
US[302]	DJ	0 (292)	------------------	100
US[317]	Nurr 1	0 (372)	------------------	100
Canada[318]	Nurr 1	0.5 (202)	------------------	37
US[302]	Nurr 1	0 (292)	------------------	100

---

[22] # subjects analyzed =n
[23] EOPD=early onset PD

The GlyArg mutation was not observed in healthy individuals of the Portuguese and Italian populations or Brazilian patients with early-onset PD. The Gly504 residue is highly conserved in the known mammalian, homologues the ATP13A2 protein suggesting that mutations in the ATP13A2 gene might be relevant for young onset PD [223]. Mutation of this gene have been recently shown to underlie the autosomal recessive, l-dopa-responsive, pallido-pyramidal disease Kufor-Rakeb syndrome [224, 225].

APOE is the only gene that has been exclusively associated with PD in Asian patients [121]. A recent study of 324 Caucasian families with PD from the US [217] showed a significant association between age of onset of PD and APOE genotypes. Age of onset was significantly earlier in those individuals with at least one ε4 allele when compared with those homozygous for the common ε3 allele [217].

Table 12. PD Prevalence in Australia

Region	Design	Population size	# cases	Crude prevalence per 100,000	Age-specific prevalence
Victoria[226]	Cross-sectional	83,001	70	85	-----------
Nambour[227]	Cross-sectional	1,207	5	414	-----------
Sydney (Randwick)[229]	Door-to-door	527	19	775	55-59:2,899 60-69:1,685 70-79:3,960 >80:7,792
Syndey (Bankstown)[228]	Door-to-door	501	17	776	60-69:599 70-79:3,941 >80:1039
Queensland[319]	GP survey[24]			146	--------------
Sydney[230]	Cross-sectional and longitudinal	3,509	3,509	104	>50:362

V. Parkinson's Disease in the Australian Population

Australia is a country in the Southern Hemisphere comprising the mainland of the world's smallest continent. The Australian mainland has been inhabited for more than 42,000 years by indigenous Australians. Today, Australia consists of six states, two major mainland territories, and other minor territories with a population of 20.8 million people, concentrated in the mainland state capitals of Sydney, Melbourne, Brisbane, Perth, and Adelaide [48, 155]. Australia's present day population are predominantly Anglo-Celtic in origin. Only 2 percent of the population is indigenous—Aborigines and Torres Strait Islanders. The fastest growing

---

[24] GP=general practioner

ethnic group is the category of people who are of mixed ethnic origins. Many Australians consider themselves to be of mixed ancestry [48]. The 1975 Racial Discrimination Act made the use of racial criteria for any official purpose illegal, so further data is somewhat limited.

Prevalence of PD: An Australian epidemiological study published in 1966 [226] reported that the prevalence of PD was quite low at 85/100,000, but a later study in the rural town of Nambour [227] revealed a prevalence of 414/100,000 leading the authors to suggest that the high prevalence of PD here may be due to rural residency. The most significant risk factor for the development of PD was a positive family history with 19% of PD patients having a positive family history of PD and 11% with a first-degree relative with PD. The most recent studies conducted in Sydney [228, 229] found a very high crude prevalence (776/100,000) indicating that Sydney has one of the highest prevalence estimates of PD in the developed world. This may be explained by predominantly the European ancestry of the Sydney population since estimated prevalence has been lower in other Australian regions [230].

Genetic studies: The frequency of the LRRK2 mutations in patients with PD in Australian studies is summarized in Table. 13. Mutations in the LRRK2 gene are less common in Australian patients with PD when compared to other Caucasian populations. Australian G2019S mutation carriers share the same cofounder as European carriers [221].

Alpha-synuclein: This allele is less common in Australian patients compared to controls. A combined analysis including all previously published ancestral European Rep1data found a highly significant association between this allele and a reduced risk for PD [231].

Table 13. Frequency of LRRK2 mutations in Australia

Mutation	Frequency % (n)[25]
G2019S[221]	0.96 (830)
R1441H[221]	0.25 (830)
A1442P[221]	0.12 (830)
A14429[320]	0.90 (109)

Parkin: Investigations of the effect of the -258 T/G SNP on the age at disease onset in an Australian idiopathic PD cohort revealed that the GG genotype was over-represented in the early-onset group. These data suggest that reduced expression of normal parkin protein may result in an earlier manifestation of PD symptoms [232]. A study of the prevalence of mtDNA haplogroups J and K in patients with PD in the Australian community did not find significant differences in the prevalence of the mtDNA haplogroup J or K in PD patients compared to control subjects [230]. Results of the study of the cys282Tyr SNP as a genetic risk factor for PD in two distinct and separately collected cohorts of Australian PD patients and controls suggest that possession of the 282Tyr allele may offer some protection against the development of PD [233].

---

[25] # subjects analyzed=n

Considerations

Idiopathic PD occurs worldwide in all major ethnic groups and genetic studies demonstrate that one or more PD-linked gene mutations can be found in many populations. The prevalence of the disease and the frequency of PD-linked gene mutations display great variability in various ethnic groups, but we are still a long way from a full understanding of the reasons for this variability.

It is currently postulated that PD is probably not a single nosological entity. The clinical manifestations of the disease in patients with PD linked gene mutations are indistinguishable from those in idiopathic PD (where no mutations have been demonstrated to date). There is a pressing need to understand how the diverse mutations identified to date lead to the degeneration of dopaminergic neurons in the substantia nigra *pars compacta* and how this determines the manifestation of the main symptoms of PD.

Neither the demonstration of associated gene mutations nor the demonstration of genotype-phenotype correlations can fully explain the degeneration of key neurons. At present it is clear that no one single gene dysfunction is the cause of PD and it is likely that many more mutations will be discovered in the future.

According to the "out of Africa" hypothesis, modern human populations dispersed from Africa to other parts of Asia and Europe through a genetic bottleneck. The variety of PD-associated mutations in African vs. non-African PD patients does not support the idea of a common founder effect. The genetic tree of PD-associated mutations in a sense constitutes a road-map of the phylogeny of the substantia nigra pars compacta in human evolution. The prevalence of PD reflects the ontogeny of the substantia nigra pars compacta in as much as its biochemical make-updetermines its ability to withstand the effects of other determinants of late-onset neuronal degeneration.

In that similar mutations are found throughout the human phylogenetic tree in high-incidence (non-African) and low-incidence (African) populations, there is no evidence yet of a phylogenetic-ontogenic correlation, though further work may reveal it if it turns out that some mutations are more important than others. At present it seems that the genetic determinants of PD interact with other determinants specific to each ethnic group or population to determine the precise clinical manifestations in an individual.

There appear to be racial and ethnic differences in the genetic determinants of cell death in the basal ganglia. These diverse genetic determinants did not arise at the same time in evolution, yet they predispose to an essentially common pathological process of SN neuronal death. Given the diversity of PD mutations in different ethnic groups, it is highly unlikely that a common ancestor gave rise to the first case of PD.

More likely these genetic determinants developed independently in European and Asian populations, and migrations of people led to the admixture of diverse genetic determinants. Whether there is a selection pressure which confers some survival advantage on these mutations in children or younger adults is as yet unknown.

Acknowledgments

We would like to thank Dr Paul Kelly, MD, FRCP, Institute of Cell and Molecular Science Barts and The London School of Medicine, for useful discussion regarding this topic. Thanks also to Jill Remenar and Natalie Organek of Michigan State University for assistance in literature search and citations management.

References

[1]   Broussolle E, Thobois S. [Genetic and environmental factors of Parkinson's disease]. *Rev. Neurol.* (Paris). 2002;158(122):11-23.

[2]   Bonifati V. Genetics of Parkinson's disease. *Minerva Med.* 2005 Jun;96(3):175-86.

[3]   Hardy J, Cai H, Cookson MR, Gwinn-Hardy K, Singleton A. Genetics of Parkinson's disease and parkinsonism. *Ann. Neurol.* 2006 Oct;60(4):389-98.

[4]   Mizuno Y, Hattori N, Yoshino H, Hatano Y, Satoh K, Tomiyama H, et al. Progress in familial Parkinson's disease. *J. Neural. Transm. Suppl.* 2006(70):191-204.

[5]   Hardy J, Myers A. Genetic variability in expression of proteins and the risk of sporadic neurologic diseases. *Neurology.* 2007 Feb 27;68(9):632-3.

[6]   Wirdefeldt K, Gatz M, Schalling M, Pedersen NL. No evidence for heritability of Parkinson disease in Swedish twins. *Neurology.* 2004 Jul 27;63(2):305-11.

[7]   Marras C, Tanner C. *Parkinson's Disease: Genetic Epidemiology and Overview. Genetics of Movement Disorders.* London: Elsevier; 2003. p. 273-86.

[8]   Hardy J, Singleton A, Gwinn-Hardy K. Ethnic differences and disease phenotypes. *Science.* 2003 May 2;300(5620):739-40.

[9]   Karter AJ. Race and ethnicity: vital constructs for diabetes research. *Diabetes Care.* 2003 Jul;26(7):2189-93.

[10] Karter AJ. Commentary: Race, genetics, and disease--in search of a middle ground. *Int. J. Epidemiol.* 2003 Feb;32(1):26-8.

[11] Tishkoff SA, Reed FA, Ranciaro A, Voight BF, Babbitt CC, Silverman JS, et al. Convergent adaptation of human lactase persistence in Africa and Europe. *Nat. Genet.* 2007 Jan;39(1):31-40.

[12] A haplotype map of the human genome. *Nature.* 2005 Oct 27;437(7063):1299-320.

[13] The use of racial, ethnic, and ancestral categories in human genetics research. *Am. J. Hum. Genet.* 2005 Oct;77(4):519-32.

[14] Burchard EG, Ziv E, Coyle N, Gomez SL, Tang H, Karter AJ, et al. The importance of race and ethnic background in biomedical research and clinical practice. *N. Engl. J. Med.* 2003 Mar 20;348(12):1170-5.

[15] Cooper RS, Kaufman JS, Ward R. Race and genomics. *N. Engl. J. Med.* 2003 Mar 20;348(12):1166-70.

[16] Phimister EG. Medicine and the racial divide. *N. Engl. J. Med.* 2003 Mar 20;348(12):1081-2.

[17] Schwartz RS. Racial profiling in medical research. *N. Engl. J. Med.* 2001 May 3;344(18):1392-3.

[18] Cooper RS. Race, genes, and health--new wine in old bottles? *Int. J. Epidemiol.* 2003 Feb;32(1):23-5.

[19] Kaufman JS, Cooper RS. Commentary: considerations for use of racial/ethnic classification in etiologic research. *Am. J. Epidemiol.* 2001 Aug 15;154(4):291-8.

[20] Bamshad M, Wooding S, Salisbury BA, Stephens JC. Deconstructing the relationship between genetics and race. *Nat. Rev. Genet.* 2004 Aug;5(8):598-609.

[21] Tishkoff SA, Kidd KK. Implications of biogeography of human populations for 'race' and medicine. *Nat. Genet.* 2004 Nov;36(11 Suppl):S21-7.

[22] Williams SM, Templeton AR. Race and genomics. *N. Engl. J. Med.* 2003 Jun 19;348(25):2581-2; author reply -2.

[23] Kosoko-Lasaki O, Gong G, Haynatzki G, Wilson MR. Race, ethnicity and prevalence of primary open-angle glaucoma. *J. Natl. Med. Assoc.* 2006 Oct;98(10):1626-9.

[24] Kurian AK, Cardarelli KM. Racial and ethnic differences in cardiovascular disease risk factors: a systematic review. *Ethn. Dis.* 2007 Winter;17(1):143-52.

[25] Low NC, Hardy J. Psychiatric disorder criteria and their application to research in different racial groups. *BMC Psychiatry.* 2007;7:1.

[26] McEvoy B, Beleza S, Shriver MD. The genetic architecture of normal variation in human pigmentation: an evolutionary perspective and model. *Hum. Mol. Genet.* 2006 Oct 15;15 Spec No 2:R176-81.

[27] O'Leary A, Fisher HH, Purcell DW, Spikes PS, Gomez CA. Correlates of Risk Patterns and Race/Ethnicity among HIV-Positive Men who have Sex with Men. *AIDS Behav.* 2007 Sep;11(5):706-15.

[28] Todorov T. On Human Diversity. Cambridge, MA: Harvard University Press; 1993.

[29] Risch N. Dissecting racial and ethnic differences. *N. Engl. J. Med.* 2006 Jan 26;354(4):408-11.

[30] Modern Human Variation: Models of Classification. 2007.

[31] Risch N, Burchard E, Ziv E, Tang H. Categorization of humans in biomedical research: genes, race and disease. *Genome Biol.* 2002 Jul 1;3(7):comment2007.

[32] Stajich JE, Hahn MW. Disentangling the effects of demography and selection in human history. *Mol. Biol. Evol.* 2005 Jan;22(1):63-73.

[33] Rebbeck TR, Sankar P. Ethnicity, ancestry, and race in molecular epidemiologic research. *Cancer Epidemiol Biomarkers Prev.* 2005 Nov;14(11 Pt 1):2467-71.

[34] Population statistics for Africa. 2007.

[35] Templeton A. A genetic and evolutionary prospective. *American Anthropology.* 2007;100:632-50.

[36] Bosch E, Calafell F, Perez-Lezaun A, Comas D, Mateu E, Bertranpetit J. Population history of north Africa: evidence from classical genetic markers. *Hum. Biol.* 1997 Jun;69(3):295-311.

[37] Lovell A, Moreau C, Yotova V, Xiao F, Bourgeois S, Gehl D, et al. Ethiopia: between Sub-Saharan Africa and western Eurasia. *Ann. Hum. Genet.* 2005 May;69(Pt 3):275-87.

[38] Ostrer H. A genetic profile of contemporary Jewish populations. *Nat. Rev. Genet.* 2001 Nov;2(11):891-8.

[39] Harich N, Esteban E, Chafik A, Lopez-Alomar A, Vona G, Moral P. Classical polymorphisms in Berbers from Moyen Atlas (Morocco): genetics, geography, and

historical evidence in the Mediterranean peoples. *Ann. Hum. Biol.* 2002 Sep-Oct;29(5):473-87.

[40]   Lefevre-Witier P, Aireche H, Benabadji M, Darlu P, Melvin K, Sevin A, et al. Genetic structure of Algerian populations. *Am. J. Hum. Biol.* 2006 Jul-Aug;18(4):492-501.

[41]   Okubadejo NU, Bower JH, Rocca WA, Maraganore DM. Parkinson's disease in Africa: A systematic review of epidemiologic and genetic studies. *Mov. Disord.* 2006 Dec;21(12):2150-6.

[42]   Chaudhuri KR, Hu MT, Brooks DJ. Atypical parkinsonism in Afro-Caribbean and Indian origin immigrants to the UK. *Mov. Disord.* 2000 Jan;15(1):18-23.

[43]   Eastham JH, Lacro JP, Jeste DV. Ethnicity and movement disorders. *Mt Sinai J. Med.* 1996 Oct-Nov;63(5-6):314-9.

[44]   McInerney-Leo A, Gwinn-Hardy K, Nussbaum RL. Prevalence of Parkinson's disease in populations of African ancestry: a review. *J. Natl. Med. Assoc.* 2004 Jul;96(7):974-9.

[45]   Kessler, II. Epidemiologic studies of Parkinson's disease. 3. A community-based survey. *Am. J. Epidemiol.* 1972 Oct;96(4):242-54.

[46]   Paddison RM, Griffith RP. Occurrence of Parkinson's disease in black patients at Charity Hospital in New Orleans. *Neurology.* 1974 Jul;24(7):688-90.

[47]   Zhang ZX, Roman GC. Worldwide occurrence of Parkinson's disease: an updated review. *Neuroepidemiology.* 1993;12(4):195-208.

[48]   Encyclopedia Britannica. [cited June 2007]; Available from:

[49]   Schoenberg BS, Osuntokun BO, Adeuja AO, Bademosi O, Nottidge V, Anderson DW, et al. Comparison of the prevalence of Parkinson's disease in black populations in the rural United States and in rural Nigeria: door-to-door community studies. *Neurology.* 1988 Apr;38(4):645-6.

[50]   Van Den Eeden SK, Tanner CM, Bernstein AL, Fross RD, Leimpeter A, Bloch DA, et al. Incidence of Parkinson's disease: variation by age, gender, and race/ethnicity. *Am. J. Epidemiol.* 2003 Jun 1;157(11):1015-22.

[51]   Bergmann K, Salak V, Rodgers J. African Americans and Parkinson's Disease in South Carolina. *Movement Disorders.* 2006;21(Suppl13):S45.

[52]   Bower JH, Teshome M, Melaku Z, Zenebe G. Frequency of movement disorders in an Ethiopian university practice. *Mov. Disord.* 2005 Sep;20(9):1209-13.

[53]   Atadzhanov M, Zumla A, Mwaba P. Study of familial Parkinson's disease in Russia, Uzbekistan, and Zambia. *Postgrad Med. J.* 2005 Feb;81(952):117-21.

[54]   Gouider-Khouja N, Belal S, Hamida MB, Hentati F. Clinical and genetic study of familial Parkinson's disease in Tunisia. *Neurology.* 2000 Apr 25;54(8):1603-9.

[55]   Hu MT, Chaudhuri KR, Jarosz J, Yaguez L, Brooks DJ. An imaging study of parkinsonism among African-Caribbean and Indian London communities. *Mov. Disord.* 2002 Nov;17(6):1321-8.

[56]   Shulman L, Griber-Baldini A, Anderson K. Racial and socioeconomic disparities in patients with parkinsonism. *Neurology.* 2007;68(12 (Suppl1)):A104.

[57]   Ishihara L, Gibson RA, Warren L, Amouri R, Lyons K, Wielinski C, et al. Screening for Lrrk2 G2019S and clinical comparison of Tunisian and North American Caucasian Parkinson's disease families. *Mov. Disord.* 2007 Jan;22(1):55-61.

[58] Jenner P, Olanow CW. The pathogenesis of cell death in Parkinson's disease. *Neurology*. 2006 May 23;66(10 Suppl 4):S24-36.

[59] Muthane UB, Chickabasaviah YT, Henderson J, Kingsbury AE, Kilford L, Shankar SK, et al. Melanized nigral neuronal numbers in Nigerian and British individuals. *Mov. Disord*. 2006 Aug;21(8):1239-41.

[60] Calafell F, Shuster A, Speed WC, Kidd JR, Kidd KK. Short tandem repeat polymorphism evolution in humans. *Eur. J. Hum. Genet*. 1998 Jan;6(1):38-49.

[61] Mellars P. Why did modern human populations disperse from Africa ca. 60,000 years ago? A new model. *Proc. Natl. Acad Sci. USA*. 2006 Jun 20;103(25):9381-6.

[62] Tishkoff SA, Verrelli BC. Patterns of human genetic diversity: implications for human evolutionary history and disease. *Annu. Rev. Genomics Hum. Genet*. 2003;4:293-340.

[63] Ouyang C, Krontiris TG. Identification and functional significance of SNPs underlying conserved haplotype frameworks across ethnic populations. *Pharmacogenet Genomics*. 2006 Sep;16(9):667-82.

[64] Ely B, Wilson JL, Jackson F, Jackson BA. African-American mitochondrial DNAs often match mtDNAs found in multiple African ethnic groups. *BMC Biol*. 2006;4:34.

[65] Salas A, Carracedo A, Richards M, Macaulay V. Charting the ancestry of African Americans. *Am. J. Hum. Genet*. 2005 Oct;77(4):676-80.

[66] Gouider-Khouja N, Larnaout A, Amouri R, Sfar S, Belal S, Ben Hamida C, et al. Autosomal recessive parkinsonism linked to parkin gene in a Tunisian family. Clinical, genetic and pathological study. *Parkinsonism Relat Disord*. 2003 Jun;9(5):247-51.

[67] Lucking CB, Abbas N, Durr A, Bonifati V, Bonnet AM, de Broucker T, et al. Homozygous deletions in parkin gene in European and North African families with autosomal recessive juvenile parkinsonism. The European Consortium on Genetic Susceptibility in Parkinson's Disease and the French Parkinson's Disease Genetics Study Group. *Lancet*. 1998 Oct 24;352(9137):1355-6.

[68] Tassin J, Durr A, de Broucker T, Abbas N, Bonifati V, De Michele G, et al. Chromosome 6-linked autosomal recessive early-onset Parkinsonism: linkage in European and Algerian families, extension of the clinical spectrum, and evidence of a small homozygous deletion in one family. The French Parkinson's Disease Genetics Study Group, and the European Consortium on Genetic Susceptibility in Parkinson's Disease. *Am. J. Hum. Genet*. 1998 Jul;63(1):88-94.

[69] Gasser T. Genetics of Parkinson's disease. Curr Opin Neurol. 2005 Aug;18(4):363-9.

[70] Lesage S, Durr A, Tazir M, Lohmann E, Leutenegger AL, Janin S, et al. LRRK2 G2019S as a cause of Parkinson's disease in North African Arabs. *N. Engl. J. Med*. 2006 Jan 26;354(4):422-3.

[71] Paisan-Ruiz C, Jain S, Evans EW, Gilks WP, Simon J, van der Brug M, et al. Cloning of the gene containing mutations that cause PARK8-linked Parkinson's disease. *Neuron*. 2004 Nov 18;44(4):595-600.

[72] Zimprich A, Biskup S, Leitner P, Lichtner P, Farrer M, Lincoln S, et al. Mutations in LRRK2 cause autosomal-dominant parkinsonism with pleomorphic pathology. *Neuron*. 2004 Nov 18;44(4):601-7.

[73] Di Fonzo A, Rohe CF, Ferreira J, Chien HF, Vacca L, Stocchi F, et al. A frequent LRRK2 gene mutation associated with autosomal dominant Parkinson's disease. *Lancet.* 2005 Jan 29-Feb 4;365(9457):412-5.

[74] Gilks WP, Abou-Sleiman PM, Gandhi S, Jain S, Singleton A, Lees AJ, et al. A common LRRK2 mutation in idiopathic Parkinson's disease. *Lancet.* 2005 Jan 29-Feb 4;365(9457):415-6.

[75] Nichols WC, Pankratz N, Hernandez D, Paisan-Ruiz C, Jain S, Halter CA, et al. Genetic screening for a single common LRRK2 mutation in familial Parkinson's disease. *Lancet.* 2005 Jan 29-Feb 4;365(9457):410-2.

[76] Clark LN, Wang Y, Karlins E, Saito L, Mejia-Santana H, Harris J, et al. Frequency of LRRK2 mutations in early- and late-onset Parkinson disease. *Neurology.* 2006 Nov 28;67(10):1786-91.

[77] Krygowska-Wajs A, Kachergus JM, Hulihan MM, Farrer MJ, Searcy JA, Booij J, et al. Clinical and genetic evaluation of 8 Polish families with levodopa-responsive parkinsonism. *J. Neural. Transm.* 2005 Nov;112(11):1487-502.

[78] Lesage S, Leutenegger AL, Ibanez P, Janin S, Lohmann E, Durr A, et al. LRRK2 haplotype analyses in European and North African families with Parkinson disease: a common founder for the G2019S mutation dating from the 13th century. *Am. J. Hum. Genet.* 2005 Aug;77(2):330-2.

[79] Deng H, Xie W, Guo Y, Le W, Jankovic J. Gene dosage analysis of alpha-synuclein (SNCA) in patients with Parkinson's disease. *Mov. Disord.* 2006 May;21(5):728-9.

[80] Goldwurm S, Di Fonzo A, Simons EJ, Rohe CF, Zini M, Canesi M, et al. The G6055A (G2019S) mutation in LRRK2 is frequent in both early and late onset Parkinson's disease and originates from a common ancestor. *J. Med. Genet.* 2005 Nov;42(11):e65.

[81] Zabetian CP, Morino H, Ujike H, Yamamoto M, Oda M, Maruyama H, et al. Identification and haplotype analysis of LRRK2 G2019S in Japanese patients with Parkinson disease. *Neurology.* 2006 Aug 22;67(4):697-9.

[82] Lesage S, Ibanez P, Lohmann E, Pollak P, Tison F, Tazir M, et al. G2019S LRRK2 mutation in French and North African families with Parkinson's disease. *Ann. Neurol.* 2005 Nov;58(5):784-7.

[83] Ozelius LJ, Senthil G, Saunders-Pullman R, Ohmann E, Deligtisch A, Tagliati M, et al. LRRK2 G2019S as a cause of Parkinson's disease in Ashkenazi Jews. *N. Engl. J. Med.* 2006 Jan 26;354(4):424-5.

[84] Jackson BA, Wilson JL, Kirbah S, Sidney SS, Rosenberger J, Bassie L, et al. Mitochondrial DNA genetic diversity among four ethnic groups in Sierra Leone. *Am. J. Phys. Anthropol.* 2005 Sep;128(1):156-63.

[85] Clark LN, Afridi S, Mejia-Santana H, Harris J, Louis ED, Cote LJ, et al. Analysis of an early-onset Parkinson's disease cohort for DJ-1 mutations. *Mov. Disord.* 2004 Jul;19(7):796-800.

[86] Amouri R, Yahmed S, Kefi M. Novel mutation in PINK1 gene causing autosomal recessive parkinsonism in a large Tunisian family. *Neurology.* 2007;68(12 (Suppl1)):A323.

[87] Carr J, Bardien S. Investigation of the molecular etiology of South African patients with Parkinson's Disease. *Neurology.* 2007;22 (Suppl16):S133.

[88]   Canada WUSo. 2006 [cited October 7, 2006]; Available from: http://www.wusc.ca/expertise/worldwide/asia

[89]   Omura K. Asian Race. [cited; Available from: http://kennethomura.tripod.com/asian_race/

[90]   Color Q World: Clarifying the definition of Asian. 2005 [cited October 1, 2006]; Available from: http://www.colorq.org/PetSins/article.asp?y=2005andm=5x=5_7

[91]   The Asian Internet Statistics. [cited March 10, 2007]; Available from: www.internet worldstats.com

[92]   Woo J, Lau E, Ziea E, Chan DK. Prevalence of Parkinson's disease in a Chinese population. *Acta Neurol. Scand.* 2004 Mar;109(3):228-31.

[93]   Chan DK, Cordato D, Bui T, Mellick G, Woo J. Comparison of environmental and genetic factors for Parkinson's disease between Chinese and Caucasians. *Neuroepidemiology.* 2004 Jan-Apr;23(1-2):13-22.

[94]   Chen RC, Chang SF, Su CL, Chen TH, Yen MF, Wu HM, et al. Prevalence, incidence, and mortality of PD: a door-to-door survey in Ilan county, Taiwan. *Neurology.* 2001 Nov 13;57(9):1679-86.

[95]   de Rijk MC, Launer LJ, Berger K, Breteler MM, Dartigues JF, Baldereschi M, et al. Prevalence of Parkinson's disease in Europe: A collaborative study of population-based cohorts. Neurologic Diseases in the Elderly Research Group. *Neurology.* 2000;54(11 Suppl 5):S21-3.

[96]   Kim JS, Sohn YH. Current status of Parkinson's disease treatment in Korea. *Parkinsonism Relat. Disord.* 2003 Aug;9 Suppl 2:S99-104.

[97]   Harada H, Nishikawa S, Takahashi K. Epidemiology of Parkinson's disease in a Japanese city. *Arch. Neurol.* 1983 Mar;40(3):151-4.

[98]   Yamawaki M, Kusumi M, Nukashima K. Epidemiological study of Parkinson's Disease in a Japanese city, the changes for quarter century. *Mov. Disord.* 2006;21(Suppl 15):S479.

[99]   Abbott RD, Ross GW, White LR, Sanderson WT, Burchfiel CM, Kashon M, et al. Environmental, life-style, and physical precursors of clinical Parkinson's disease: recent findings from the Honolulu-Asia Aging Study. *J. Neurol.* 2003 Oct;250 Suppl 3:III30-9.

[100] Bharucha NE, Bharucha EP, Bharucha AE, Bhise AV, Schoenberg BS. Prevalence of Parkinson's disease in the Parsi community of Bombay, India. *Arch. Neurol.* 1988 Dec;45(12):1321-3.

[101] Ragothaman M, Murgod UA, Gururaj G, Kumaraswamy SD, Muthane U. Lower risk of Parkinson's disease in an admixed population of European and Indian origins. *Mov. Disord.* 2003 Aug;18(8):912-4.

[102] Anca M, Paleacu D, Shabtai H, Giladi N. Cross-sectional study of the prevalence of Parkinson's disease in the Kibbutz movement in Israel. *Neuroepidemiology.* 2002 Jan-Feb;21(1):50-5.

[103] Inzelberg R, Masarwa M, Strugatsky R. Prevalence of sporadic Parkinson's disease in Arabic villages in Isreal: a door-to-door study. *Mov. Disord.* 2007;22(Suppl16):S248.

[104] Chung EJ, Ki CS, Lee WY, Kim IS, Kim JY. Clinical features and gene analysis in Korean patients with early-onset Parkinson disease. *Arch. Neurol.* 2006 Aug;63(8):1170-4.

[105] Tan EK, Chai A, Teo YY, Zhao Y, Tan C, Shen H, et al. Alpha-synuclein haplotypes implicated in risk of Parkinson's disease. *Neurology.* 2004 Jan 13;62(1):128-31.

[106] Tiqva P, Hassin-Baer S, Gan R. Clinical characteristics of Parkinson's disease among Jewish ethnic groups in Isreal. *Neurology.* 2007;68(12):A257.

[107] Fearnley JM, Lees AJ. Ageing and Parkinson's disease: substantia nigra regional selectivity. *Brain.* 1991 Oct;114 (Pt 5):2283-301.

[108] Bennett DA, Beckett LA, Murray AM, Shannon KM, Goetz CG, Pilgrim DM, et al. Prevalence of parkinsonian signs and associated mortality in a community population of older people. *N. Engl. J. Med.* 1996 Jan 11;334(2):71-6.

[109] Ross OA, Toft M, Whittle AJ, Johnson JL, Papapetropoulos S, Mash DC, et al. Lrrk2 and Lewy body disease. *Ann. Neurol.* 2006 Feb;59(2):388-93.

[110] Huang YW, Jeng JS, Tsai CF, Chen LL, Wu RM. Transcranial imaging of substantia nigra hyperechogenicity in a Taiwanese cohort of Parkinson's disease. *Mov. Disord.* 2007 Mar 15;22(4):550-5.

[111] Chu JY, Huang W, Kuang SQ, Wang JM, Xu JJ, Chu ZT, et al. Genetic relationship of populations in China. *Proc. Natl. Acad. Sci. USA.* 1998 Sep 29;95(20):11763-8.

[112] Basu A, Mukherjee N, Roy S, Sengupta S, Banerjee S, Chakraborty M, et al. Ethnic India: a genomic view, with special reference to peopling and structure. *Genome Res.* 2003 Oct;13(10):2277-90.

[113] Majumder PP. Ethnic populations of India as seen from an evolutionary perspective. *J. Biosci.* 2001 Nov;26(4 Suppl):533-45.

[114] Sahoo S, Kashyap VK. Phylogeography of mitochondrial DNA and Y-chromosome haplogroups reveal asymmetric gene flow in populations of Eastern India. *Am. J. Phys. Anthropol.* 2006 Sep;131(1):84-97.

[115] Wood-Kaczmar A, Gandhi S, Wood NW. Understanding the molecular causes of Parkinson's disease. *Trends Mol. Med.* 2006 Nov;12(11):521-8.

[116] Kubo S, Hattori N, Mizuno Y. Recessive Parkinson's disease. *Mov. Disord.* 2006 Jul;21(7):885-93.

[117] Olanow CW, McNaught KS. Ubiquitin-proteasome system and Parkinson's disease. *Mov. Disord.* 2006 Nov;21(11):1806-23.

[118] Tan EK, Chan DK, Ng PW, Woo J, Teo YY, Tang K, et al. Effect of MDR1 haplotype on risk of Parkinson disease. *Arch. Neurol.* 2005 Mar;62(3):460-4.

[119] Tang G, Xie H, Xu L, Hao Y, Lin D, Ren D. Genetic study of apolipoprotein E gene, alpha-1 antichymotrypsin gene in sporadic Parkinson disease. *Am. J. Med. Genet.* 2002 May 8;114(4):446-9.

[120] Benmoyal-Segal L, Soreq H. Gene-environment interactions in sporadic Parkinson's disease. *J. Neurochem.* 2006 Jun;97(6):1740-55.

[121] Pchelina SN, Yakimovskii AF, Ivanova ON, Emelianov AK, Zakharchuk AH, Schwarzman AL. G2019S LRRK2 mutation in familial and sporadic Parkinson's disease in Russia. *Mov. Disord.* 2006 Dec;21(12):2234-6.

[122] Clark LN, Nicolai A, Afridi S, Harris J, Mejia-Santana H, Strug L, et al. Pilot association study of the beta-glucocerebrosidase N370S allele and Parkinson's disease in subjects of Jewish ethnicity. *Mov. Disord.* 2005 Jan;20(1):100-3.

[123] Djaldetti R, Yust-Katz S, Kolianov V, Melamed E, Dabby R. The effect of duloxetine on primary pain symptoms in Parkinson disease. *Clin. Neuropharmacol.* 2007 Jul-Aug;30(4):201-5.

[124] Punia S, Behari M, Govindappa ST, Swaminath PV, Jayaram S, Goyal V, et al. Absence/rarity of commonly reported LRRK2 mutations in Indian Parkinson's disease patients. *Neurosci. Lett.* 2006 Dec 1;409(2):83-8.

[125] Lu CS, Simons EJ, Wu-Chou YH, Fonzo AD, Chang HC, Chen RS, et al. The LRRK2 I2012T, G2019S, and I2020T mutations are rare in Taiwanese patients with sporadic Parkinson's disease. *Parkinsonism Relat. Disord.* 2005 Dec;11(8):521-2.

[126] Fung HC, Chen CM, Hardy J, Hernandez D, Singleton A, Wu YR. Lack of G2019S LRRK2 mutation in a cohort of Taiwanese with sporadic Parkinson's disease. *Mov. Disord.* 2006 Jun;21(6):880-1.

[127] Fung HC, Chen CM, Hardy J, Singleton AB, Lee-Chen GJ, Wu YR. Analysis of the PINK1 gene in a cohort of patients with sporadic early-onset parkinsonism in Taiwan. *Neurosci. Lett.* 2006 Feb 6;394(1):33-6.

[128] Tan E, Zhao Y, Tan L. LRRK Glu2385Arg in Parkinson's disease patients of non-Chinese Asian ethnicity. *Mov. Disord.* 2007;22(Suppl 16):S131.

[129] Cho J, Kim H, Park S, Jeon B. The G2019S LRRK2 mutation is rare in Korean patients with Parkinson's Disease. *Mov. Disord.* 2006;21(Suppl 15):S402.

[130] Berg D, Niwar M, Maass S, Zimprich A, Moller JC, Wuellner U, et al. Alpha-synuclein and Parkinson's disease: implications from the screening of more than 1,900 patients. *Mov. Disord.* 2005 Sep;20(9):1191-4.

[131] Bialecka M, Hui S, Klodowska-Duda G, Opala G, Tan EK, Drozdzik M. Analysis of LRRK 2 G 2019 S and I 2020 T mutations in Parkinson's disease. *Neurosci. Lett.* 2005 Dec 16;390(1):1-3.

[132] Di Fonzo A, Wu-Chou YH, Lu CS, van Doeselaar M, Simons EJ, Rohe CF, et al. A common missense variant in the LRRK2 gene, Gly2385Arg, associated with Parkinson's disease risk in Taiwan. *Neurogenetics.* 2006 Jul;7(3):133-8.

[133] Tan EK. Identification of a common genetic risk variant (LRRK2 Gly2385Arg) in Parkinson's disease. *Ann. Acad. Med. Singapore.* 2006 Nov;35(11):840-2.

[134] Paisan-Ruiz C, Lang AE, Kawarai T, Sato C, Salehi-Rad S, Fisman GK, et al. LRRK2 gene in Parkinson disease: mutation analysis and case control association study. *Neurology.* 2005 Sep 13;65(5):696-700.

[135] Hardy J, Orr H. The genetics of neurodegenerative diseases. *J. Neurochem.* 2006 Jun;97(6):1690-9.

[136] Kobayashi H, Ujike H, Hasegawa J, Yamamoto M, Kanzaki A, Sora I. Identification of a risk haplotype of the alpha-synuclein gene in Japanese with sporadic Parkinson's disease. *Mov. Disord.* 2006 Dec;21(12):2157-64.

[137] Kim Y, Woo M, Choi J. Analysis of PARKIN, PINK1 and DJ-1 mutation in an early onset Parkinson's Disease Korean cohort. *Mov. Disord.* 2006;21(Suppl 15):S406.

[138] Kim Y, Woo M, Choi J. Analysis of PARK gene mutations in an early onset Parkinson's disease Korean cohort. *Neurology.* 2007;68(12 (Suppl 1)):A325.

[139] Kitada T, Asakawa S, Hattori N, Matsumine H, Yamamura Y, Minoshima S, et al. Mutations in the parkin gene cause autosomal recessive juvenile parkinsonism. *Nature.* 1998 Apr 9;392(6676):605-8.

[140] Foroud T, Uniacke SK, Liu L, Pankratz N, Rudolph A, Halter C, et al. Heterozygosity for a mutation in the parkin gene leads to later onset Parkinson disease. *Neurology.* 2003 Mar 11;60(5):796-801.

[141] Hattori N, Kitada T, Matsumine H, Asakawa S, Yamamura Y, Yoshino H, et al. Molecular genetic analysis of a novel Parkin gene in Japanese families with autosomal recessive juvenile parkinsonism: evidence for variable homozygous deletions in the Parkin gene in affected individuals. *Ann. Neurol.* 1998 Dec;44(6):935-41.

[142] Madegowda RH, Kishore A, Anand A. Mutational screening of the parkin gene among South Indians with early onset Parkinson's disease. *J. Neurol. Neurosurg. Psychiatry.* 2005 Nov;76(11):1588-90.

[143] Biswas A, Gupta A, Naiya T, Das G, Neogi R, Datta S, et al. Molecular pathogenesis of Parkinson's disease: identification of mutations in the Parkin gene in Indian patients. *Parkinsonism Relat. Disord.* 2006 Oct;12(7):420-6.

[144] Wang M, Hattori N, Matsumine H, Kobayashi T, Yoshino H, Morioka A, et al. Polymorphism in the parkin gene in sporadic Parkinson's disease. *Ann. Neurol.* 1999 May;45(5):655-8.

[145] Satoh J, Kuroda Y. Association of codon 167 Ser/Asn heterozygosity in the parkin gene with sporadic Parkinson's disease. *Neuroreport.* 1999 Sep 9;10(13):2735-9.

[146] Li X, Kitami T, Wang M, Mizuno Y, Hattori N. Geographic and ethnic differences in frequencies of two polymorphisms (D/N394 and L/I272) of the parkin gene in sporadic Parkinson's disease. *Parkinsonism Relat. Disord.* 2005 Dec;11(8):485-91.

[147] Hatano Y, Li Y, Sato K, Asakawa S, Yamamura Y, Tomiyama H, et al. Novel PINK1 mutations in early-onset parkinsonism. *Ann. Neurol.* 2004 Sep;56(3):424-7.

[148] Klein C, Schlossmacher MG. The genetics of Parkinson disease: Implications for neurological care. *Nat. Clin. Pract. Neurol.* 2006 Mar;2(3):136-46.

[149] Rogaeva E, Johnson J, Lang AE, Gulick C, Gwinn-Hardy K, Kawarai T, et al. Analysis of the PINK1 gene in a large cohort of cases with Parkinson disease. *Arch. Neurol.* 2004 Dec;61(12):1898-904.

[150] Healy DG, Abou-Sleiman PM, Gibson JM, Ross OA, Jain S, Gandhi S, et al. PINK1 (PARK6) associated Parkinson disease in Ireland. *Neurology.* 2004 Oct 26;63(8):1486-8.

[151] Valente EM, Salvi S, Ialongo T, Marongiu R, Elia AE, Caputo V, et al. PINK1 mutations are associated with sporadic early-onset parkinsonism. *Ann. Neurol.* 2004 Sep;56(3):336-41.

[152] Rohe CF, Montagna P, Breedveld G, Cortelli P, Oostra BA, Bonifati V. Homozygous PINK1 C-terminus mutation causing early-onset parkinsonism. *Ann. Neurol.* 2004 Sep;56(3):427-31.

[153] Lockhart PJ, Bounds R, Hulihan M, Kachergus J, Lincoln S, Lin CH, et al. Lack of mutations in DJ-1 in a cohort of Taiwanese ethnic Chinese with early-onset parkinsonism. *Mov. Disord.* 2004 Sep;19(9):1065-9.

[154] Encyclopedia Britannica; 2007.

[155] Europe: Internet World Stats. [cited May 2, 2007]; Available from: http://en.wikipedia.org/wiki/Europe

[156] de Lau LM, Breteler MM. Epidemiology of Parkinson's disease. *Lancet Neurol.* 2006 Jun;5(6):525-35.

[157] Chalmanov VN. Epidemiological studies of parkinsonism in Sofia. *Neuroepidemiology.* 1986;5(3):171-7.

[158] Milanov I, Kmetska K, Karakolev B, Nedialkov E. Prevalence of Parkinson's disease in Bulgaria. *Neuroepidemiology.* 2001 Aug;20(3):212-4.

[159] Milanov I, Kmetski TS, Lyons KE, Koller WC. Prevalence of Parkinson's disease in Bulgarian Gypsies. *Neuroepidemiology.* 2000 Jul-Aug;19(4):206-9.

[160] The World Factbook. In: *Agency CI,* editor.: Washington, DC.; 2007.

[161] Wermuth L, Joensen P, Bunger N, Jeune B. High prevalence of Parkinson's disease in the Faroe Islands. *Neurology.* 1997 Aug;49(2):426-32.

[162] Wermuth L, Pakkenberg H, Jeune B. High age-adjusted prevalence of Parkinson's disease among Inuits in Greenland. *Neurology.* 2002 May 14;58(9):1422-5.

[163] Wermuth L, von Weitzel-Mudersbach P, Jeune B. A two-fold difference in the age-adjusted prevalences of Parkinson's disease between the island of Als and the Faroe Islands. *Eur. J. Neurol.* 2000 Nov;7(6):655-60.

[164] Svenson LW, Platt GH, Woodhead SE. Geographic variations in the prevalence rates of Parkinson's disease in Alberta. *Can. J. Neurol. Sci.* 1993 Nov;20(4):307-11.

[165] INSEE. [cited October 12, 2007]; Available from: http://www.insee.fr/en/home/home_page.asp

[166] Munoz M, Boutros-Toni F, Preux PM, Chartier JP, Ndzanga E, Boa F, et al. Prevalence of neurological disorders in Haute-Vienne department (Limousin region-France). *Neuroepidemiology.* 1995;14(4):193-8.

[167] Trenkwalder C, Schwarz J, Gebhard J, Ruland D, Trenkwalder P, Hense HW, et al. Starnberg trial on epidemiology of Parkinsonism and hypertension in the elderly. Prevalence of Parkinson's disease and related disorders assessed by a door-to-door survey of inhabitants older than 65 years. *Arch. Neurol.* 1995 Oct;52(10):1017-22.

[168] Vieregge P, Kleinhenz J, Fassl H, Jorg J, Kompf D. Epidemiology and out-patient care in Parkinson's disease--results from a pilot-study in northern Germany (Schleswig-Holstein). *J. Neural. Transm Suppl.* 1991;33:115-8.

[169] Columbia Encyclopedia; 2007.

[170] Gudmundsson KR. A clinical survey of parkinsonism in Iceland. *Acta Neurol. Scand.* 1967;43:Suppl 33:1-61.

[171] van de Vijver DA, Stricker BH, Breteler MM, Roos RA, Porsius AJ, de Boer A. Evaluation of antiparkinsonian drugs in pharmacy records as a marker for Parkinson's disease. *Pharm. World Sci.* 2001 Aug;23(4):148-52.

[172] de Rijk MC, Tzourio C, Breteler MM, Dartigues JF, Amaducci L, Lopez-Pousa S, et al. Prevalence of parkinsonism and Parkinson's disease in Europe: the

EUROPARKINSON Collaborative Study. European Community Concerted Action on the Epidemiology of Parkinson's disease. *J. Neurol. Neurosurg. Psychiatry.* 1997 Jan;62(1):10-5.

[173] Bekkelund SI, Selseth B, Mellgren SI. [Parkinson's disease in a population group in northern Norway]. *Tidsskr Nor. Laegeforen.* 1989 Feb 20;109(5):561-3.

[174] Wender M, Pruchnik D, Kowal P, Florczak J, Zalejski M. [Epidemiology of Parkinson disease in the Pozna'n province]. *Przegl. Epidemiol.* 1989;43(2):150-5.

[175] Dias JA, Felgueiras MM, Sanchez JP, Goncalves JM, Falcao JM, Pimenta ZP. The prevalence of Parkinson's disease in Portugal. A population approach. *Eur. J. Epidemiol.* 1994 Dec;10(6):763-7.

[176] Sutcliffe RL, Prior R, Mawby B, McQuillan WJ. Parkinson's disease in the district of the Northampton Health Authority, United Kingdom. A study of prevalence and disability. *Acta Neurol. Scand.* 1985 Oct;72(4):363-79.

[177] Mutch WJ, Dingwall-Fordyce I, Downie AW, Paterson JG, Roy SK. Parkinson's disease in a Scottish city. *Br. Med. J. (Clin. Res. Ed).* 1986 Feb 22;292(6519):534-6.

[178] Hobson P, Gallacher J, Meara J. Cross-sectional survey of Parkinson's disease and parkinsonism in a rural area of the United Kingdom. *Mov. Disord.* 2005 Aug;20(8):995-8.

[179] Schrag A, Ben-Shlomo Y, Quinn NP. Cross sectional prevalence survey of idiopathic Parkinson's disease and Parkinsonism in London. *Bmj.* 2000 Jul 1;321(7252):21-2.

[180] Wermuth L, Bunger N, von Weitzel-Mudersback P, Pakkenberg H, Jeune B. Clinical characteristics of Parkinson's disease among Inuit in Greenland and inhabitants of the Faroe Islands and Als (Denmark). *Mov. Disord.* 2004 Jul;19(7):821-4.

[181] Schapira AH, Cooper JM, Dexter D, Clark JB, Jenner P, Marsden CD. Mitochondrial complex I deficiency in Parkinson's disease. *J. Neurochem.* 1990 Mar;54(3):823-7.

[182] Hattori N. [Etiology and pathogenesis of Parkinson's disease: from mitochondrial dysfunctions to familial Parkinson's disease]. Rinsho Shinkeigaku. 2004 Apr-May;44(4-5):241-62.

[183] Lesage S, Janin S, Lohmann E, Leutenegger AL, Leclere L, Viallet F, et al. LRRK2 exon 41 mutations in sporadic Parkinson disease in Europeans. *Arch. Neurol.* 2007 Mar;64(3):425-30.

[184] Gaig C, Ezquerra M, Marti MJ, Munoz E, Valldeoriola F, Tolosa E. LRRK2 mutations in Spanish patients with Parkinson disease: frequency, clinical features, and incomplete penetrance. *Arch. Neurol.* 2006 Mar;63(3):377-82.

[185] Ferreira JJ, Guedes LC, Rosa MM, Coelho M, van Doeselaar M, Schweiger D, et al. High prevalence of LRRK2 mutations in familial and sporadic Parkinson's disease in Portugal. *Mov. Disord.* 2007 Jun 15;22(8):1194-201.

[186] Goldwurm S, Zini M, Di Fonzo A, De Gaspari D, Siri C, Simons EJ, et al. LRRK2 G2019S mutation and Parkinson's disease: a clinical, neuropsychological and neuropsychiatric study in a large Italian sample. *Parkinsonism Relat. Disord.* 2006 Oct;12(7):410-9.

[187] Belin A, Westerlund M, Sydow O. LRRK2 mutations in a Swedish Parkinson's cohort and health nonagenarians. *Mov. Disord.* 2006;21(10):1731-4.

[188] Infante J, Rodriguez E, Combarros O, Mateo I, Fontalba A, Pascual J, et al. LRRK2 G2019S is a common mutation in Spanish patients with late-onset Parkinson's disease. *Neurosci. Lett.* 2006 Mar 13;395(3):224-6.

[189] Bras JM, Guerreiro RJ, Ribeiro MH, Januario C, Morgadinho A, Oliveira CR, et al. G2019S dardarin substitution is a common cause of Parkinson's disease in a Portuguese cohort. *Mov. Disord.* 2005 Dec;20(12):1653-5.

[190] Encyclopedia O. [cited October 12, 2007]; Available from: http://encyclopedia. jrank.org/I27_INV/IBERIANS_Iberi_I_3r7Aes_.html

[191] Masso J, Paisan-Ruiz C, Simon J. Parkinson's disease related to the Basque dardarin mutation. *Neurology.* 2005;2005(64 (6)):A148.

[192] Simon-Sanchez J, Marti-Masso JF, Sanchez-Mut JV, Paisan-Ruiz C, Martinez-Gil A, Ruiz-Martinez J, et al. Parkinson's disease due to the R1441G mutation in Dardarin: a founder effect in the Basques. *Mov. Disord.* 2006 Nov;21(11):1954-9.

[193] Mata IF, Taylor JP, Kachergus J, Hulihan M, Huerta C, Lahoz C, et al. LRRK2 R1441G in Spanish patients with Parkinson's disease. *Neurosci. Lett.* 2005 Jul 15;382(3):309-11.

[194] Giordana MT, D'Agostino C, Albani G, Mauro A, Di Fonzo A, Antonini A, et al. Neuropathology of Parkinson's disease associated with the LRRK2 Ile1371Val mutation. *Mov. Disord.* 2007 Jan 15;22(2):275-8.

[195] McInerney-Leo A, Hadley DW, Gwinn-Hardy K, Hardy J. Genetic testing in Parkinson's disease. *Mov. Disord.* 2005 Jan;20(1):1-10.

[196] Klein C, Lohmann-Hedrich K, Rogaeva E, Schlossmacher MG, Lang AE. Deciphering the role of heterozygous mutations in genes associated with parkinsonism. *Lancet Neurol.* 2007 Jul;6(7):652-62.

[197] Zarranz JJ, Alegre J, Gomez-Esteban JC, Lezcano E, Ros R, Ampuero I, et al. The new mutation, E46K, of alpha-synuclein causes Parkinson and Lewy body dementia. Ann Neurol. 2004 Feb;55(2):164-73.

[198] Hedrich K, Eskelson C, Wilmot B, Marder K, Harris J, Garrels J, et al. Distribution, type, and origin of Parkin mutations: review and case studies. *Mov. Disord.* 2004 Oct;19(10):1146-57.

[199] Bonifati V, Rizzu P, van Baren MJ, Schaap O, Breedveld GJ, Krieger E, et al. Mutations in the DJ-1 gene associated with autosomal recessive early-onset parkinsonism. *Science.* 2003 Jan 10;299(5604):256-9.

[200] Budget UOoMa. Revisions of the standards for the classification of federal data on race and ethnicity. 1997 [cited November 29, 2003]; Available from: http://www.white house.gov/omb/redreg/obbdir15.html

[201] Sorensen A, Wood B, Prince E. Race and Ethnicity: Developing a common language for public health surveillence in Hawaii. *California Journal for Health Promotion.* 2003;Special Issue 1:91-104.

[202] Zhang ZX, Anderson DW, Huang JB, Li H, Hong X, Wei J, et al. Prevalence of Parkinson's disease and related disorders in the elderly population of greater Beijing, China. *Mov. Disord.* 2003 Jul;18(7):764-72.

[203] Bergmann K, Rodgers J, Salak V. Diversity in Parkinson's disease among elder South Carolinians. *Mov. Disord.* 2007;22(Suppl 16):S172.

[204] Schoenberg BS, Anderson DW, Haerer AF. Prevalence of Parkinson's disease in the biracial population of Copiah County, Mississippi. *Neurology*. 1985 Jun;35(6):841-5.

[205] Hirtz D, Thurman DJ, Gwinn-Hardy K, Mohamed M, Chaudhuri AR, Zalutsky R. How common are the "common" neurologic disorders? *Neurology*. 2007 Jan 30;68(5):326-37.

[206] Mayeux R, Marder K, Cote LJ, Denaro J, Hemenegildo N, Mejia H, et al. The frequency of idiopathic Parkinson's disease by age, ethnic group, and sex in northern Manhattan, 1988-1993. *Am. J. Epidemiol.* 1995 Oct 15;142(8):820-7.

[207] Racette B, Good L, Kissel A. A population-based study of parkinsonism in an Amish community. *Neurology*. 2006;66(5 (Suppl2)):A383.

[208] Melcon MO, Anderson DW, Vergara RH, Rocca WA. Prevalence of Parkinson's disease in Junin, Buenos Aires Province, Argentina. *Mov. Disord.* 1997 Mar;12(2):197-205.

[209] Nicoletti A, Sofia V, Bartoloni A, Bartalesi F, Gamboa Barahon H, Giuffrida S, et al. Prevalence of Parkinson's disease: a door-to-door survey in rural Bolivia. *Parkinsonism Relat. Disord.* 2003 Oct;10(1):19-21.

[210] Barbosa MT, Caramelli P, Maia DP, Cunningham MC, Guerra HL, Lima-Costa MF, et al. Parkinsonism and Parkinson's disease in the elderly: a community-based survey in Brazil (the Bambui study). *Mov. Disord.* 2006 Jun;21(6):800-8.

[211] Sanchez JL, Buritica O, Pineda D, Uribe CS, Palacio LG. Prevalence of Parkinson's disease and parkinsonism in a Colombian population using the capture-recapture method. *Int. J. Neurosci.* 2004 Feb;114(2):175-82.

[212] Ketzoian C, Chuza C. Estudio piloto de prevalencia da las principales enfermedades neurologicas en una poblacion semirural del Uraguay. *Proc. 5th Panamerican symposium of Neuroepidemiology;* 1991; Montevideo; 1991. p. 214.

[213] Kang GA, Bronstein JM, Masterman DL, Redelings M, Crum JA, Ritz B. Clinical characteristics in early Parkinson's disease in a central California population-based study. *Mov. Disord.* 2005 Sep;20(9):1133-42.

[214] Swarztrauber K, Anau J, Peters D. Identifying and distinguishing cases of parkinsonism and Parkinson's disease using ICD-9 CM codes and pharmacy data. *Mov. Disord.* 2005 Aug;20(8):964-70.

[215] Nichols W, Pauciulo M, Elsaesser V. Screening for known LRRK2 mutations in familial Parkinson's disease. *Mov. Disord.* 2006;21(Suppl 13):S57.

[216] Pankratz N, Byder L, Halter C, Rudolph A, Shults CW, Conneally PM, et al. Presence of an APOE4 allele results in significantly earlier onset of Parkinson's disease and a higher risk with dementia. *Mov. Disord.* 2006 Jan;21(1):45-9.

[217] Camargos S, Cardosa F, Dormas L. Familial parkinsonism and early onset Parkinson's disease: phenotypic and genotypic characertization in a Brazilian populations. *Mov. Disord.* 2007;22(Suppl 16):S136.

[218] Reider CR, Halter CA, Castelluccio PF, Oakes D, Nichols WC, Foroud T. Reliability of reported age at onset for Parkinson's disease. *Mov. Disord.* 2003 Mar;18(3):275-9.

[219] Bertoli-Avella AM, Giroud-Benitez JL, Akyol A, Barbosa E, Schaap O, van der Linde HC, et al. Novel parkin mutations detected in patients with early-onset Parkinson's disease. *Mov. Disord.* 2005 Apr;20(4):424-31.

[220] Huang Y, Halliday GM, Vandebona H, Mellick GD, Mastaglia F, Stevens J, et al. Prevalence and clinical features of common LRRK2 mutations in Australians with Parkinson's disease. *Mov. Disord.* 2007 May 15;22(7):982-9.

[221] Kasaten M, Pramstaller P, Koenig I. Substantia nigra hyperechogenicity correlates with clinical and genetic status. *Mov. Disord.* 2005;20(Suppl 10):S85.

[222] Di Fonzo A, Chien HF, Socal M, Giraudo S, Tassorelli C, Iliceto G, et al. ATP13A2 missense mutations in juvenile parkinsonism and young onset Parkinson disease. *Neurology.* 2007 May 8;68(19):1557-62.

[223] Najim al-Din AS, Wriekat A, Mubaidin A, Dasouki M, Hiari M. Pallido-pyramidal degeneration, supranuclear upgaze paresis and dementia: Kufor-Rakeb syndrome. *Acta Neurol. Scand.* 1994 May;89(5):347-52.

[224] Lees AJ, Singleton AB. Clinical heterogeneity of ATP13A2 linked disease (Kufor-Rakeb) justifies a PARK designation. *Neurology.* 2007 May 8;68(19):1553-4.

[225] Jenkins AC. Epidemiology of parkinsonism in Victoria. *Med. J. Aust.* 1966 Sep 10;2(11):496-502.

[226] McCann SJ, LeCouteur DG, Green AC, Brayne C, Johnson AG, Chan D, et al. The epidemiology of Parkinson's disease in an Australian population. *Neuroepidemiology.* 1998;17(6):310-7.

[227] Chan DK, Cordato D, Karr M, Ong B, Lei H, Liu J, et al. Prevalence of Parkinson's disease in Sydney. *Acta Neurol. Scand.* 2005 Jan;111(1):7-11.

[228] Chan DK, Dunne M, Wong A, Hu E, Hung WT, Beran RG. Pilot study of prevalence of Parkinson's disease in Australia. *Neuroepidemiology.* 2001 May;20(2):112-7.

[229] Mehta P, Kifley A, Wang J. Populations prevalence and incidnece of Parkinson's disease in an Australian community. *Internal. Med. J.* 2007;1:1-3.

[230] Mellick GD, Maraganore DM, Silburn PA. Australian data and meta-analysis lend support for alpha-synuclein (NACP-Rep1) as a risk factor for Parkinson's disease. *Neurosci. Lett.* 2005 Feb 28;375(2):112-6.

[231] Sutherland G, Mellick G, Sue C, Chan DK, Rowe D, Silburn P, et al. A functional polymorphism in the parkin gene promoter affects the age of onset of Parkinson's disease. *Neurosci. Lett.* 2007 Mar 6;414(2):170-3.

[232] Buchanan DD, Silburn PA, Chalk JB, Le Couteur DG, Mellick GD. The Cys282Tyr polymorphism in the HFE gene in Australian Parkinson's disease patients. *Neurosci. Lett.* 2002 Jul 19;327(2):91-4.

[233] Richards M, Chaudhuri KR. Parkinson's disease in populations of African origin: a review. *Neuroepidemiology.* 1996;15(4):214-21.

[234] Osuntokun BO, Adeuja AO, Schoenberg BS, Bademosi O, Nottidge VA, Olumide AO, et al. Neurological disorders in Nigerian Africans: a community-based study. *Acta Neurol. Scand.* 1987 Jan;75(1):13-21.

[235] Ashok PP, Radhakrishnan K, Sridharan R, Mousa ME. Epidemiology of Parkinson's disease in Benghazi, North-East Libya. *Clin. Neurol. Neurosurg.* 1986;88(2):109-13.

[236] Attia Romdhane N, Ben Hamida M, Mrabet A, Larnaout A, Samoud S, Ben Hamda A, et al. Prevalence study of neurologic disorders in Kelibia (Tunisia). *Neuroepidemiology.* 1993;12(5):285-99.

[237] Tekle-Haimanot R, Abebe M, Gebre-Mariam A, Forsgren L, Heijbel J, Holmgren G, et al. Community-based study of neurological disorders in rural central Ethiopia. *Neuroepidemiology*. 1990;9(5):263-77.

[238] Balogou AA, Doh A, Grunitzky KE. [Neurological disorders and endemic goiter: comparative analysis of 2 provinces in Togo]. *Bull. Soc. Pathol. Exot.* 2001 Dec;94(5):406-10.

[239] Haddock D. Neurological disorders in Ghana. In: Spillane J, editor. *Tropical Neurology*. London: Oxford University Press; 1973. p. 143-60.

[240] Harries J. Neurological disorders in Kenya. In: Spillane J, editor. *Tropical Neurology*. London: Oxford University Press; 1973.

[241] Rahman I. Neurological disorders in Rhodesia. In: Spillane J, editor. *Tropical Neurology*. London: Oxford University Press; 1973. p. 237-46.

[242] Li SC, Schoenberg BS, Wang CC, Cheng XM, Rui DY, Bolis CL, et al. A prevalence survey of Parkinson's disease and other movement disorders in the People's Republic of China. *Arch. Neurol.* 1985 Jul;42(7):655-7.

[243] Wang Y, Shi Y, Wu S. The incidence and prevalence of Parkinson's Diseasein the People's Republic of China. *Proc. Natl. Symp. Neurol. Dis. Aging.* 1990:1.

[244] Zhang L, Nie ZY, Liu Y, Chen W, Xin SM, Sun XD, et al. The prevalence of PD in a nutritionally deficient rural population in China. *Acta Neurol. Scand.* 2005 Jul;112(1):29-35.

[245] Wang SJ, Fuh JL, Teng EL, Liu CY, Lin KP, Chen HM, et al. A door-to-door survey of Parkinson's disease in a Chinese population in Kinmen. *Arch. Neurol.* 1996 Jan;53(1):66-71.

[246] Okada K, Kobayashi S, Tsunematsu T. Prevalence of Parkinson's disease in Izumo City, Japan. *Gerontology.* 1990;36(5-6):340-4.

[247] Muthane U, Jain S, Gururaj G. Hunting genes in Parkinson's disease from the roots. *Med. Hypotheses.* 2001 Jul;57(1):51-5.

[248] Ragothaman M, Murgod U, Gopalakrishna G. High occurrence and low recognician of Parkinson's Disease in elderly homes in Bangalore, India. *Mov. Disord.* 2006;21(Suppl 15):S495.

[249] Bademomosi O, Al-Rnjeh S, Ismail H. *Prevalence of PD in an Arab community.* Congres de Neurologic Tropicale: Tropicale Presse; 1991. p. 27.

[250] Herishanu YO, Goldsmith JR, Abarbanel JM, Weinbaum Z. Clustering of Parkinson's disease in southern Israel. *Can. J. Neurol. Sci.* 1989 Nov;16(4):402-5.

[251] Shanker V, Halipern S, Ozelius L. Clinical expression of the LRRK2 G2019s mutation in Ashkenazi Jews. *Neurology.* 2007;68(12(Suppl1)):A324.

[252] Orr-Urtreger A, Shifrin C, Rozovski U. The frequency of the LRRK2 G2019S mutation in Ashkenazi and non-Ashkenazi jews with Parkinson's disease in Isreal. *Mov. Disord.* 2007;22(Suppl16):S135.

[253] Tan EK, Shen H, Tan LC, Farrer M, Yew K, Chua E, et al. The G2019S LRRK2 mutation is uncommon in an Asian cohort of Parkinson's disease patients. *Neurosci. Lett.* 2005 Aug 26;384(3):327-9.

[254] Tan EK, Skipper L, Tan L, Liu JJ. LRRK2 G2019S founder haplotype in the Chinese population. *Mov. Disord.* 2007 Jan;22(1):105-7.

[255] Bagyeva G, Illarioshkin S, Slominsky P. Frequency of the LRRK2 G2019S mutation in patients with Parkinson's disease in a Russian populations. *Mov. Disord.* 2006;21(Suppl 15):S407.

[256] Skipper L, Shen H, Chua E, Bonnard C, Kolatkar P, Tan LC, et al. Analysis of LRRK2 functional domains in nondominant Parkinson disease. *Neurology.* 2005 Oct 25;65(8):1319-21.

[257] Zabetian C, Ujike H, Morino H. Comprehensive analysis of the LRRK2 gene in Japanese patients with Parkinson's disease. *Neurology.* 2007;68 12 (Suppl1)(A305).

[258] Ahn T, Cho J, Park S. Alpha-synuclein gene duplication in a Korean patient with Parkinson's disease. *Mov. Disord.* 2006;21(Suppl 15):S469.

[259] Shyu WC, Lin SZ, Chiang MF, Pang CY, Chen SY, Hsin YL, et al. Early-onset Parkinson's disease in a Chinese population: 99mTc-TRODAT-1 SPECT, Parkin gene analysis and clinical study. *Parkinsonism. Relat. Disord.* 2005 May;11(3):173-80.

[260] Tan EK, Yew K, Chua E, Puvan K, Shen H, Lee E, et al. PINK1 mutations in sporadic early-onset Parkinson's disease. *Mov. Disord.* 2006 Jun;21(6):789-93.

[261] Tan EK, Tan C, Zhao Y, Yew K, Shen H, Chandran VR, et al. Genetic analysis of DJ-1 in a cohort Parkinson's disease patients of different ethnicity. *Neurosci. Lett.* 2004 Aug 26;367(1):109-12.

[262] Dupont E. *Epidemiology of Parkinsonism: The Parkinson Investigation.* In: Worm-Petersen J, Bottcher L, editors. Symposium on Parkinsonism; 1977; Copenhagen; 1977. p. 65-7.

[263] Marttila RJ, Rinne UK. Epidemiology of Parkinson's disease in Finland. *Acta Neurol. Scand.* 1976 Feb;53(2):81-102.

[264] Fender P, Paita M, Ganay D, Benech JM. [Prevalence of thirty long term disorders for French health insurance members in 1994]. *Rev. Epidemiol. Sante Publique.* 1997 Dec;45(6):454-64.

[265] Rosati G, Granieri E, Pinna L, Aiello I, Tola R, De Bastiani P, et al. The risk of Parkinson disease in Mediterranean people. *Neurology.* 1980 Mar;30(3):250-5.

[266] Rocca W, Morgante L, Grigoletto F. Prevalence of Parkinson's disease: A door-to-door survey in two Sicilian communities. *Neurology.* 1990;40(Suppl 1):422.

[267] D'Alessandro R, Gamberini G, Granieri E, Benassi G, Naccarato S, Manzaroli D. Prevalence of Parkinson's disease in the Republic of San Marino. *Neurology.* 1987 Oct;37(10):1679-82.

[268] Casetta I, Granieri E, Govoni V, Tola MR, Paolino E, Monetti VC, et al. Epidemiology of Parkinson's disease in Italy. A descriptive survey in the U.S.L. of Cento, province of Ferrara, Emilia-Romagna. *Acta Neurol.* (Napoli). 1990 Aug;12(4):284-91.

[269] Granieri E, Carreras M, Casetta I, Govoni V, Tola MR, Paolino E, et al. Parkinson's disease in Ferrara, Italy, 1967 through 1987. *Arch. Neurol.* 1991 Aug;48(8):854-7.

[270] Chio A, Magnani C, Schiffer D. Prevalence of Parkinson's disease in Northwestern Italy: comparison of tracer methodology and clinical ascertainment of cases. *Mov. Disord.* 1998 May;13(3):400-5.

[271] Totaro R, Marini C, Pistoia F, Sacco S, Russo T, Carolei A. Prevalence of Parkinson's disease in the L'Aquila district, central Italy. *Acta Neurol. Scand.* 2005 Jul;112(1):24-8.

[272] Artazcoz Sanz MT, Vines Rueda JJ. [The estimation of prevalence of Parkinson disease in Navarra. An epidemiological study of the consumption of anti-parkinsonian drugs]. *Rev. Esp. Salud Publica.* 1995 Nov-Dec;69(6):479-85.

[273] Criado-Alvarez JJ, Romo-Barrientos C, Martinez-Hernandez J, Gonzalez-Solana I. [Use of antiparkinsonian agents in Castilla-La Mancha. Estimate of prevalence of Parkinson disease]. *Rev. Neurol.* 1998 Sep;27(157):405-8.

[274] Errea JM, Ara JR, Aibar C, de Pedro-Cuesta J. Prevalence of Parkinson's disease in lower Aragon, Spain. *Mov. Disord.* 1999 Jul;14(4):596-604.

[275] Martinez-Suarez MM, Blazquez-Menes B. [Estimation of the prevalence of Parkinson's disease in Asturia, Spain. A pharmacoepidemiological study of the consumption of antiparkinson drugs]. *Rev. Neurol.* 2000 Dec 1-15;31(11):1001-6.

[276] Claveria LE, Duarte J, Sevillano MD, Perez-Sempere A, Cabezas C, Rodriguez F, et al. Prevalence of Parkinson's disease in Cantalejo, Spain: a door-to-door survey. *Mov. Disord.* 2002 Mar;17(2):242-9.

[277] Benito-Leon J, Bermejo-Pareja F, Rodriguez J, Molina JA, Gabriel R, Morales JM. Prevalence of PD and other types of parkinsonism in three elderly populations of central Spain. *Mov. Disord.* 2003 Mar;18(3):267-74.

[278] Bergareche A, De La Puente E, Lopez de Munain A, Sarasqueta C, de Arce A, Poza JJ, et al. Prevalence of Parkinson's disease and other types of Parkinsonism. A door-to-door survey in Bidasoa, Spain. *J. Neurol.* 2004 Mar;251(3):340-5.

[279] Seijo-Martinez M, Rio Md, Sobrido-Gomez M. Prevalence of parkinsonism and Parkinson's disease in the elderly population of the Arosa Islands (Spain). *Neurology.* 2007;12(Suppl 1):A224.

[280] de Pedro J. Tracers for paralysis agitans in epidemiological research. V. Prevalence of the disease in Swedish counties. *Neuroepidemiology.* 1986;5(4):207-19.

[281] Fall PA, Axelson O, Fredriksson M, Hansson G, Lindvall B, Olsson JE, et al. Age-standardized incidence and prevalence of Parkinson's disease in a Swedish community. *J. Clin. Epidemiol.* 1996 Jun;49(6):637-41.

[282] Duzcan F, Zencir M, Ozdemir F, Cetin GO, Bagci H, Heutink P, et al. Familial influence on parkinsonism in a rural area of Turkey (Kizilcaboluk-Denizli): a community-based case-control study. *Mov. Disord.* 2003 Jul;18(7):799-804.

[283] Sutcliffe RL, Meara JR. Parkinson's disease epidemiology in the Northampton District, England, 1992. *Acta Neurol. Scand.* 1995 Dec;92(6):443-50.

[284] Marongiu R, Ghezzi D, Ialongo T, Soleti F, Elia A, Cavone S, et al. Frequency and phenotypes of LRRK2 G2019S mutation in Italian patients with Parkinson's disease. *Mov. Disord.* 2006 Aug;21(8):1232-5.

[285] Squillaro T, Cambi F, Ciacci G, Rossi S, Ulivelli M, Malandrini A, et al. Frequency of the LRRK2 G2019S mutation in Italian patients affected by Parkinson's disease. *J. Hum. Genet.* 2007;52(3):201-4.

[286] Cossu G, van Doeselaar M, Deriu M, Melis M, Molari A, Di Fonzo A, et al. LRRK2 mutations and Parkinson's disease in Sardinia--A Mediterranean genetic isolate. *Parkinsonism Relat. Disord.* 2007 Feb;13(1):17-21.

[287] Mir P, Gao L, Diaz F. LRRK2 mutations in patients with Parkinson's disease in southern Spain. *Mov. Disord.* 2007;22(Suppl 16):S129.

[288] Lewthwaite A, Lambert T, Wood N. Screening for LRRK2 mutations in UK familial Parkinson's disease patients. *Mov. Disord.* 2007;22(Suppl 16):S102.

[289] Funalot B, Nichols WC, Perez-Tur J, Mercier G, Lucotte G. Genetic screening for two LRRK2 mutations in French patients with idiopathic Parkinson's disease. *Genet Test.* 2006 Winter;10(4):290-3.

[290] Riviere J, Dupre N, Allard M. LRRK2 is not a significant cause of Parkinson's disease in French-Canadian founder populations. *Neurology.* 2007 A324;2007(68):12 (Suppl1).

[291] Bialecka M, Hui S, Klodowska-Duda G. G2019S and 12020T mutations of LRRK2 genes are rare causes of Parkinson's disease in the Polish populations. *Mov. Disord.* 2006;21(Suppl 13):S56.

[292] Illarioshkin S, Klyushnikov S, Slominsky P. Molecular screening of the LRRK2 and parkin genes in a large cohort of Russian patients with Parkinson's disease. *Mov. Disord.* 2007;22(sUPPL 16):s193.

[293] Aasly JO, Toft M, Fernandez-Mata I, Kachergus J, Hulihan M, White LR, et al. Clinical features of LRRK2-associated Parkinson's disease in central Norway. *Ann. Neurol.* 2005 May;57(5):762-5.

[294] Kachergus J, Mata IF, Hulihan M, Taylor JP, Lincoln S, Aasly J, et al. Identification of a novel LRRK2 mutation linked to autosomal dominant parkinsonism: evidence of a common founder across European populations. *Am. J. Hum. Genet.* 2005 Apr;76(4):672-80.

[295] Xiromerisiou G, Hadjigeorgiou GM, Gourbali V, Johnson J, Papakonstantinou I, Papadimitriou A, et al. Screening for SNCA and LRRK2 mutations in Greek sporadic and autosomal dominant Parkinson's disease: identification of two novel LRRK2 variants. *Eur. J. Neurol.* 2007 Jan;14(1):7-11.

[296] Papapetropoulos S, Adi N, Shehadeh N. Is the G2019S LRRK2 mutation common in all southern European populations? *Mov. Disord.* 2007;22(Suppl 16):S133.

[297] Haubenberger D, Bonelli S, Leitner P. Detection of a novel LRRK2 mutations in an Austrian cohort of patients with Parkinson's disease. 21. 2006;Suppl 15:S408.

[298] Berg D, Schweitzer K, Leitner P, Zimprich A, Lichtner P, Belcredi P, et al. Type and frequency of mutations in the LRRK2 gene in familial and sporadic Parkinson's disease*. *Brain.* 2005 Dec;128(Pt 12):3000-11.

[299] Pirkevi C, Lesage S, Brice A, Basak A. Parkinson's Disease in Turkish patients: Molecular analysis of parkin and LRRK2 genes in familial and isolated cases. *Mov. Disord.* 2007;22(Suppl 16):S135.

[300] Toft M, Mata IF, Ross OA, Kachergus J, Hulihan MM, Haugarvoll K, et al. Pathogenicity of the Lrrk2 R1514Q substitution in Parkinson's disease. *Mov. Disord.* 2007 Feb 15;22(3):389-92.

[301] Karamohamed S, Golbe L, Mark M, Lazzarini A, Suchowersky O, Labelle N. Absence of previously reported variants in the SCNA, NR4A2 and DJ-1 genes in familial Parkinson's Disease. *Mov. Disord.* 2005;9:1188-91.

[302] Snow B, Wiens M, Hertzman C, Calne D. A community survey of Parkinson's disease. *Cmaj.* 1989 Sep 1;141(5):418-22.

[303] Djarmati A, Hedrich K, Svetel M, Lohnau T, Schwinger E, Romac S, et al. Heterozygous PINK1 mutations: a susceptibility factor for Parkinson disease? *Mov. Disord.* 2006 Sep;21(9):1526-30.

[304] Strickland D, Bertoni J. Parinson's prevalence estimated by a state registry. *Mov. Disord.* 2004;18(3):318-23.

[305] Moghal S, Rajput AH, D'Arcy C, Rajput R. Prevalence of movement disorders in elderly community residents. *Neuroepidemiology.* 1994;13(4):175-8.

[306] Guttman M, Slaughter PM, Theriault ME, DeBoer DP, Naylor CD. Burden of parkinsonism: a population-based study. *Mov. Disord.* 2003 Mar;18(3):313-9.

[307] Raggio V, Dieguez E, Aljanati R. Sporadic and familial Parkinson's disease in Uruguay. *Mov. Disord.* 2007;22(Suppl 16):S135.

[308] Giroud Benitez JL, Collado-Mesa F, Esteban EM. [Prevalence of Parkinson disease in an urban area of the Ciudad de La Habana province, Cuba. Door-to-door population study]. *Neurologia.* 2000 Aug-Sep;15(7):269-73.

[309] Zabetian CP, Samii A, Mosley AD, Roberts JW, Leis BC, Yearout D, et al. A clinic-based study of the LRRK2 gene in Parkinson disease yields new mutations. *Neurology.* 2005 Sep 13;65(5):741-4.

[310] Farrer M, Stone J, Mata IF, Lincoln S, Kachergus J, Hulihan M, et al. LRRK2 mutations in Parkinson disease. *Neurology.* 2005 Sep 13;65(5):738-40.

[311] Pankratz N, Pauciulo MW, Elsaesser VE, Marek DK, Halter CA, Rudolph A, et al. Mutations in LRRK2 other than G2019S are rare in a north American-based sample of familial Parkinson's disease. *Mov. Disord.* 2006 Dec;21(12):2257-60.

[312] Kay DM, Zabetian CP, Factor SA, Nutt JG, Samii A, Griffith A, et al. Parkinson's disease and LRRK2: frequency of a common mutation in U.S. movement disorder clinics. *Mov. Disord.* 2006 Apr;21(4):519-23.

[313] Deng H, Le WD, Zhang X, Pan TH, Jankovic J. G309D and W437OPA PINK1 mutations in Caucasian Parkinson's disease patients. *Acta Neurol. Scand.* 2005 Jun;111(6):351-2.

[314] Keen J, Scholz S, Guo Y. Genetic and clinical identification of Parkinson's disease patients with LRRK2 G2019S mutation. *Ann. Neurol.* 2005;57:933-4.

[315] Goldman S, Tanner C, Schuele B. Failure to detect sequence variants associated with monogenic parkinsonism genes in twins. *Neurology.* 2007;68(12 (Suppl1)):A192.

[316] Nichols WC, Uniacke SK, Pankratz N, Reed T, Simon DK, Halter C, et al. Evaluation of the role of Nurr1 in a large sample of familial Parkinson's disease. *Mov. Disord.* 2004 Jun;19(6):649-55.

[317] Grimes DA, Han F, Panisset M, Racacho L, Xiao F, Zou R, et al. Translated mutation in the Nurr1 gene as a cause for Parkinson's disease. *Mov. Disord.* 2006 Jul;21(7):906-9.

[318] Peters CM, Gartner CE, Silburn PA, Mellick GD. Prevalence of Parkinson's disease in metropolitan and rural Queensland: a general practice survey. *J. Clin. Neurosci.* 2006 Apr;13(3):343-8.

[319] Mastaglia F, Huang Y, Halliday G. Novel LRRK2 mutations in the Roc domain in a Western Australian family with autosomal dominant late onset Parkinson's Disease. *Mov. Disord.* 2007;22(Suppl 16):S224.

In: New Research on Parkinson's Disease
Editors: T. F. Hahn, J. Werner

ISBN: 978-1-60456-601-7
© 2008 Nova Science Publishers, Inc.

Chapter IV

Inflammation in Parkinson's Disease

R. Lee Mosley[*], *Eric J. Benner, Irena Kadiu,*
Mark Thomas and Howard E. Gendelman
Center for Neurovirology and Neurodegenerative Disorders, Department of
Pharmacology and Experimental Neuroscience, University of Nebraska Medical Center,
Omaha, NE

1. Introduction

Parkinson's disease (PD) is the most common movement disorder and second, only to Alzheimer's disease as a cause of age-linked neurodegeneration [1-3]. The primary pathological characteristics of PD are the progressive loss of dopaminergic neurons in the substantia nigra pars compacta (SNpc) and reductions in their terminals within the dorsal striatum [4]. These lead to profound and irreversible striatal dopamine loss. Indeed, extrapolated cell modeling data [5] demonstrate that 100–200 SNpc neurons degenerate per day during the course of PD [6]. However, the SNpc is not the sole site for neuronal damage involving, in measure, the locus coeruleus, raphe nuclei, and the nucleus basalis of Meynert. Nonetheless, progressive degeneration of the nigrostriatal pathway is the predominant mediator for clinical manifestations of PD including rigidity, resting tremor, slowness of voluntary movement and postural instability, and in some cases, dementia [2].

In regards to disease epidemiology, the mean age of PD onset is 55. This increases dramatically with time [7]. While the cause of PD is not known, data obtained from familial disease and from animal models of PD support a pathogenic process that is closely linked to mitochondrial dysfunction and oxidative stress. Indeed, oxidative stress is an acknowledged central component of PD pathogenesis [7-9] and is strongly linked to dopaminergic neuronal

* Corresponding author: R. Lee Mosley, PhD Center for Neurovirology and Neurodegenerative Disorders Department of Pharmacology and Experimental Neuroscience 985800 Nebraska Medical Center University of Nebraska Medical Center Omaha, NE 68198-5800 Email: rlmosley@unmc.edu; phone 402-559-2510; fax: 402-559-7495

apoptosis. Moreover, increased risk of localized oxidative damage for dopaminergic neurons is linked to dopamine metabolism itself [8]. With the exception of rare familial forms, the majority of PD cases are sporadic and due, in part, to mitochondrial defects at complex I [7, 10]. Indeed, complex I inhibitors (for example, rotenone) recapitulate many of the pathological features of disease [7]. Moreover, the presence of ubiquitinated and misfolded proteins suggests the dysregulation of protein assembly or defects in protein degradation pathway as a critical part of disease pathogenesis. Misfolding and abnormal degradation of brain proteins are linked to dopaminergic neuronal death [11].

A key player in the pathogenesis of PD is the microglial cell, largely believed to represent the brain's resident macrophage population. Phagocytic function is clearly only one of the roles this cell utilizes to maintain tissue homeostasis. Indeed, macrophages orchestrate other cellular processes, including but not limited to, intracellular killing of pathogenic microbes, antigen presentation, and secretion of biologically active factors, as well as mediation of pathological processes. Underlying such cellular functions is inflammation; the same type that often proves detrimental in localized and systemic diseases, including those of the brain and in PD. Inflammation is the frontline defense of multi-cellular organisms against infection and its absence is incompatible with life. Inflammation enables the host to fend off various disease-causing microbes including bacteria, viruses, and parasites.

However, inflammatory responses can also prove deadly to tissue and to the host. Inflammatory responses are closely linked to a number of degenerative states including, but not limited to, cancer, arthritis, cardiovascular disease, and autoimmune diseases. With regards to the nervous system, recent data suggests that neuroinflammation perpetrated through activation of brain mononuclear phagocytes (MP; perivascular and parenchymal macrophages and microglia), other glial elements including astrocytes and to a lesser degree endothelial cells may act in concert as a central pathway in a diverse set of neurodegenerative diseases (Figure 1). These include PD as well as Alzheimer's and Huntington's diseases (AD and HD), HIV-1-associated dementia (HAD), and more recently, spongiform encephalopathies or prion-mediated neurodegeneration. Central nervous system (CNS) inflammatory infiltrates are complex and multifaceted. The initial responders or the MP cell elements of innate immunity set up a cascade, which later involve the activation and recruitment of the adaptive immune system and ultimately neurodegeneration. Microglia are the primary MPs in the CNS that respond to injury [12] and whose principal function is brain defense. As professional phagocytes, they scavenge microbes, serve as effectors of innate immune responses, and coordinate adaptive immune responses within the CNS. Activated microglia participate in inflammatory processes linked to neurodegeneration by producing neurotoxic factors including quinolinic acid, superoxide anions, matrix metalloproteinases (MMP), nitric oxide, arachidonic acid and its metabolites, chemokines, pro-inflammatory cytokines and excitotoxins including glutamate. On the other hand, neuroprotective functions of microglia have been suggested through their abilities to produce neurotrophins and to eliminate excitotoxins present in the extracellular spaces [13]. In particular, evidence indicates that under certain circumstances microglia may also promote neuronal survival after brain injury [14, 15].

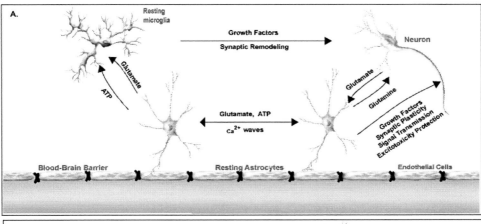

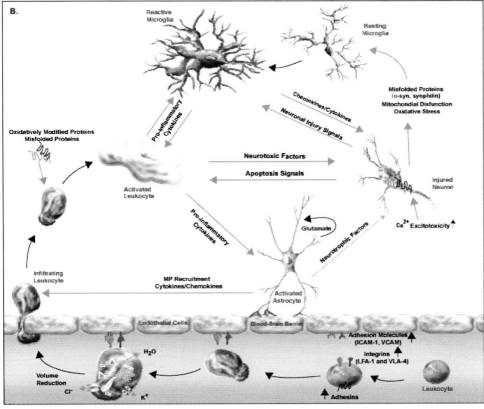

Figure 1. Brain mononuclear phagocytes (MP; perivascular macrophages and microglia) in nervous system during health and disease. (A, top panel) Under steady state conditions, microglia secrete neurotrophic factors and engage other glial elements to promote tissue homeostasis. (B, bottom panel) During disease states (for example, Parkinson's and Alzheimer's disease), MP inflammatory responses damage the BBB, increase oxidative stress and release pro-inflammatory and pro-apoptotic cytokines and other neurotoxic factors that affect neuronal damage or dropout. The damage and stress signals enhance microglial activation, resulting in positive feedback in the release of chemokines and cytotoxic cytokines that cause further ingress of immune cells into the brain and expand inflammatory responses.

Thus, during PD-associated neurodegeneration, a spectrum of environmental cues affects glial function, serving to accelerate the tempo of neurotoxic processes. These lead to neuronal excitotoxicity, synaptic dysfunction, and cell death (apoptosis and/or necrosis). Whether the environmental cues are dysregulated or misfolded proteins or toxic/metabolic events, the inevitable amplification of primary disease processes results in the disruption of CNS homeostasis. In all, whether responding to or directly secreting toxic factors as a result of environmental cues, microglia can affect the evolving stages of neurodegeneration. This review articulates specific features of the inflammation that occur in response to or as part of the PD process.

2. Microglial Cells: Structure and Function in Health and Disease

Microglia are bone marrow-derived myeloid-lineage cells that enter the brain early during embryogenesis and develop in parallel with the maturation of the nervous system. They are the resident phagocytes of the CNS and can react promptly in response to brain insults of various natures, ranging from pathogens to aggregated proteins and to more subtle alterations in their micro-environment such as alterations in ion homeostasis that can affect pathological processes [12]. For these processes, microglia possess macrophage-like functions and remove infected or damaged cells, thus serving as a sensor in the brain. In the normal brain, microglial cells are in a resting state as shown in Figure 1A; their cell bodies barely visible and only few fine ramified processes are detectable. However, in pathological settings (Figure 1B), resting microglial cells quickly proliferate, become hypertrophic, and increase or express *de novo* a large number of marker molecules such as CD11b and major histocompatibility complex (MHC) antigens transforming to macrophage-like cells [12, 16, 17]. Activated microglia, now readily visible, increase their numbers at the affected site and exhibit a "spider-like" or macrophage-like appearance. Ramified microglia change appearance by means of retracted processes and enlarged cell bodies. Within the damaged area, the maximal density of activated microglia is located at the epicenter of the lesion, close to injured cells (e.g., degenerating neurons). Following activation and during tissue regeneration, microglia gradually return to a ramified morphology exhibited prior to injury or insult. While such changes are clearly implicated in neurodegenerative processes of the CNS, the innate immune system has also been tasked with alternative functions. In addition to guarding the nervous system from invading pathogens, this system is involved in many physiological functions such as tissue remodeling during development or after damage [18, 19], transportation of blood lipids [19, 20], and scavenging apoptotic cells [21]. Neuroprotective responses are elicited through elimination of the ongoing infectious agents by innate immune activities and subsequently through adaptive immune functions orchestrated in the CNS by microglia and other antigen presenting cells (see below). All together MP, including macrophages and microglia, are the Dr. Jekyll and Mr. Hyde of the nervous system. In health, they support critical regulatory immune and homeostatic functions, whereas in disease their roles progress from supportive, to reactive, and ultimately to destructive. The functional transformations of brain MP from neurotrophic to neurotoxic phenotypes and the common pathways of MP activation and inflammatory responses in neurodegenerative diseases are believed to underlie the pathogenesis in PD. Indeed, harnessing the protective and nourishing capabilities of brain's MP is believed a key element towards developing novel therapeutic treatments and preventive measures in PD.

3. Microglia and Neuroinflammatory Responses in PD

As noted, the key cell element in neuroinflammatory responses is the brain MP. Supporting this idea, PD is characterized by activation of microglial cells found in and around degenerating neurons [22-26]. Evidence for a neuroinflammatory role in disease onset and progression is significant and profound from several independent lines of investigation [26-31]. *First*, reactive microglia are commonly seen within the SNpc of PD brains investigated at autopsy [22, 25, 26]. A six-fold increase in numbers of reactive microglia has been shown phagocytosing dopaminergic neurons [32] and correlates with the deposition of α-synuclein [22]. Such microglia are reactive and over-express a variety of inflammatory markers including, HLA-DR of the human MHC II complex [22, 26], complement receptor type 3 (CR3, Cd11b/CD18, Mac-1, Mo 1) [17, 33], CD68 (EMB11) [17, 22], CD23 (Fc receptor for IgE) [31], ferritin [33], CD11a (LFA-1) and CD54 (ICAM-1) [34]. These reactive microglia are functionally active and secrete a plethora of proinflammatory cytokines such as interferon-γ (IFN-γ) tumor necrosis factor-α (TNF-α) [30, 31], interleukin 1-β (IL-1β) [31], and upregulate enzymes such as inducible nitric oxide synthase (iNOS) [31, 35], and cyclooxygenase (COX) 1 and 2 [23, 35]. Although the SN is relatively rich in microglia when compared to other brain regions [36], the total number of MHC class II positive microglia are also significantly increased in the putamen, hippocampus, transentorhinal cortex, cingulate cortex and temporal cortex of the PD brain [34]. *Second*, microglia activation is strongly associated with dopaminergic neuronal cell death in PD, suggesting that reactive microglia may be a sensitive biomarker for disease. Indeed, reactive microglia serve as *in vivo* indicators of neuroinflammatory responses and contribute significantly to progressive degenerative processes. This is supported by early-stage PD imaging tests, where PK11195 binding to benzodiazepine receptors present on reactive midbrain microglia inversely correlates with binding of 2-beta-carbomethoxy-3beta-(4-fluorophenyl) tropane (CFT) to the dopamine transporter (DAT) in the putamen as a measure of surviving dopaminergic termini. These observations also correlate with the severity of motor impairment [22]. *Third*, epidemiological data demonstrates that the use of nonsteroidal anti-inflammatory agents decreases the risk of PD [37]. *Fourth*, biochemical and histological evidence for oxidative stress in PD abounds and includes observed increased levels of carbonyl and nitrotyrosine protein modifications, lipid peroxidation, DNA damage, and reduction of glutathione and ferritin [38]. Indeed, nicotinamide adenine dinucleotide phosphate (NADPH) oxidase, a primary producer of reactive oxygen species (ROS), is upregulated in PD and its expression coincides with activated microglia. Postmortem samples of SNpc from sporadic PD patients show elevated levels of the protein gp91^{phox} [39], the main transmembrane component of NADPH-oxidase [40], which colocalizes with microglia.

Likewise, in 1-methyl-4-phenyl-1,2,3,6-tetrahydropyridine (MPTP)-treated mice, large increases in gp91[phox] immunoreactivity also colocalize in the SNpc with activated (Mac-1 immunopositive) microglia, but not with astrocytes or neurons [39]. Thus, microglia in the vicinity of dopaminergic neurons in disease appear to have an upregulated capacity for ROS production, consistent with an activated state leading to a continuous cycle of neuronal injury and neuroimmune activation. *Fifth*, a robust microglial response occurs in the midbrains of MPTP-intoxicated animals [41], one of the foremost model systems for human PD. Studies of post-mortem brains from three human subjects who injected MPTP and developed a parkinsonian syndrome [42], demonstrated the accumulation of activated microglial cells around dopaminergic neurons [43]. Thus, the initial acute insult to dopaminergic neurons likely leads to a secondary and perpetuated neuroinflammatory response. This neuroinflammatory reaction, serves to alter homeostatic neural mechanisms or to exacerbate disease process by the production of proinflammatory factors.

4. Adaptive Immunity

While naïve T cells are precluded from CNS entry, neuroinflammation aggressively recruits activated components of the adaptive immune system to sites of active neurodegeneration by increasing expression of cellular adhesion molecules and inducing chemokine gradients [44]. Moreover, glial cells secrete toxic factors that disrupt blood brain barrier function. Nonetheless, much evidence indicates a far more complex relationship between the CNS and immunological systems than previously thought. For example, immune molecules such as Thy-1, interleukins, and chemokines are expressed at high levels in neurons and surrounding glia and may be involved in direct communication between the CNS and immune cells [45]. Signaling between neurons and glia during neuronal injury incite inflammatory responses and leukocyte migration [44]. Interestingly, molecules mediating specific antigen recognition by T lymphocytes, including MHC class I and CD3ζ molecules, also have a role in axonal guidance, activity-dependent remodeling, and plasticity in the developing and mature mammalian CNS [46]. Within the neuronal synapse, MHC class I molecules may participate in the refinement or elimination of synaptic connections. The cognate receptor for MHC class I peptide complexes is the $\alpha\beta$ T cell receptor (TCR) expressed on T cells. It was recently determined that neurons, particularly in the developing neonatal CNS, express mRNA transcripts for unrearranged β subunit of the TCR [47, 48]. Functional cooperation between these two molecules in neuronal populations has yet to be determined. Interestingly, during inflammatory states, MHC class I molecules are up-regulated on neuronal surfaces yet there is no direct evidence of cytotoxic T lymphocyte (CTL) mediated neuronal damage in common neurodegenerative disorders [49, 50]. However, MHC class I molecules alone are unstable and must associate with proteasome-derived peptides and β2-microglobulin to form stable complexes at the cell surface. Altered peptide profiles presented at the neuronal synapse during neuronal degeneration may, therefore also affect neuronal plasticity and remodeling during disease states.

Further challenging this view of the "immune privileged" status of the CNS are animal model systems where immune deficiencies translate into exacerbated neuronal loss following traumatic injuries [51-54]. Such injuries are corrected in animals that receive immune reconstitution prior to experimental injury. Rodents and humans that have sustained CNS injuries also have expanded T cell repertoires against myelin-associated antigens, yet do not appear to be at increased risk for the development of CNS autoimmunity. Any functional consequence of such T cell responses against CNS antigens following injury remains to be determined.

CD8$^+$ T cells have been reported in close proximity to activated microglia and degenerating neurons within the SN of PD patients; however, those numbers are consistently low in frequency [26]. Whether these T cells are activated, antigen-specific or migrating in response to microglial inflammation has yet to be determined; however the presence of one major T cell subset in ratios exceeding those typically found in the periphery suggests a more profound function in PD than surveillance [12, 55-57]. Numerous aberrations in peripheral lymphocyte subsets have also been detected in PD patients [58-60]. In both drug-naïve and treated PD patient cohorts compared to age-matched controls, numbers of total lymphocytes were shown to be diminished by 17%, while CD19$^+$ B cells were diminished by 35% and CD3$^+$ T cells were diminished by 22% [58]. Among CD3$^+$ T cells, numbers of CD4$^+$ T cells were diminished by 31%; whereas, numbers of CD8$^+$ T cells were not significantly changed. The frequencies of cells within CD4$^+$ T cell subsets are differentially diminished, with a greater loss of naïve helper T cells (CD45RA+) and either unchanged or increased effector/memory helper T cell subset (CD29$^+$ or CD45RO+) [58, 60]. Increased mutual co-expression of CD4 and CD8 by CD45RO$^+$ T cells [59] as well as upregulation of CD25 (α-chain of the IL-2 receptor) [58], TNF-α receptors [61], and significant downregulation of IFN-γ receptors [62, 63] indicate that at least some T cell subsets from PD patients are activated; however, evaluation of these parameters to assess whether activated T cell phenotypes are derived from any one T cell subset or many have yet to be incorporated into one study. Interestingly, a significantly greater number of micronuclei and unrepaired single strand DNA breaks, which have been shown to result from exposure to higher levels of ROS and inflammation [64], are detected in lymphocytes and activated T cells from PD patients compared to age-matched controls [65, 66].

5. Pathways and Mechanisms for Neuroinflammation

5.1 Cytokines

As microglia and peripheral macrophages share the same cell surface markers, it is difficult to distinguish the cell types in postmortem PD brain tissues. Lipopolysaccharide (LPS) stimulated peripheral macrophages from PD patients produce less TNF-α, IL-1β, IFN-γ, and IL-6 than healthy controls and their levels correlate inversely with disability, thus suggesting that impaired cytokine production may progress with disease [66]. In contrast levels of several cytokines, including TNFα, IL-1β, IL-3 and IL-6 are increased in the postmortem striatum, SN and cerebral spinal fluid (CSF) of PD patients [29, 67-70] and elevated levels of TNF-α receptor R1 (TNF-R1, p55), bcl-2, soluble Fas (sFas), caspase-1 and caspase-3 [29] support the existence of a proinflammatory/apoptotic microenvironment in PD patients. However, other regulatory cytokines, including IL-4, transforming growth factor (TGF)-α, TGF-β1, and TGF-β2 are also increased [29], which may indicate an attempt to regulate the predominantly proinflammatory environment. Additionally, hippocampal tissues from PD patients bind increased levels of IL-2 compared to controls indicating that IL-2 receptors (IL-2R) on cells contained within the hippocampus are also upregulated in PD patients [71]. Although likely expressed by both neuronal and glial cells, the localization of IL-2 and IL-2R primarily to the frontal cortex, septum, striatum, hippocampal formation, hypothalamus, locus coeruleus, cerebellum, and the pituitary and fiber tracts of the corpus callosum suggests possible regulatory interactions between peripheral tissues and the CNS [72]. Most likely, IL-2 acts in an auto- and paracrine fashion in the brain as in the peripheral immune system, but exhibits characteristics of a neuroendocrine modulator under different physiological conditions. For instance, IL-2 regulates neuronal and glial growth and differentiation during development, but has pleiotropic effects in the mature brain being involved in modulation of sleep/arousal, memory and cognition, locomotion, and neuroendocrine activities [72].

5.2 ROS and Nigrostriatal Degeneration

Once microglia are activated, they can produce noxious factors including pro-inflammatory cytokines, chemokines, quinolinic acid, arachidonic acid and its metabolites and excitatory amino acids among others. Importantly, large amounts of ROS production, known as a respiratory burst [73, 74], may have disastrous effects on delicate neuronal networks in the CNS. Indeed, oxidative stress is implicated as a major cause of neuronal injury in a wide range of neurological diseases including PD, however whether oxidative stress is causal or consequential is unclear. Altered configuration of proteins including aggregation may trigger aberrant cellular processes such as oxidative phosphorylation resulting in the accumulation of reactive oxygen and nitrogen byproducts, which are typically produced by microglia and serve to destroy invading microorganisms. ROS include superoxide, hydrogen peroxide and hydroxyl free radicals as well as nitrogen intermediates (nitric oxide and peroxynitrite) and can cause damage to neurons if produced in excess as occurs during prolonged neuroinflammatory responses. Much of the microglial-derived ROS such as superoxide cannot efficiently traverse cellular membranes [75], making it unlikely that these extracellular ROS gain access to dopaminergic neurons and trigger intraneuronal toxic events [39]. However, superoxide can rapidly react with NO in the extracellular space to form a more stable oxidant, peroxynitrite [39], which can readily cross cell membranes and damage intracellular components in neighboring neurons. Nitrated species have been associated with the disruption of mitochondrial electron transport chain, lipid peroxidation, DNA damage, and the nitration of tyrosine residues in cellular proteins. This suggests that microglial-derived superoxide, by contributing to peroxynitrite formation, is a significant contributor to the pathogenesis of PD. NADPH-oxidase is a large multi-subunit complex and is the main enzyme known to produce ROS in activated macrophages and microglia. Moreover, genetic deletion of gp91, an essential subunit of NAPDH oxidase, mitigates neuronal loss in numerous models of neurodegeneration including the MPTP model of PD [39].

NO is a biological messenger molecule that has numerous physiological roles in the CNS. In addition, NO plays an important role in innate immunity and is associated with tumoricidal and bactericidal activities of macrophages [76, 77]. Three distinct forms of nitric oxide synthase (NOS) have been identified to date and are designated neuronal NOS (nNOS), inducible NOS (iNOS), and endothelial NOS (eNOS). In contrast to the physiological roles of normal NO levels, excessive NO produced under pathological settings can act as a potent neurotoxin in a number of neurodegenerative models [78-81]. For example, nNOS and iNOS are both upregulated in sporadic PD and some animal models; however, genetic ablation or pharmacological inhibition of excess NO production is neuroprotective in the MPTP model [81, 82]. Although NO may generate much of its toxicity through the formation of peroxynitrite, it also reacts with sulfur containing cysteine residues in protein (S-nitrosylation), which may modify protein structural conformations or enzymatic activities [83].

Production of ROS and NO in neurons is buffered primarily by the glutathione system, which is compromised in the brain of PD patients, leading to an imbalance in redox homeostasis and consequent oxidative stress. The tripeptide glutathione (GSH; gamma-L-glutamyl-L-cysteinylglycine) is the major cellular thiol present in brain tissue, and the most important redox buffer in mammalian cells [84]. This antioxidant molecule cycles between reduced glutathione (GSH) and oxidized glutathione disulfide (GSSG) and serves as a vital sink for control of ROS levels in cells. GSH reacts directly with oxygen and nitrogen free radicals nonenzmatically and donates electrons in the enzyme-catalyzed reduction of peroxides [85, 86]. Determination of the relative levels of glutathione and glutathione-related enzymes in neuronal and glial compartments is incompletely understood and remains an active area of research in our laboratories.

GSH content in the SNpc of PD patients is decreased by 40-50%, but not in other regions of the brain, nor in age-matched controls or patients with other diseases affecting dopaminergic neurons [87-89], This diminution continues with progression and severity of disease, suggesting a correlation with concomitant increases in reactive species [88-92]. GSH depletion has been suggested as the first indicator of oxidative stress during PD progression, possibly occurring prior to other hallmarks of PD including the decreased activity of mitochondrial complex I [8, 92-94]. Also, elevated GSSG/GSH ratios in PD patients [87, 95] argue strongly for a role of oxidative stress in this disease [84]. An increase in glutathione peroxidase immunoreactivity, exclusive to glial cells surrounding surviving dopaminergic neurons, has also been observed in PD brains [96]. Interestingly, the SN and striatum have lower levels of GSH relative to other regions of the brain, which include, in increasing order: SN, striatum, hippocampus, cerebellum, and cortex [97-99]. Although varying in different regions of the brain, all GSH levels diminish by about 30% in the elderly [99], suggesting a possible link with the age associated risk factor for PD. GSH depletion cannot be explained by increased oxidation of GSH to GSSG as levels of both are diminished in the nigra of PD patients [87, 99]. Diminished GSH levels do not appear to be caused from failure of GSH synthesis as γ-glutamylcysteine synthetase is unaltered as are glutathione peroxidase and glutathione transferase activities [95]. Other possibilities for diminished levels include increased removal of GSH from cells by γ-glutamyltranspeptidase [95] or formation of adducts of the glutamyl and cysteinyl peptides of GSH with dopamine [100-102]. Nevertheless, depletion of GSH may render cells more sensitive to toxic effects of oxidative stress and potentiate the toxic effects of reactive microglia [103, 104].

Inflammatory responses induced by reactive microglia, macrophages, and proinflammatory T cells, provide a primary source of free radicals, ROS ($O_2^-\cdot$, H_2O_2, $\cdot OH$, HOCl, ferryl, peroxyl, and alkoxyl) and reactive nitrogen species [nitric acid (NO$\cdot$), peroxynitrite (ONOO$^-$) and peroxynitrous acid (ONOOH)] with the capacity to modify proteins, lipids, and nucleic acids (Figure 2). This induces a condition of oxidative stress whereby the increased production of highly reactive species and decreased scavenging of free radicals results in increased modification and damage of biomolecules, and decreased clearance of those damaged macromolecules that are potentially toxic for neurons. The highly reactive nature and short half-lives of reactive species, combined with the restrictive nature of the neuroinflammatory foci to clinical sampling, preclude the direct measurement in disease processes of these reactive species. However, modifications of proteins, lipids and nucleic acids provide surrogate biomarkers, which can be directly measured as indirect assessments of the extent of oxidative stress. Postmortem analyses of PD patients have consistently demonstrated the increased presence of these biomarkers for oxidative stress. Protein modifications are among the many biomarkers detected in the brains of PD patients. Compared to brains from control donors, elevated levels of nitrated proteins are found in brains and CSF of PD patients [105, 106]. Most notable are modifications of proteins that comprise Lewy bodies (LB), which are neuronal inclusions that consist primarily of α-synuclein, ubiquitin, and lipids, and considered hallmarks of PD. In LB cores from PD patients, increased 3-nitrotyrosine immunoreactivity, primarily due to the presence of a nitrated form of α-synuclein identifies peroxynitrite modifications of tyrosine moieties [107-109] suggesting the participation of inflammatory responses; however, whether those modifications occur before or after inclusion into LB remain unclear. Also S-nitrosylated forms of parkin, an E3 ubiquitin ligase involved in protein ubiquitination have been isolated from the temporal cortex from 4 PD patients, but not from brains of Huntington's or AD patients [110]. *In vitro* and *in vivo*, S-nitrosylation of parkin induces an initial increase in ligase activity leading to autoubiquitination of parkin [110], eventual inhibition of ubiquitin ligase activity, and decreased activity in the E3 ligase-ubiquitin-proteasome degradative pathway [83, 110]. Carbonyl modifications, which are reflective of protein oxidation, are increased by greater than 2-fold in the SN compared to the basal ganglia and prefrontal cortex of normal subjects [111]. Increases in protein carbonyls have been found in substantia nigra, basal ganglia, globus pallidus, substantia innominata, cerebellum and frontal pole, but not in patients with incidental LB disease (ILBD), a putatively presymptomatic PD disorder [112]. The involvement of the latter two brain regions are unexpected based on the restricted neuropathology of PD, but may reflect a consequence of L-DOPA treatment or a more global consequence of the inflammatory spread of oxidative stress in PD. Other evidence for oxidative damage to proteins in PD is the increased expression of neural heme oxygenase-1 [113] and increased immunostaining of glycosylated proteins on nigral neurons [114].

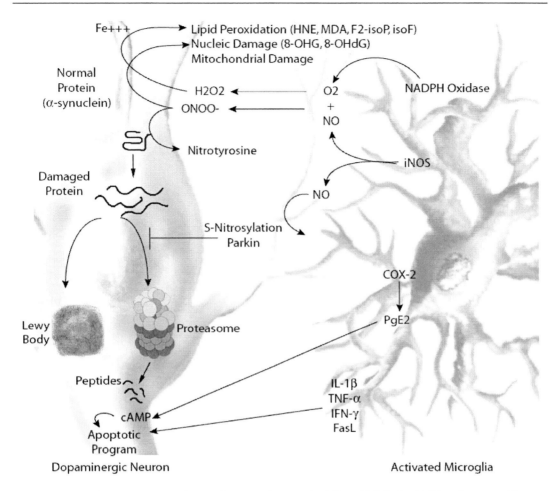

Figure 2. Neuroinflammatory pathways in PD pathogenesis. Microglial derived NO and superoxide species react in extracellular spaces to form peroxynitrite. Peroxynitrite readily crosses cell membranes where it contributes to lipid peroxidation, DNA damage and nitrotyrosine formation in α-synuclein and other cellular proteins. Damaged proteins are targeted to cellular proteosomes for degradation via the ubiquitination pathway. Excess NO produced by activated microglia can lead to S-nitrosylation of cellular proteins, including parkin. Such modifications may diminish E3 ubiquitin ligase activity necessary for efficient protein turnover by proteosomes. Excessive protein damage caused by oxidants and disruptions in the ubiquitin pathways may overload or inhibit protein degradation quality control measures leading to the accumulation of damaged proteins in cells.

5.3 Free Radicals and Nucleic Acid Modifications

Modification of nucleic acids by free radicals and reactive species can induce chromosomal aberrations with a high efficiency [64], suggesting that chromosomal damage exhibited in neurons of PD patients might be related to an abnormally high oxidative stress. Among the most promising biomarkers of oxidative damage to nucleic acids is nucleoside 8-hydroxyguanosine (8-OHG) for RNA or 8-hydroxy-2'-deoxyguanosine (8-OHdG) for DNA. 8-OHG is an oxidized base produced by free radical attack on DNA by C-8 hydroxylation of guanine and is one of the most frequent nucleic acid modifications observed under conditions of oxidative stress [115]. In PD patients, levels of 8-OHG nucleic acid modifications are commonly increased in the caudate and SN compared to age-matched controls [116-119]. Immunohistochemical characterization of these modifications indicates that the highest levels of 8-OHG modifications are found in neurons of the SN and to a lesser extent in neurons of the nucleus raphe dorsalis and oculomotor nucleus, and occasionally in glial cells [118]. That 8-OHG nucleic acid modifications are rarely detected in the nuclear area and mostly restricted to the cytoplasm, and that immunoreactivity is diminished by RNase or DNase and ablated with both enzymes [118], suggest that targets of oxidative attack include both cytoplasmic RNA and mitochondrial DNA. Of particular interest are the findings that concentrations of 8-OHG in CSF of PD patients are higher than in age-matched controls; however, serum concentrations of 8-OHG appear highly variable [120, 121].

5.4 Lipid Peroxidation

4-Hydroxy-2-nonenal (HNE) is a reactive α,β unsaturated aldehyde that is one of the major products during the oxidation of membrane lipid polyunsaturated fatty acids, and forms stable adducts with nucleophilic groups on proteins such as thiols and amines [122, 123]. Thus, HNE modification of membrane proteins forms can be used as biomarkers of cellular damage due to oxidative stress [123]. Immunochemical staining for HNE modified proteins on melanized nigral neurons in the midbrains of PD patients show 58% of remaining nigral neurons exhibit positive HNE-modified proteins compared to only 9% in control subjects, weak or no staining on oculomotor neurons in the same midbrain sections from PD patients [124], and are detected in LB from PD and diffuse LB disease patients, but not age-matched controls [125]. HNE species are typically more stable than oxygen species, thus can spread from site of production to effect modifications at a distant site [126]. HNE modifications of DNA, RNA, and proteins have various adverse biological effects such as interference with enzymatic reactions and induction of heat shock proteins, and are considered to be largely responsible for cytotoxic effects under conditions of oxidative stress [122, 127, 128]. The cytotoxic effects of HNE modifications may be founded in part due to inhibition of complexes I and II of the mitochondrial respiratory chain [129]; induction of caspase-8, -9, and -3; cleavage of poly(ADP-ribose) polymerase (PARP) with subsequent DNA fragmentation [130]; inhibition of NF-κB mediated signaling pathways [131]; and diminution of glutathione levels [130]. Consistent with an abundance of data showing the dysregulation of proteasomal function in PD, direct binding of HNE to the proteasome also inhibits the processing of ubiquinated proteins [132]. Concentrations that induce no acute change in cell viability *in vitro,* initially cause a decrease in the proteasomal catalytic activity to the extent that it induces accumulation of ubiquinated and nitrated proteins, reductions in glutathione levels and mitochondrial activity, and increased levels of oxidative damage to DNA, RNA, proteins, and lipids [132-134].

Another reactive aldehyde species produced from the peroxidation of lipids is malonyldialdehyde (MDA), which is formed from the breakdown of endoperoxides during the last stages of the oxidation of polyunsaturated fatty acids; particularly susceptible are those containing three or more double bonds [122, 135, 136]. MDA can exist as free aldehydes or react with primary amine groups of macromolecules to form adducts with cellular structures [122, 137, 138]. Evidence of increased levels of MDA-modified proteins in the SN [139, 140] and CSF [141] of PD patients, but not in controls is indicative of increased lipid peroxidation and supports the existence of chronic inflammatory responses in those patients.

F2-isoprostanes (F2-IsoP) and isofurans (IsoF) are other products of lipid peroxidation and both are well-established as specific biomarkers of *in vivo* oxidative stress [142-144]. Under conditions of relatively low oxygen tension, the F2-IsoP species is favored; whereas, under higher oxygen tensions, IsoF is heavily favored [142]. Increased F2-IsoP concentrations in affected tissues from patients of most neurodegenerative disorders have provided general support for the role of inflammation and oxidative stress in those disorders [143], but the failure to detect similar levels in tissues from PD patients was particularly perplexing [145]. However comparison of tissues for IsoF as well as F2-IsoP has shown that levels of IsoF, but not F2-IsoP in the SN of patients with PD and dementia with LB are significantly higher than those of controls [142]. This preferential increase in IsoF in PD patients indicates that the microenvironmental oxygen tension is typically greater in PD than other disorders, and suggests a unique mode of oxidant injury in PD, which may be indicative of an increased intracellular oxygen tension resulting from mitochondrial dysfunction or a greater intensity of inflammatory response in PD. These data certainly indicate that oxidative stress in the SNpc region is elevated in PD, but whether microglial and astroglial (*i.e.* innate immune) activation during the progression of PD shifts the balance towards increased protection from ROS damage or towards exacerbation of ROS damage, and whether this dynamic changes as the disease progresses remains to be determined.

5.5 Iron and Oxidative Stress

Investigators using a variety of methods have provided a consensus that iron levels naturally increase with age and are significantly increased (reported from 25% - 100%) in the SN and CSF of postmortem PD patients compared to age-matched controls [90, 146-158]. Iron in its ferrous (Fe^{2+}) form catalyzes the formation of strong oxidants and ferric iron (Fe^{3+}). With disease progression, levels of Fe^{3+} increase within the SN suggesting an increased state of oxidative stress [159]. Although most of the total iron in healthy brains is stored in ferritin, and levels are typically depleted under inflammatory conditions, ferric ions are readily released after damage to neuronal tissues by yet unknown mechanisms, making those ions available for oxidative catalysis [160]. In PD, proteins such as transferrin, ferritin, and iron regulatory proteins (IRP), which control iron homeostasis, could be modified by ROS and lose their regulatory capacity. Indeed, *in vitro* and *in vivo* nitrosylation of IRP2 leads to rapid ubiquitination and degradation of IRP2 in the proteasome [161]. Additionally, IRP knockout mice exhibit high levels of iron and ferritin with an extensive axonopathy in the white matter tracts and reactive microglia and vacuoles SN [162]. These mice also manifest motor impairments when axonopathy is prominent, however dopaminergic cell loss is minimal.

6. Genetics and Immunity

Recent evidence has shown that genetics may contribute to the onset of neurodegenerative disorders [163]. Linkages to the age at onset (AAO) for PD have been identified on chromosomes 1 and 10. The latter is significantly associated with glutathione s-transferase omega-1 (GSTO1) [164]; a provocative finding since GSTO1 is thought to be involved in the post-translation modification of IL-1, a major component in the regulation of inflammatory responses [165-167]. One factor associated with the chromosome 1p peak is the ELAVL4 gene [168], a human homologue of the Drosophila ELAV (embryonic lethal abnormal vision) [169] and essential for temporal and spatial gene expression during CNS development. Additionally, ELAVL gene products are known to bind to AU-rich response elements (ARE) in the 3'-untranslated region (3'UTR) of inflammation-associated factors [169]. Interestingly, PD patients homozygotic for allele 1 at position -511 of the IL-1β gene have an earlier onset of the disease than those homozygotic for allele 2, which produces higher amounts of IL-1. Thus, higher production of IL-1β might provide some neuroprotective effect for dopaminergic neurons [170, 171].

The generalized toxicity of these inflammatory responses provides very little insight into the selective neurodegeneration patterns observed in various disease states. However, it is tempting to speculate that the shared phenotype of multiple genetic mutations identified in familial forms of PD suggests the dysregulation of a common pathway may be involved. Consistent with aberrant protein accumulation in PD, malfunction of the ubiquitin-proteasome system appears to be a common link in these familial forms of PD. Indeed, many of the genes identified are linked to protein misfolding and/or degradation pathways [11, 172]. While these genetic mutations offer insight into common pathways involved in familial forms of PD, the information they offer for sporadic forms of the disease in individuals who lack these genetic lesions are not completely understood. Interestingly, recent data suggests that some of these PD associated genes are active targets of reactive nitrogen and oxygen species both of which are generated during chronic inflammation.

In keeping with this notion, three missense mutations (A53T, A30P, and E46K) have been identified in the gene encoding α-synuclein leading to an autosomal dominant inheritance of PD. Moreover, genomic triplication of the α-synuclein gene is associated with familial PD [173]. Transgenic overexpression of wild-type or mutant forms of α-synuclein in mice produces intraneuronal aggregates [174], while in *Drosophila*, this resulted in both aggregate formation as well as dopaminergic neuronal cell death [175]. In sporadic PD, recent studies support a role for oxidative and/or nitrative stress in α-synuclein modification and aggregation [108]. Nitrating agents such as peroxynitrite can readily nitrate α-synuclein at tyrosine residues, and generate highly stable *o,o'*-dityrosine oligomers (Figure 2). These biochemical lesions enhance fibril formation *in vitro*, similar to the biophysical properties of α-synuclein isolated from PD brains [176]. Aberrant protein conformations of modified α-synuclein can potentially overload cellular proteasome and by doing so, may increase cellular stress associated with the accumulation of misfolded proteins in affected neurons [177].

Parkin is another gene associated with familial PD whose protein product may be a target of nitrosative stress-associated protein modifications. Parkin is an ubiquitin E3 ligase responsible for the addition of ubiquitin to protein substrates marked for degradation by cellular proteasomes including α-synuclein and its interacting protein, synphilin-1 [178]. Over expression of parkin in α-synuclein transgenic flies rescues neurons from degeneration [179]. Mutations in parkin result in the loss of ubiquitin E3 ligase activity and are found in juvenile PD in an autosomal recessive fashion [180]. The posttranslational modification (S-nitrosylation) of parkin also abolishes its E3 ligase activity and inhibits the ability to rescue cells from α-synuclein/synphilin coexpression in the presence of proteasome inhibition (Figure 2) [83, 110]. Nitrosylation modifications on parkin were found in sporadic cases of PD in affected brain regions, as well as in both MPTP and rotenone animal models. Animal studies reveal that nitrosylation of parkin is dependent on both nNOS, as well as microglial-derived iNOS [83]. Thus, it is conceivable that inflammation contributes to oxidative modifications in parkin, which in turn predispose affected neurons to cytotoxic stress caused by altered protein catabolism.

7. Experimental Models of PD: Neuroinflammation and Disease

The prevalence of reactive microglia and biomarkers of inflammatory responses in PD necessitates the inclusion of an inflammatory component in most models of PD. Although reactive microglia in PD may have an initial function to scavenge dead or dying neurons after the primary etiological event, evidence of a more adverse role in neuroinflammation and neurodegeneration emerges from animal models of PD. Several models of PD exist that induce significant inflammatory responses as evidenced by reactive microglia and degeneration of dopaminergic neurons along the nigrostiatal axis, and include 1-methyl-4-phenyl-1,2,5,6-tetrahydropyridine (MPTP), 6-hydroxydopamine (6-OHDA), rotenone, paraquat, LPS, and trisialoganglioside GT1b [81, 181-188].

Arguably, of great importance among the compounds used to model PD is MPTP, the only agent reported to have dopaminergic effects in humans. MPTP is a neurotoxin that was discovered after induction of irreversible parkinsonian syndrome in addicts following injection of MPTP as a contaminant of illicitly and poorly synthesized meperidine [42, 43]. Postmortem examination of several patients ranging from 3 to 16 years post-exposure and onset of parkinsonism, revealed not only evidence of progressive neurodegeneration, but also reactive microglial clusters surrounding nerve cells. This ongoing inflammatory reaction years after the original toxic exposure supports the notion of a self-perpetuating process of neurodegeneration mediated by localized inflammatory processes within the nigrostriatal axis. However, that many of these patients self-administered drugs both before and after MPTP exposure, and that only a few were affected from an estimated 300 individuals exposed to MPTP, warrants caution about extrapolating these data to extremes.

Among several animal models of PD, MPTP can reproduce many characteristics of the disease when administered to mice [189] and primates [41]. MPTP is converted to 1-methyl-4-phenylpyridinium (MPP+) in astrocytes, which is taken up by dopaminergic neurons where it inhibits mitochondrial electron transport complex I, resulting in decreased ATP production and cell death. This toxin has proven to be valuable for the study of PD pathology, both in murine and primate animal models and *in vitro* culture systems. MPTP induces peak microglia activation within 2 days after acute MPTP intoxication and produces a proinflammatory environment in the substantia nigra and striatum with predominant production of TNFα, IL-1β, and IL-6, and upregulation of iNOS, COX-2, and MMP-9 [23, 31, 190-194]. In addition to increased reactive microglia in the MPTP model, a minor, but consistent T cell infiltrate occurs soon after MPTP treatment, but before peak neuronal loss, and is comprised mostly of CD8+ T cells with fewer CD4+ T cells [181, 182]. These T cells express LFA-1 and CD44 suggesting they are an effector/memory phenotype and may be activated.

However, MPTP is not the only valid model of PD. Intrastriatal injection of 6-OHDA induces increased numbers of reactive microglia in striatum and SN, as evidenced by increased expression of MHC II, Mac-1 and peripheral benzodiazepine receptors by day 1 after exposure, which peak after 6 to 10 days post injection, and gradually resolve 20-30 days thereafter [183, 195-197]. Proinflammatory cytokines are also implicated in 6-OHDA-induced neurodegeneration as levels of TNF-α are elevated in striatum and CSF of treated rats [67]. Signs of inflammation remain after one month post-intoxication as shown by significantly increased levels of mRNA for IL-1α and IL-1β in lesioned tissues, however significant amounts of those cytokine proteins have not been demonstrated [197] suggesting a role for post-transcriptional regulation in regulation of the inflammatory response.

Rotenone is a lipophilic herbicide that causes a chronic, systemic defect of mitochondrial complex 1 and release of superoxide free radicals, inducing selective degeneration of nigrostriatal dopaminergic neurons along the nigrastriatal axis and leading to hypokinesia and rigidity [184, 185, 198]. However, behavioral abnormalities occur even in the absence of detectable dopaminergic neurodegeneration, suggesting that other systems may be affected by rotenone [199, 200]. Additionally, neurons from treated rats accumulate fibrillary inclusions comprised of ubiquitin and α-synuclein. Rotenone induces a prominent inflammatory response of Mac-1+ reactive microglia in the striatum and substantia nigra, even in the absence of detectable dopaminergic neurodegeneration [185, 199].

Paraquat (PQ, 1,1'-dimethyl-4,4'-bypyridinium) is a herbicide that induces selective degeneration of dopaminergic neurons along the nigrostriatal axis [201-205]; thus PQ exposure is implicated as a putative risk factor for PD [203]. PQ induces nigral astrocytosis and microgliosis; the latter showing a reactive phenotype with increased numbers of Mac-1 immunoreactive cells [203, 206]. Co-culture with microglia is necessary to induce PQ-mediated degeneration of dopaminergic neurons in vitro [207]. Additionally, PQ mediates the accumulation of α-synuclein inclusions and 4-HNE modifications by nigral dopaminergic neurons [204, 205], suggesting increased oxidative stress may contribute to proteasomal dysregulation.

To assess the role of microglial inflammation on dopaminergic neurodegeneration, known inducers of inflammation have been introduced intrastriatally. Of those, LPS is a most potent activator of microglia. Injection of LPS into the nigrostiratal area induces a strong reactive microglial response that precedes a delayed and progressive dopaminergic neuronal loss along that axis [184, 186, 187, 208], whereas injection into other brain regions, such as the hippocampus or cortex, has no detectable deleterious affect on neurons in those areas [187]. Injection of LPS between the subtantia nigra and ventral tegmental area (VTA) affects only those neuronal bodies within the SN as similarly observed with dopaminergic-specific neurotoxins. Progression of neurodegeneration without an overt neurotoxin, but in the presence of LPS-induced reactive microglia suggests that reactive microglia are a primary neurodegenerative agent for dopaminergic neurons. LPS-induced neuronal death is subsequent to upregulation by nigral microglia of iNOS, TNFα, and IL-1β, and increased production of NO and superoxide [186, 187, 208-211]. While LPS does not induce any detectable adverse effects to purified dopaminergic neurons *in vitro*, the presence of reactive microglia, but not astrocytes, is essential for LPS-induced neurodegeneration [186, 212, 213]. Inhibition of LPS binding to its cognate receptor inhibits activation of microglia, subsequent production and release of all proinflammatory factors and protection of dopaminergic neurons in culture [209]. Interestingly, inhibition of proinflammatory cytokines by neutralizing antibodies is also neuroprotective [211]. Thus, the salient features of these models are that prominent inflammatory responses precede a progressive dopaminergic neuronal degeneration, and a critical role for microglia and the products of inflammation in dopaminergic neurodegeneration exists.

8. Inhibition of Inflammation in PD and Experimental Models

Various sources of evidence suggest that long-known inflammatory changes in the parkinsonian brain, rather than mere secondary scavenging affects, may participate more actively in the neurodegenerative processes. Of greatest interest is the finding in a large cohort of health care professionals, that daily administration of nonsteroidal anti-inflammatory drugs (NSAIDs) reduces the risk for PD by 45% compared to those that did not routinely take NSAIDS [37]. Additionally, evidence for the role of neuroinflammation is provided in several intoxicant models of neuroinflammation; whereby, attenuation of the inflammatory component protects subsequent dopaminergic neurodegeneration along the nigrostriatal axis.

As an inducible proinflammatory enzyme, iNOS is thought to play a major role in dopaminergic neurodegeneration. Ablation by genetic manipulation or inhibition with specific pharmaceutical agents protects nigral neurodegeneration induced by MPTP [81, 214, 215], LPS [208] or 6-OHDA [183], but is less active at protecting striatal termini [81, 214]. Interesting, not all microglia express iNOS and inhibition of iNOS does not attenuate all reactive microglia suggesting that only a subpopulation of reactive microglia may participate in neurodegeneration [81, 214].

Minocycline is a long-acting second generation tetracycline shown to have a high capability to penetrate the brain parenchyma and CSF. Minocycline acts on activated microglia to prevent upregulation of iNOS, inhibit phosphorylation of p38 mitogen-activated protein (MAP) kinase, and reduce IL-1β converting enzyme (ICE) and IL-1β production [216-222]. In the MPTP model, the effects of minocycline have a combined effect to reduce reactive microglia and inhibit neurodegeneration of the dopaminergic neuronal bodies of the nigra as well as the termini in the striatum in a dose-dependent fashion, but does not effect the conversion of MPTP by astrocyes [183, 219, 220]. Similarly, in 6-OHDA treated animals, minocycline reduces the number of reactive microglia and protects dopaminergic neurons in the SN [183].

Similarly ablation or inhibition of COX-2, the rate-limiting enzyme in prostaglandin E2 synthesis markedly diminishes dopaminergic neurodegeneration along the nigrostriatal axis after treatment with MPTP [23, 223-227], or 6-OHDA [228]. *In vitro* data shows that inhibition of COX-2 is more efficacious in 6-OHDA-induced toxicity compared to that induced with MPP$^+$ suggesting that MPTP-induced dopaminergic neurodegeneration may be COX independent [229]. Indeed, in MPTP/MPP+ induced toxicity, COX-2 inhibition does not entirely attenuate microglia activation, but rather prevents the formation of reactive oxygen/nitrogen species [23, 230].

On a more general level, MMPs are a class of extracellular soluble or membrane bound cysteine proteases involved in remodeling of the extracellular matrix and are regulated by tissue inhibitors of metalloproteinases (TIMPs). Both classes of proteins have been implicated in a range of neurodegenerative diseases including HAD, AD, PD and stoke. Indeed, consistent with the possibility that alterations in MMPs/TIMPs may contribute to disease pathogenesis, samples from PD patients show levels of MMP-2, expressed primarily by microglia and astrocytes that are significantly reduced in the SN compared to age-matched controls, but remain unchanged in cortex and hippocampus [231]. Gu and colleagues reported that S-nitrosylation of N-terminal cysteine residues within proMMP-9 leads to the subsequent activation of MMP-9 protease activity, which identifies an extracellular proteolysis mechanism putatively involved in neuronal cell death in which S-nitrosylation activates MMPs [232]. Additionally, an increase in MMP-9 expression has been determined in the MPTP model and pharmacological inhibition of MMP-9 was neuroprotective [193].

9. Therapeutic Immunoregulation

To establish a disease diagnosis at earlier stages, as well as designing rational therapeutic modalities for this disease, efforts have been made in recent years to identify the neuropathological, biochemical, and genetic biomarkers of PD. α-Synuclein-containing LB and altered DAT imaging for PD are the most eminent biomarkers. Several potential markers of oxidative stress such as malondialdehyde, superoxide radicals, the coenzyme Q10 redox ratio, and 8-OHdG from RNA oxidation have been measured in blood and the levels of these markers tend to be higher in PD compared with control groups [233]. Thus, therapeutic approaches to PD may target a number of factors that play a role in disease onset, inflammation and neurodegenerative progression

Studies involving pro-apoptotic proteins in PD animal models indicate that their suppression may lead to decreased rates of neuronal loss. Fas, a member of the TNF receptor family, shows pro-apoptotic and inflammatory functions, and is upregulated in the SNpc of both PD patients and MPTP mouse models [234]. However, Fas blockage with dominant-negative c-Jun adenovirus indicates that Fas deficiency does not significantly prevent the reduction of dopaminergic terminal fibers within the striatum or attenuate the activation of striatal microglia [234]. Numerous studies have demonstrated that Bax is a pro-apoptotic factor required for the programmed death of several types of neurons in the peripheral and central nervous systems [235]. Bax is upregulated in the SNpc of MPTP mice, and its ablation alleviates SNpc neuronal apoptosis, indicating that targeting Bax may provide a protective benefit in PD [236].

The role of neurotrophins in reducing neurodegeneration and promotion of neuroregenerative processes presents an exciting possibility for therapeutic benefit to PD. A study of lentiviral delivery of glial cell line-derived neurotrophic factor (GDNF) showed trophic effects on degenerating nigrostriatal neurons in a primate model of PD [237]. Results indicated augmented dopaminergic function in aged monkeys and reversal of functional deficits with complete prevention of nigrostriatal degeneration in MPTP-treated monkeys. These data indicate that GDNF delivery using a lentiviral vector system can prevent nigrostriatal degeneration and potentially induce regeneration in primate models of PD, showing the potential for a viable therapeutic strategy for PD patients. However, recent clinical trials of intraputamenally infused GDNF in PD patients are controversial with one 2-year phase I trial showing improved activity scores and no untoward effects in a limited cohort [238], while phase II trials were halted after six months due to lack of efficacy and adverse effects in patients and nonhuman primates .

Immune suppression through receptor modulation has been another approach attempting to alleviate or reverse PD progression. For example, agonists of peroxisome proliferator-activated receptor-γ (PPAR-γ), a nuclear receptor involved in carbohydrate and lipid metabolism, have been shown to inhibit inflammatory responses in a variety of cell lines, including monocyte/macrophages and microglial cells [239]. *In vivo* administration of PPAR-γ agonists modulate inflammatory responses in the brain. Pioglitazone, a PPAR-γ agonist used currently as an anti-diabetic agent, has been shown to have anti-inflammatory effects in animal models of autoimmune disease, attenuate glial activation, and inhibit dopaminergic cell loss in the SN of MPTP treated mice [239]. However, pioglitazone treatment had little effect on MPTP-induced changes in the striatum. This result seems to indicate that in the MPTP mouse model of PD, mechanisms regulating glial activation in the dopaminergic terminals compared with the dopaminergic cell bodies are PPAR-γ independent [239].

Another potential therapeutic avenue for PD may involve T cell mediated immune responses. Activation of T cells directed against antigens expressed at the injured areas of the CNS has been shown to be neuroprotective under acute and chronic neurodegenerative conditions [240-242]. However, immunization with such antigens might lead to development of an autoimmune disease. Immunization with Copolymer-1 (Cop-1, glatiramer acetate) or passive transfer of Cop-1 specific T cells has been shown to be beneficial for protecting neurons from secondary degeneration after injurious conditions [243]. Cop-1 reactive T cells have partial cross-reactivity with myelin basic protein (MBP) and other self-antigens expressed in the brain [244]. Therefore, immunization with Cop-1 leads to increased accumulation of T lymphocytes in areas of injury within the brain and spinal cord and is neuroprotective without causing any adverse effects; however, the molecular mechanism of this response is not fully understood. T cells reactive to Cop-1 could be a source of brain-derived neurotrophic factor (BDNF) and other neurotrophic factors [243] or can induce production of neurotrophins by microglial or astroglial cells.

Recently, the neuroprotective effect of immunization with Cop-1 was tested in the MPTP model of PD and demonstrated that adoptive transfer of Cop-1-specific T cells, but not ovalbumin-specifc T cells, into MPTP-intoxicated mice attenuates reactive microglia neuroinflammation and inhibits dopaminergic neurodegeneration in both the SNpc and the striatum [245]. Additionally, by determination with quantitative proton magnetic resonance spectroscopic imaging (^{1}H MRSI), adoptive transfer of those T cells protect the loss of nigral N-acetylaspartate (NAA) levels associated with MPTP-induced neurodegeneration [246], Additionally, suppression of microglial-associated inflammation was associated with T cell accumulation within the SNpc, induction of a TH$_2$ phenotypic T cell response with production of anti-inflammatory cytokines (IL-4, IL-10), and increased expression of GDNF by astrocytes, but not by infiltrating T cells or microglia [245]. These data suggest a putative mechanism for which regulatory T cells, induced by vaccination with cross-reactive epitopes, extravasate in response to neuroinflammation from neurodegenerative processes; secrete anti-inflammatory cytokines in response to cross-reactive self-epitopes (e.g. myelin basic protein) to attenuate reactive microglia; suppress the inflammatory response; induce a neurotrophic response by T cells and/or other glia, which can interdict ensuing neurodegenerative processes (Figure 3). This therapeutic vaccine approach using Cop-1 represents a potential interdictory modality for slowing or halting the progression of neuroinflammation and secondary neurodegeneration, and could be considered in strategies with other anti-inflammatory or anti-oxidant therapies for a combinatorial modality to protect against neuroinflammation and consequent neurodegeneration in PD.

10. Summary

Evidence for the role of inflammatory processes in the pathogenesis of Parkinson's disease (PD) is significant. Epidemiologic, animal, human autopsy studies, and immune-based therapeutics all support the presence of an inflammatory cascade, whereby microglial cells play center stage affecting disease processes through secretory neurotoxic and antigen presentation activities. In steady state, microglia, a cell type with a diverse functional repertoire, protect the nervous system acting as debris scavengers, killers of microbial pathogens, and regulators of immune responses. In neurodegenerative diseases, activated microglia can mediate cell injury and death through production of reactive oxygen species, mobilization of adaptive immunity, and cell chemotaxis. This induces tissue remodeling and blood-brain barrier dysfunction. As the disease progresses, inflammatory secretions engage neighboring cells including the recruitment of the adaptive immune system in a vicious cycle of autocrine and paracrine amplification of inflammation, leading to tissue injury and ultimately destruction. Such pathogenic processes contribute to neurodegeneration in PD. Research from others and our own laboratories seek to develop therapeutic interventions that harness inflammatory processes and block disease processes.

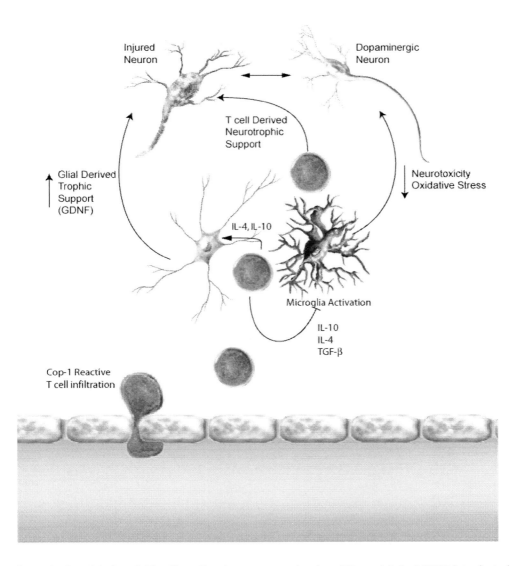

Figure 3. Cop-1 induced, T cell-mediated neuroprotection in a PD model. In MPTP-intoxicated mice, regulatory T cells infiltrate the inflamed nigrostriatal pathway where they encounter cross-reactive self-antigens (myelin basic protein) presented in the context of MHC by resident microglial cells. Activated T cells secrete anti-inflammatory cytokines such as IL-4, IL-10, and TGF-β that suppress toxic microglial activities. Neurotrophin expression may occur directly from T cells or T cell derived IL-4 and IL-10 may induce neurotrophin production in neighboring glia. These activities lead to neuroprotection indirectly by suppression of microglial responses and directly through the local delivery of neurotrophins.

Acknowledgments

The authors wish to thank Ms. Robin Taylor for excellent graphic and administrative assistance. The National Institutes of Health (NIH) grants that supported this work included R21 NS049264 (to R.L.M.) and P01 NS31492, R01 NS34239, P01 NS043985, and R37 NS36136 and P01 MH64570-03 (to H.E.G.).

References

[1]   Mayeux R. Epidemiology of neurodegeneration. *Annu Rev Neurosci* 2003;26:81-104.
[2]   Fahn S, *Przedborski S. Merritt's Neurology*. New York: Lippincott Williams & Wilkins; 2000.
[3]   Fahn S, Sulzer D. Neurodegeneration and neuroprotection in Parkinson disease. *NeuroRx* 2004;1:139-54.
[4]   Hornykiewicz O, Kish SJ. Biochemical pathophysiology of Parkinson's disease. *Adv Neurol* 1987;45:19-34.
[5]   Clarke G, Collins RA, Leavitt BR, Andrews DF, Hayden MR, Lumsden CJ, et al. A one-hit model of cell death in inherited neuronal degenerations. *Nature* 2000;406:195-9.
[6]   Orr CF, Rowe DB, Halliday GM. An inflammatory review of Parkinson's disease. *Prog Neurobiol* 2002;68:325-40.
[7]   Dauer W, Przedborski S. Parkinson's disease: mechanisms and models. *Neuron* 2003;39:889-909.
[8]   Andersen JK. Oxidative stress in neurodegeneration: cause or consequence? *Nat Med* 2004;10 Suppl:S18-25.
[9]   Przedborski S, Jackson-Lewis V, Vila M, Wu du C, Teismann P, Tieu K, et al. Free radical and nitric oxide toxicity in Parkinson's disease. *Adv Neurol* 2003;91:83-94.
[10]   Dawson TM, Dawson VL. Molecular pathways of neurodegeneration in Parkinson's disease. *Science* 2003;302:819-22.
[11]   Vila M, Przedborski S. Genetic clues to the pathogenesis of Parkinson's disease. *Nat Med* 2004;10 Suppl:S58-62.
[12]   Kreutzberg GW. Microglia: a sensor for pathological events in the CNS. *Trends Neurosci* 1996;19:312-8.
[13]   Schwartz M, Shaked I, Fisher J, Mizrahi T, Schori H. Protective autoimmunity against the enemy within: fighting glutamate toxicity. *Trends Neurosci* 2003;26:297-302.
[14]   Batchelor PE, Porritt MJ, Martinello P, Parish CL, Liberatore GT, Donnan GA, et al. Macrophages and microglia produce local trophic gradients that stimulate axonal sprouting toward but not beyond the wound edge. *Mol Cell Neurosci* 2002;21:436-53.
[15]   Batchelor PE, Liberatore GT, Wong JY, Porritt MJ, Frerichs F, Donnan GA, et al. Activated macrophages and microglia induce dopaminergic sprouting in the injured striatum and express brain-derived neurotrophic factor and glial cell line-derived neurotrophic factor. *J Neurosci* 1999;19:1708-16.

[16]   McGeer PL, McGeer EG. Innate immunity, local inflammation, and degenerative disease. *Sci Aging Knowledge Environ* 2002;2002:re3.

[17]   Banati RB, Daniel SE, Blunt SB. Glial pathology but absence of apoptotic nigral neurons in long-standing Parkinson's disease. *Mov Disord* 1998;13:221-7.

[18]   Wahl LM, Shankavaram U, Zhang Y. Role of macrophages in vascular tissue remodelling. *Transpl Immunol* 1997;5:173-6.

[19]   Takeda K, Kaisho T, Akira S. Toll-like receptors. *Annu Rev Immunol* 2003;21:335-76.

[20]   Wang PY, Munford RS. CD14-dependent internalization and metabolism of extracellular phosphatidylinositol by monocytes. *J Biol Chem* 1999;274:23235-41.

[21]   Callahan MK, Halleck MS, Krahling S, Henderson AJ, Williamson P, Schlegel RA. Phosphatidylserine expression and phagocytosis of apoptotic thymocytes during differentiation of monocytic cells. *J Leukoc Biol* 2003;74:846-56.

[22]   Croisier E, Moran LB, Dexter DT, Pearce RK, Graeber MB. Microglial inflammation in the parkinsonian substantia nigra: relationship to alpha-synuclein deposition. *J Neuroinflammation* 2005;2:14.

[23]   Teismann P, Tieu K, Choi DK, Wu DC, Naini A, Hunot S, et al. Cyclooxygenase-2 is instrumental in Parkinson's disease neurodegeneration. *Proc Natl Acad Sci U S A* 2003;100:5473-8.

[24]   Vila M, Jackson-Lewis V, Guegan C, Wu DC, Teismann P, Choi DK, et al. The role of glial cells in Parkinson's disease. *Curr Opin Neurol* 2001;14:483-9.

[25]   Yamada T, McGeer PL, McGeer EG. Lewy bodies in Parkinson's disease are recognized by antibodies to complement proteins. *Acta Neuropathol (Berl)* 1992;84:100-4.

[26]   McGeer PL, Itagaki S, Boyes BE, McGeer EG. Reactive microglia are positive for HLA-DR in the substantia nigra of Parkinson's and Alzheimer's disease brains. *Neurology* 1988;38:1285-91.

[27]   Hunot S, Hirsch EC. Neuroinflammatory processes in Parkinson's disease. *Ann Neurol* 2003;53 Suppl 3:S49-58; discussion S58-60.

[28]   Mogi M, Harada M, Kondo T, Riederer P, Nagatsu T. Brain beta 2-microglobulin levels are elevated in the striatum in Parkinson's disease. *J Neural Transm Park Dis Dement Sect* 1995;9:87-92.

[29]   Nagatsu T, Mogi M, Ichinose H, Togari A. Changes in cytokines and neurotrophins in Parkinson's disease. *J Neural Transm Suppl* 2000:277-90.

[30]   Boka G, Anglade P, Wallach D, Javoy-Agid F, Agid Y, Hirsch EC. Immunocytochemical analysis of tumor necrosis factor and its receptors in Parkinson's disease. *Neurosci Lett* 1994;172:151-4.

[31]   Hunot S, Dugas N, Faucheux B, Hartmann A, Tardieu M, Debre P, et al. FcepsilonRII/CD23 is expressed in Parkinson's disease and induces, in vitro, production of nitric oxide and tumor necrosis factor-alpha in glial cells. *J Neurosci* 1999;19:3440-7.

[32]   McGeer PL, Itagaki S, Akiyama H, McGeer EG. Rate of cell death in parkinsonism indicates active neuropathological process. *Ann Neurol* 1988;24:574-6.

[33] Mirza B, Hadberg H, Thomsen P, Moos T. The absence of reactive astrocytosis is indicative of a unique inflammatory process in Parkinson's disease. *Neuroscience* 2000;95:425-32.

[34] Imamura K, Hishikawa N, Sawada M, Nagatsu T, Yoshida M, Hashizume Y. Distribution of major histocompatibility complex class II-positive microglia and cytokine profile of Parkinson's disease brains. *Acta Neuropathol (Berl)* 2003;106:518-26.

[35] Knott C, Stern G, Wilkin GP. Inflammatory regulators in Parkinson's disease: iNOS, lipocortin-1, and cyclooxygenases-1 and -2. *Mol Cell Neurosci* 2000;16:724-39.

[36] Lawson LJ, Perry VH, Dri P, Gordon S. Heterogeneity in the distribution and morphology of microglia in the normal adult mouse brain. *Neuroscience* 1990;39:151-70.

[37] Chen H, Zhang SM, Hernan MA, Schwarzschild MA, Willett WC, Colditz GA, et al. Nonsteroidal anti-inflammatory drugs and the risk of Parkinson disease. *Arch Neurol* 2003;60:1059-64.

[38] Hald A, Lotharius J. Oxidative stress and inflammation in Parkinson's disease: is there a causal link? *Exp Neurol* 2005;193:279-90.

[39] Wu DC, Teismann P, Tieu K, Vila M, Jackson-Lewis V, Ischiropoulos H, et al. NADPH oxidase mediates oxidative stress in the 1-methyl-4-phenyl-1,2,3,6-tetrahydropyridine model of Parkinson's disease. *Proc Natl Acad Sci U S A* 2003;100:6145-50.

[40] Babior BM. NADPH oxidase: an update. *Blood* 1999;93:1464-76.

[41] Hurley SD, O'Banion MK, Song DD, Arana FS, Olschowka JA, Haber SN. Microglial response is poorly correlated with neurodegeneration following chronic, low-dose MPTP administration in monkeys. *Exp Neurol* 2003;184:659-68.

[42] Langston JW, Ballard P, Tetrud JW, Irwin I. Chronic Parkinsonism in humans due to a product of meperidine-analog synthesis. *Science* 1983;219:979-80.

[43] Langston JW, Forno LS, Tetrud J, Reeves AG, Kaplan JA, Karluk D. Evidence of active nerve cell degeneration in the substantia nigra of humans years after 1-methyl-4-phenyl-1,2,3,6-tetrahydropyridine exposure. *Ann Neurol* 1999;46:598-605.

[44] Babcock AA, Kuziel WA, Rivest S, Owens T. Chemokine expression by glial cells directs leukocytes to sites of axonal injury in the CNS. *J Neurosci* 2003;23:7922-30.

[45] Wyss-Coray T, Mucke L. Inflammation in neurodegenerative disease--a double-edged sword. *Neuron* 2002;35:419-32.

[46] Huh GS, Boulanger LM, Du H, Riquelme PA, Brotz TM, Shatz CJ. Functional requirement for class I MHC in CNS development and plasticity. *Science* 2000;290:2155-9.

[47] Syken J, Shatz CJ. Expression of T cell receptor beta locus in central nervous system neurons. *Proc Natl Acad Sci U S A* 2003;100:13048-53.

[48] Nishiyori A, Hanno Y, Saito M, Yoshihara Y. Aberrant transcription of unrearranged T-cell receptor beta gene in mouse brain. *J Comp Neurol* 2004;469:214-26.

[49] Foster JA, Quan N, Stern EL, Kristensson K, Herkenham M. Induced neuronal expression of class I major histocompatibility complex mRNA in acute and chronic inflammation models. *J Neuroimmunol* 2002;131:83-91.

[50] Cabarrocas J, Bauer J, Piaggio E, Liblau R, Lassmann H. Effective and selective immune surveillance of the brain by MHC class I-restricted cytotoxic T lymphocytes. *Eur J Immunol* 2003;33:1174-82.

[51] Schori H, Yoles E, Wheeler LA, Raveh T, Kimchi A, Schwartz M. Immune-related mechanisms participating in resistance and susceptibility to glutamate toxicity. *Eur J Neurosci* 2002;16:557-64.

[52] Kipnis J, Yoles E, Schori H, Hauben E, Shaked I, Schwartz M. Neuronal survival after CNS insult is determined by a genetically encoded autoimmune response. *J Neurosci* 2001;21:4564-71.

[53] Serpe CJ, Kohm AP, Huppenbauer CB, Sanders VM, Jones KJ. Exacerbation of facial motoneuron loss after facial nerve transection in severe combined immunodeficient (scid) mice. *J Neurosci* 1999;19:1-5.

[54] Stalder AK, Carson MJ, Pagenstecher A, Asensio VC, Kincaid C, Benedict M, et al. Late-onset chronic inflammatory encephalopathy in immune-competent and severe combined immune-deficient (SCID) mice with astrocyte-targeted expression of tumor necrosis factor. *Am J Pathol* 1998;153:767-83.

[55] Ransohoff RM, Kivisakk P, Kidd G. Three or more routes for leukocyte migration into the central nervous system. *Nat Rev Immunol* 2003;3:569-81.

[56] Aloisi F, Ambrosini E, Columba-Cabezas S, Magliozzi R, Serafini B. Intracerebral regulation of immune responses. *Ann Med* 2001;33:510-5.

[57] Wekerle H, Linington C, Lassmann H, Meyermann R. Cellular immune reactivity within the CNS. *Trends Neurosci* 1986;9:271-7.

[58] Bas J, Calopa M, Mestre M, Mollevi DG, Cutillas B, Ambrosio S, et al. Lymphocyte populations in Parkinson's disease and in rat models of parkinsonism. *J Neuroimmunol* 2001;113:146-52.

[59] Hisanaga K, Asagi M, Itoyama Y, Iwasaki Y. Increase in peripheral CD4 bright+ CD8 dull+ T cells in Parkinson disease. *Arch Neurol* 2001;58:1580-3.

[60] Fiszer U, Mix E, Fredrikson S, Kostulas V, Link H. Parkinson's disease and immunological abnormalities: increase of HLA-DR expression on monocytes in cerebrospinal fluid and of CD45RO+ T cells in peripheral blood. *Acta Neurol Scand* 1994;90:160-6.

[61] Bongioanni P, Castagna M, Maltinti S, Boccardi B, Dadone F. T-lymphocyte tumor necrosis factor-alpha receptor binding in patients with Parkinson's disease. *J Neurol Sci* 1997;149:41-5.

[62] Bongioanni P, Mondino C, Borgna M, Boccardi B, Sposito R, Castagna M. T-lymphocyte immuno-interferon binding in parkinsonian patients. *J Neural Transm* 1997;104:199-207.

[63] Bernabei P, Allione A, Rigamonti L, Bosticardo M, Losana G, Borghi I, et al. Regulation of interferon-gamma receptor (INF-gammaR) chains: a peculiar way to rule the life and death of human lymphocytes. *Eur Cytokine Netw* 2001;12:6-14.

[64] Cerutti PA. Prooxidant states and tumor promotion. *Science* 1985;227:375-81.

[65] Petrozzi L, Lucetti C, Scarpato R, Gambaccini G, Trippi F, Bernardini S, et al. Cytogenetic alterations in lymphocytes of Alzheimer's disease and Parkinson's disease patients. *Neurol Sci* 2002;23 Suppl 2:S97-8.

[66] Migliore L, Petrozzi L, Lucetti C, Gambaccini G, Bernardini S, Scarpato R, et al. Oxidative damage and cytogenetic analysis in leukocytes of Parkinson's disease patients. *Neurology* 2002;58:1809-15.

[67] Mogi M, Harada M, Riederer P, Narabayashi H, Fujita K, Nagatsu T. Tumor necrosis factor-alpha (TNF-alpha) increases both in the brain and in the cerebrospinal fluid from parkinsonian patients. *Neurosci Lett* 1994;165:208-10.

[68] Blum-Degen D, Muller T, Kuhn W, Gerlach M, Przuntek H, Riederer P. Interleukin-1 beta and interleukin-6 are elevated in the cerebrospinal fluid of Alzheimer's and de novo Parkinson's disease patients. *Neurosci Lett* 1995;202:17-20.

[69] Mogi M, Harada M, Kondo T, Riederer P, Inagaki H, Minami M, et al. Interleukin-1 beta, interleukin-6, epidermal growth factor and transforming growth factor-alpha are elevated in the brain from parkinsonian patients. *Neurosci Lett* 1994;180:147-50.

[70] Muller T, Blum-Degen D, Przuntek H, Kuhn W. Interleukin-6 levels in cerebrospinal fluid inversely correlate to severity of Parkinson's disease. *Acta Neurol Scand* 1998;98:142-4.

[71] Araujo DM, Lapchak PA. Induction of immune system mediators in the hippocampal formation in Alzheimer's and Parkinson's diseases: selective effects on specific interleukins and interleukin receptors. *Neuroscience* 1994;61:745-54.

[72] Hanisch UK, Quirion R. Interleukin-2 as a neuroregulatory cytokine. *Brain Res Brain Res Rev* 1995;21:246-84.

[73] Locksley RM, Wilson CB, Klebanoff SJ. Increased respiratory burst in myeloperoxidase-deficient monocytes. *Blood* 1983;62:902-9.

[74] Sankarapandi S, Zweier JL, Mukherjee G, Quinn MT, Huso DL. Measurement and characterization of superoxide generation in microglial cells: evidence for an NADPH oxidase-dependent pathway. *Arch Biochem Biophys* 1998;353:312-21.

[75] Ischiropoulos H, Beckman JS. Oxidative stress and nitration in neurodegeneration: cause, effect, or association? *J Clin Invest* 2003;111:163-9.

[76] MacMicking JD, North RJ, LaCourse R, Mudgett JS, Shah SK, Nathan CF. Identification of nitric oxide synthase as a protective locus against tuberculosis. *Proc Natl Acad Sci U S A* 1997;94:5243-8.

[77] MacMicking J, Xie QW, Nathan C. Nitric oxide and macrophage function. *Annu Rev Immunol* 1997;15:323-50.

[78] Dawson VL, Dawson TM. Nitric oxide in neurodegeneration. *Prog Brain Res* 1998;118:215-29.

[79] Samdani AF, Dawson TM, Dawson VL. Nitric oxide synthase in models of focal ischemia. *Stroke* 1997;28:1283-8.

[80] Brown GC, Bal-Price A. Inflammatory neurodegeneration mediated by nitric oxide, glutamate, and mitochondria. *Mol Neurobiol* 2003;27:325-55.

[81] Liberatore GT, Jackson-Lewis V, Vukosavic S, Mandir AS, Vila M, McAuliffe WG, et al. Inducible nitric oxide synthase stimulates dopaminergic neurodegeneration in the MPTP model of Parkinson disease. *Nat Med* 1999;5:1403-9.

[82] Przedborski S, Jackson-Lewis V, Yokoyama R, Shibata T, Dawson VL, Dawson TM. Role of neuronal nitric oxide in 1-methyl-4-phenyl-1,2,3,6-tetrahydropyridine (MPTP)-induced dopaminergic neurotoxicity. *Proc Natl Acad Sci U S A* 1996;93:4565-71.

[83] Chung KK, Thomas B, Li X, Pletnikova O, Troncoso JC, Marsh L, et al. S-nitrosylation of parkin regulates ubiquitination and compromises parkin's protective function. *Science* 2004;304:1328-31.

[84] Dringen R. Glutathione metabolism and oxidative stress in neurodegeneration. *Eur J Biochem* 2000;267:4903.

[85] Winterbourn CC, Metodiewa D. The reaction of superoxide with reduced glutathione. *Arch Biochem Biophys* 1994;314:284-90.

[86] Chance B, Sies H, Boveris A. Hydroperoxide metabolism in mammalian organs. *Physiol Rev* 1979;59:527-605.

[87] Sian J, Dexter DT, Lees AJ, Daniel S, Agid Y, Javoy-Agid F, et al. Alterations in glutathione levels in Parkinson's disease and other neurodegenerative disorders affecting basal ganglia. *Ann Neurol* 1994;36:348-55.

[88] Sofic E, Lange KW, Jellinger K, Riederer P. Reduced and oxidized glutathione in the substantia nigra of patients with Parkinson's disease. *Neurosci Lett* 1992;142:128-30.

[89] Perry TL, Yong VW. Idiopathic Parkinson's disease, progressive supranuclear palsy and glutathione metabolism in the substantia nigra of patients. *Neurosci Lett* 1986;67:269-74.

[90] Riederer P, Sofic E, Rausch WD, Schmidt B, Reynolds GP, Jellinger K, et al. Transition metals, ferritin, glutathione, and ascorbic acid in parkinsonian brains. *J Neurochem* 1989;52:515-20.

[91] Jenner P. Altered mitochondrial function, iron metabolism and glutathione levels in Parkinson's disease. *Acta Neurol Scand Suppl* 1993;146:6-13.

[92] Pearce RK, Owen A, Daniel S, Jenner P, Marsden CD. Alterations in the distribution of glutathione in the substantia nigra in Parkinson's disease. *J Neural Transm* 1997;104:661-77.

[93] Bharath S, Hsu M, Kaur D, Rajagopalan S, Andersen JK. Glutathione, iron and Parkinson's disease. *Biochem Pharmacol* 2002;64:1037-48.

[94] Nakamura J, Bannai S. Glutathione alters the mode of calcium-mediated regulation of adenylyl cyclase in membranes from mouse brain. *Biochim Biophys Acta* 1997;1339:239-46.

[95] Sian J, Dexter DT, Lees AJ, Daniel S, Jenner P, Marsden CD. Glutathione-related enzymes in brain in Parkinson's disease. *Ann Neurol* 1994;36:356-61.

[96] Damier P, Hirsch EC, Zhang P, Agid Y, Javoy-Agid F. Glutathione peroxidase, glial cells and Parkinson's disease. *Neuroscience* 1993;52:1-6.

[97] Kang Y, Viswanath V, Jha N, Qiao X, Mo JQ, Andersen JK. Brain gamma-glutamyl cysteine synthetase (GCS) mRNA expression patterns correlate with regional-specific enzyme activities and glutathione levels. *J Neurosci Res* 1999;58:436-41.

[98] Abbott LC, Nejad HH, Bottje WG, Hassan AS. Glutathione levels in specific brain regions of genetically epileptic (tg/tg) mice. *Brain Res Bull* 1990;25:629-31.

[99] Chen TS, Richie JP, Jr., Lang CA. The effect of aging on glutathione and cysteine levels in different regions of the mouse brain. *Proc Soc Exp Biol Med* 1989;190:399-402.

[100] Spencer JP, Jenner P, Halliwell B. Superoxide-dependent depletion of reduced glutathione by L-DOPA and dopamine. Relevance to Parkinson's disease. *Neuroreport* 1995;6:1480-4.

[101] Shen XM, Dryhurst G. Further insights into the influence of L-cysteine on the oxidation chemistry of dopamine: reaction pathways of potential relevance to Parkinson's disease. *Chem Res Toxicol* 1996;9:751-63.

[102] Spencer JP, Jenner P, Daniel SE, Lees AJ, Marsden DC, Halliwell B. Conjugates of catecholamines with cysteine and GSH in Parkinson's disease: possible mechanisms of formation involving reactive oxygen species. *J Neurochem* 1998;71:2112-22.

[103] Chen Y, Vartiainen NE, Ying W, Chan PH, Koistinaho J, Swanson RA. Astrocytes protect neurons from nitric oxide toxicity by a glutathione-dependent mechanism. *J Neurochem* 2001;77:1601-10.

[104] Ibi M, Sawada H, Kume T, Katsuki H, Kaneko S, Shimohama S, et al. Depletion of intracellular glutathione increases susceptibility to nitric oxide in mesencephalic dopaminergic neurons. *J Neurochem* 1999;73:1696-703.

[105] Aoyama K, Matsubara K, Fujikawa Y, Nagahiro Y, Shimizu K, Umegae N, et al. Nitration of manganese superoxide dismutase in cerebrospinal fluids is a marker for peroxynitrite-mediated oxidative stress in neurodegenerative diseases. *Ann Neurol* 2000;47:524-7.

[106] Shergill JK, Cammack R, Cooper CE, Cooper JM, Mann VM, Schapira AH. Detection of nitrosyl complexes in human substantia nigra, in relation to Parkinson's disease. *Biochem Biophys Res Commun* 1996;228:298-305.

[107] Good PF, Hsu A, Werner P, Perl DP, Olanow CW. Protein nitration in Parkinson's disease. *J Neuropathol Exp Neurol* 1998;57:338-42.

[108] Giasson BI, Duda JE, Murray IV, Chen Q, Souza JM, Hurtig HI, et al. Oxidative damage linked to neurodegeneration by selective alpha-synuclein nitration in synucleinopathy lesions. *Science* 2000;290:985-9.

[109] Duda JE, Giasson BI, Chen Q, Gur TL, Hurtig HI, Stern MB, et al. Widespread nitration of pathological inclusions in neurodegenerative synucleinopathies. *Am J Pathol* 2000;157:1439-45.

[110] Yao D, Gu Z, Nakamura T, Shi ZQ, Ma Y, Gaston B, et al. Nitrosative stress linked to sporadic Parkinson's disease: S-nitrosylation of parkin regulates its E3 ubiquitin ligase activity. *Proc Natl Acad Sci U S A* 2004;101:10810-4.

[111] Floor E, Wetzel MG. Increased protein oxidation in human substantia nigra pars compacta in comparison with basal ganglia and prefrontal cortex measured with an improved dinitrophenylhydrazine assay. *J Neurochem* 1998;70:268-75.

[112] Alam ZI, Daniel SE, Lees AJ, Marsden DC, Jenner P, Halliwell B. A generalised increase in protein carbonyls in the brain in Parkinson's but not incidental Lewy body disease. *J Neurochem* 1997;69:1326-9.

[113] Schipper HM, Liberman A, Stopa EG. Neural heme oxygenase-1 expression in idiopathic Parkinson's disease. *Exp Neurol* 1998;150:60-8.

[114] Castellani R, Smith MA, Richey PL, Perry G. Glycoxidation and oxidative stress in Parkinson disease and diffuse Lewy body disease. *Brain Res* 1996;737:195-200.

[115] Loft S, Poulsen HE. Cancer risk and oxidative DNA damage in man. *J Mol Med* 1996;74:297-312.

[116] Sanchez-Ramos JR, Overvik E, Ames BN. A marker of oxyradical-mediated DNA damage (8-hydroxy-2 '-deoxyguanosine) is increased in nigro-striatum of Parkinson's disease brain. *Neurodegeneration* 1994;3:197-204.

[117] Alam ZI, Jenner A, Daniel SE, Lees AJ, Cairns N, Marsden CD, et al. Oxidative DNA damage in the parkinsonian brain: an apparent selective increase in 8-hydroxyguanine levels in substantia nigra. *J Neurochem* 1997;69:1196-203.

[118] Zhang J, Perry G, Smith MA, Robertson D, Olson SJ, Graham DG, et al. Parkinson's disease is associated with oxidative damage to cytoplasmic DNA and RNA in substantia nigra neurons. *Am J Pathol* 1999;154:1423-9.

[119] Shimura-Miura H, Hattori N, Kang D, Miyako K, Nakabeppu Y, Mizuno Y. Increased 8-oxo-dGTPase in the mitochondria of substantia nigral neurons in Parkinson's disease. *Ann Neurol* 1999;46:920-4.

[120] Abe T, Isobe C, Murata T, Sato C, Tohgi H. Alteration of 8-hydroxyguanosine concentrations in the cerebrospinal fluid and serum from patients with Parkinson's disease. *Neurosci Lett* 2003;336:105-8.

[121] Kikuchi A, Takeda A, Onodera H, Kimpara T, Hisanaga K, Sato N, et al. Systemic increase of oxidative nucleic acid damage in Parkinson's disease and multiple system atrophy. *Neurobiol Dis* 2002;9:244-8.

[122] Esterbauer H, Schaur RJ, Zollner H. Chemistry and biochemistry of 4-hydroxynonenal, malonaldehyde and related aldehydes. *Free Radic Biol Med* 1991;11:81-128.

[123] Uchida K, Stadtman ER. Modification of histidine residues in proteins by reaction with 4-hydroxynonenal. *Proc Natl Acad Sci U S A* 1992;89:4544-8.

[124] Yoritaka A, Hattori N, Uchida K, Tanaka M, Stadtman ER, Mizuno Y. Immunohistochemical detection of 4-hydroxynonenal protein adducts in Parkinson disease. *Proc Natl Acad Sci U S A* 1996;93:2696-701.

[125] Castellani RJ, Perry G, Siedlak SL, Nunomura A, Shimohama S, Zhang J, et al. Hydroxynonenal adducts indicate a role for lipid peroxidation in neocortical and brainstem Lewy bodies in humans. *Neurosci Lett* 2002;319:25-8.

[126] Zarkovic K. 4-hydroxynonenal and neurodegenerative diseases. *Mol Aspects Med* 2003;24:293-303.

[127] Okamoto K, Toyokuni S, Uchida K, Ogawa O, Takenewa J, Kakehi Y, et al. Formation of 8-hydroxy-2'-deoxyguanosine and 4-hydroxy-2-nonenal-modified proteins in human renal-cell carcinoma. *Int J Cancer* 1994;58:825-9.

[128] Toyokuni S, Uchida K, Okamoto K, Hattori-Nakakuki Y, Hiai H, Stadtman ER. Formation of 4-hydroxy-2-nonenal-modified proteins in the renal proximal tubules of rats treated with a renal carcinogen, ferric nitrilotriacetate. *Proc Natl Acad Sci U S A* 1994;91:2616-20.

[129] Picklo MJ, Amarnath V, McIntyre JO, Graham DG, Montine TJ. 4-Hydroxy-2(E)-nonenal inhibits CNS mitochondrial respiration at multiple sites. *J Neurochem* 1999;72:1617-24.

[130] Liu W, Kato M, Akhand AA, Hayakawa A, Suzuki H, Miyata T, et al. 4-hydroxynonenal induces a cellular redox status-related activation of the caspase cascade for apoptotic cell death. *J Cell Sci* 2000;113:635-41.

[131] Camandola S, Poli G, Mattson MP. The lipid peroxidation product 4-hydroxy-2,3-nonenal inhibits constitutive and inducible activity of nuclear factor kappa B in neurons. *Brain Res Mol Brain Res* 2000;85:53-60.

[132] Okada K, Wangpoengtrakul C, Osawa T, Toyokuni S, Tanaka K, Uchida K. 4-Hydroxy-2-nonenal-mediated impairment of intracellular proteolysis during oxidative stress. Identification of proteasomes as target molecules. *J Biol Chem* 1999;274:23787-93.

[133] Hyun DH, Lee M, Halliwell B, Jenner P. Proteasomal inhibition causes the formation of protein aggregates containing a wide range of proteins, including nitrated proteins. *J Neurochem* 2003;86:363-73.

[134] Hyun DH, Lee MH, Halliwell B, Jenner P. Proteasomal dysfunction induced by 4-hydroxy-2,3-trans-nonenal, an end-product of lipid peroxidation: a mechanism contributing to neurodegeneration? *J Neurochem* 2002;83:360-70.

[135] Benzie IF. Lipid peroxidation: a review of causes, consequences, measurement and dietary influences. *Int J Food Sci Nutr* 1996;47:233-61.

[136] Valenzuela A. The biological significance of malondialdehyde determination in the assessment of tissue oxidative stress. *Life Sci* 1991;48:301-9.

[137] Marnett LJ. Chemistry and biology of DNA damage by malondialdehyde. *IARC Sci Publ* 1999:17-27.

[138] Bermejo P, Gomez-Serranillos P, Santos J, Pastor E, Gil P, Martin-Aragon S. Determination of malonaldehyde in Alzheimer's disease: a comparative study of high-performance liquid chromatography and thiobarbituric acid test. *Gerontology* 1997;43:218-22.

[139] Dexter DT, Carter CJ, Wells FR, Javoy-Agid F, Agid Y, Lees A, et al. Basal lipid peroxidation in substantia nigra is increased in Parkinson's disease. *J Neurochem* 1989;52:381-9.

[140] Dexter DT, Holley AE, Flitter WD, Slater TF, Wells FR, Daniel SE, et al. Increased levels of lipid hydroperoxides in the parkinsonian substantia nigra: an HPLC and ESR study. *Mov Disord* 1994;9:92-7.

[141] Ilic TV, Jovanovic M, Jovicic A, Tomovic M. Oxidative stress indicators are elevated in de novo Parkinson's disease patients. *Funct Neurol* 1999;14:141-7.

[142] Fessel JP, Hulette C, Powell S, Roberts LJ, 2nd, Zhang J. Isofurans, but not F2-isoprostanes, are increased in the substantia nigra of patients with Parkinson's disease and with dementia with Lewy body disease. *J Neurochem* 2003;85:645-50.

[143] Montuschi P, Barnes PJ, Roberts LJ, 2nd. Isoprostanes: markers and mediators of oxidative stress. *Faseb J* 2004;18:1791-800.

[144] Roberts LJ, 2nd, Fessel JP, Davies SS. The biochemistry of the isoprostane, neuroprostane, and isofuran Pathways of lipid peroxidation. *Brain Pathol* 2005;15:143-8.

[145] Pratico D, Lee VM-Y, Trojanowski JQ, Rokach J, Fitzgerald GA. Increased F2-isoprostanes in Alzheimer's disease: evidence for enhanced lipid peroxidation in vivo. *Faseb J* 1998;12:1777-83.

[146] Dexter DT, Wells FR, Agid F, Agid Y, Lees AJ, Jenner P, et al. Increased nigral iron content in postmortem parkinsonian brain. *Lancet* 1987;2:1219-20.

[147] Sofic E, Riederer P, Heinsen H, Beckmann H, Reynolds GP, Hebenstreit G, et al. Increased iron (III) and total iron content in post mortem substantia nigra of parkinsonian brain. *J Neural Transm* 1988;74:199-205.

[148] Dexter DT, Wells FR, Lees AJ, Agid F, Agid Y, Jenner P, et al. Increased nigral iron content and alterations in other metal ions occurring in brain in Parkinson's disease. *J Neurochem* 1989;52:1830-6.

[149] Hirsch EC, Brandel JP, Galle P, Javoy-Agid F, Agid Y. Iron and aluminum increase in the substantia nigra of patients with Parkinson's disease: an X-ray microanalysis. *J Neurochem* 1991;56:446-51.

[150] Olanow CW. Magnetic resonance imaging in parkinsonism. *Neurol Clin* 1992;10:405-20.

[151] Good PF, Olanow CW, Perl DP. Neuromelanin-containing neurons of the substantia nigra accumulate iron and aluminum in Parkinson's disease: a LAMMA study. *Brain Res* 1992;593:343-6.

[152] Griffiths PD, Dobson BR, Jones GR, Clarke DT. Iron in the basal ganglia in Parkinson's disease. An in vitro study using extended X-ray absorption fine structure and cryo-electron microscopy. *Brain* 1999;122:667-73.

[153] Loeffler DA, Connor JR, Juneau PL, Snyder BS, Kanaley L, DeMaggio AJ, et al. Transferrin and iron in normal, Alzheimer's disease, and Parkinson's disease brain regions. *J Neurochem* 1995;65:710-24.

[154] Griffiths PD, Crossman AR. Distribution of iron in the basal ganglia and neocortex in postmortem tissue in Parkinson's disease and Alzheimer's disease. *Dementia* 1993;4:61-5.

[155] Sofic E, Paulus W, Jellinger K, Riederer P, Youdim MB. Selective increase of iron in substantia nigra zona compacta of parkinsonian brains. *J Neurochem* 1991;56:978-82.

[156] Mann VM, Cooper JM, Daniel SE, Srai K, Jenner P, Marsden CD, et al. Complex I, iron, and ferritin in Parkinson's disease substantia nigra. *Ann Neurol* 1994;36:876-81.

[157] Jellinger K, Paulus W, Grundke-Iqbal I, Riederer P, Youdim MB. Brain iron and ferritin in Parkinson's and Alzheimer's diseases. *J Neural Transm Park Dis Dement Sect* 1990;2:327-40.

[158] Zecca L, Youdim MB, Riederer P, Connor JR, Crichton RR. Iron, brain ageing and neurodegenerative disorders. *Nat Rev Neurosci* 2004;5:863-73.

[159] Yoshida S, Ektessabi A, Fujisawa S. XANES spectroscopy of a single neuron from a patient with Parkinson's disease. *J Synchrotron Radiat* 2001;8:998-1000.

[160] Halliwell B. Role of free radicals in the neurodegenerative diseases: therapeutic implications for antioxidant treatment. *Drugs Aging* 2001;18:685-716.

[161] Kim S, Wing SS, Ponka P. S-nitrosylation of IRP2 regulates its stability via the ubiquitin-proteasome pathway. *Mol Cell Biol* 2004;24:330-7.

[162] Smith SR, Cooperman S, Lavaute T, Tresser N, Ghosh M, Meyron-Holtz E, et al. Severity of neurodegeneration correlates with compromise of iron metabolism in mice with iron regulatory protein deficiencies. *Ann N Y Acad Sci* 2004;1012:65-83.

[163] Li YJ, Scott WK, Hedges DJ, Zhang F, Gaskell PC, Nance MA, et al. Age at onset in two common neurodegenerative diseases is genetically controlled. *Am J Hum Genet* 2002;70:985-93.

[164] Li YJ, Oliveira SA, Xu P, Martin ER, Stenger JE, Scherzer CR, et al. Glutathione S-transferase omega-1 modifies age-at-onset of Alzheimer disease and Parkinson disease. *Hum Mol Genet* 2003;12:3259-67.

[165] Laliberte RE, Perregaux DG, Hoth LR, Rosner PJ, Jordan CK, Peese KM, et al. Glutathione s-transferase omega 1-1 is a target of cytokine release inhibitory drugs and may be responsible for their effect on interleukin-1beta posttranslational processing. *J Biol Chem* 2003;278:16567-78.

[166] Griffin WS, Mrak RE. Interleukin-1 in the genesis and progression of and risk for development of neuronal degeneration in Alzheimer's disease. *J Leukoc Biol* 2002;72:233-8.

[167] Grimaldi LM, Casadei VM, Ferri C, Veglia F, Licastro F, Annoni G, et al. Association of early-onset Alzheimer's disease with an interleukin-1alpha gene polymorphism. *Ann Neurol* 2000;47:361-5.

[168] Noureddine MA, Qin XJ, Oliveira SA, Skelly TJ, van der Walt J, Hauser MA, et al. Association between the neuron-specific RNA-binding protein ELAVL4 and Parkinson disease. *Hum Genet* 2005;117:27-33.

[169] Good PJ. A conserved family of elav-like genes in vertebrates. *Proc Natl Acad Sci U S A* 1995;92:4557-61.

[170] Nishimura M, Mizuta I, Mizuta E, Yamasaki S, Ohta M, Kuno S. Influence of interleukin-1beta gene polymorphisms on age-at-onset of sporadic Parkinson's disease. *Neurosci Lett* 2000;284:73-6.

[171] Mizuta I, Nishimura M, Mizuta E, Yamasaki S, Ohta M, Kuno S, et al. Relation between the high production related allele of the interferon-gamma (IFN-gamma) gene and age at onset of idiopathic Parkinson's disease in Japan. *J Neurol Neurosurg Psychiatry* 2001;71:818-9.

[172] Giasson BI, Lee VM. Are ubiquitination pathways central to Parkinson's disease? *Cell* 2003;114:1-8.

[173] Singleton AB, Farrer M, Johnson J, Singleton A, Hague S, Kachergus J, et al. alpha-Synuclein locus triplication causes Parkinson's disease. *Science* 2003;302:841.

[174] Masliah E, Rockenstein E, Veinbergs I, Mallory M, Hashimoto M, Takeda A, et al. Dopaminergic loss and inclusion body formation in alpha-synuclein mice: implications for neurodegenerative disorders. *Science* 2000;287:1265-9.

[175] Auluck PK, Chan HY, Trojanowski JQ, Lee VM, Bonini NM. Chaperone suppression of alpha-synuclein toxicity in a Drosophila model for Parkinson's disease. *Science* 2002;295:865-8.

[176] Norris EH, Giasson BI, Ischiropoulos H, Lee VM. Effects of oxidative and nitrative challenges on alpha -synuclein fibrillogenesis involve distinct mechanisms of protein modifications. *J Biol Chem* 2003;278:27230-40.

[177] Lindersson E, Beedholm R, Hojrup P, Moos T, Gai W, Hendil KB, et al. Proteasomal inhibition by alpha-synuclein filaments and oligomers. *J Biol Chem* 2004;279:12924-34.

[178] Petrucelli L, O'Farrell C, Lockhart PJ, Baptista M, Kehoe K, Vink L, et al. Parkin protects against the toxicity associated with mutant alpha-synuclein: proteasome dysfunction selectively affects catecholaminergic neurons. *Neuron* 2002;36:1007-19.

[179] Yang Y, Nishimura I, Imai Y, Takahashi R, Lu B. Parkin suppresses dopaminergic neuron-selective neurotoxicity induced by Pael-R in Drosophila. *Neuron* 2003;37:911-24.

[180] Kitada T, Asakawa S, Hattori N, Matsumine H, Yamamura Y, Minoshima S, et al. Mutations in the parkin gene cause autosomal recessive juvenile parkinsonism. *Nature* 1998;392:605-8.

[181] Kurkowska-Jastrzebska I, Wronska A, Kohutnicka M, Czlonkowski A, Czlonkowska A. MHC class II positive microglia and lymphocytic infiltration are present in the substantia nigra and striatum in mouse model of Parkinson's disease. *Acta Neurobiol Exp (Wars)* 1999;59:1-8.

[182] Kurkowska-Jastrzebska I, Wronska A, Kohutnicka M, Czlonkowski A, Czlonkowska A. The inflammatory reaction following 1-methyl-4-phenyl-1,2,3, 6-tetrahydropyridine intoxication in mouse. *Exp Neurol* 1999;156:50-61.

[183] He Y, Appel S, Le W. Minocycline inhibits microglial activation and protects nigral cells after 6-hydroxydopamine injection into mouse striatum. *Brain Res* 2001;909:187-93.

[184] Gao HM, Hong JS, Zhang W, Liu B. Distinct role for microglia in rotenone-induced degeneration of dopaminergic neurons. *J Neurosci* 2002;22:782-90.

[185] Sherer TB, Betarbet R, Kim JH, Greenamyre JT. Selective microglial activation in the rat rotenone model of Parkinson's disease. *Neurosci Lett* 2003;341:87-90.

[186] Gao HM, Jiang J, Wilson B, Zhang W, Hong JS, Liu B. Microglial activation-mediated delayed and progressive degeneration of rat nigral dopaminergic neurons: relevance to Parkinson's disease. *J Neurochem* 2002;81:1285-97.

[187] Kim WG, Mohney RP, Wilson B, Jeohn GH, Liu B, Hong JS. Regional difference in susceptibility to lipopolysaccharide-induced neurotoxicity in the rat brain: role of microglia. *J Neurosci* 2000;20:6309-16.

[188] Ryu JK, Shin WH, Kim J, Joe EH, Lee YB, Cho KG, et al. Trisialoganglioside GT1b induces in vivo degeneration of nigral dopaminergic neurons: role of microglia. *Glia* 2002;38:15-23.

[189] Przedborski S, Jackson-Lewis V, Djaldetti R, Liberatore G, Vila M, Vukosavic S, et al. The parkinsonian toxin MPTP: action and mechanism. *Restor Neurol Neurosci* 2000;16:135-142.

[190] Youdim MB, Grunblatt E, Levites Y, Maor G, Mandel S. Early and late molecular events in neurodegeneration and neuroprotection in Parkinson's disease MPTP model as assessed by cDNA microarray; the role of iron. *Neurotox Res* 2002;4:679-689.

[191] Teismann P, Tieu K, Cohen O, Choi DK, Wu du C, Marks D, et al. Pathogenic role of glial cells in Parkinson's disease. *Mov Disord* 2003;18:121-9.

[192] Grunblatt E, Mandel S, Youdim MB. Neuroprotective strategies in Parkinson's disease using the models of 6-hydroxydopamine and MPTP. *Ann N Y Acad Sci* 2000;899:262-73.

[193] Lorenzl S, Calingasan N, Yang L, Albers DS, Shugama S, Gregorio J, et al. Matrix metalloproteinase-9 is elevated in 1-methyl-4-phenyl-1,2,3,6-tetrahydropyridine-induced parkinsonism in mice. *Neuromolecular Med* 2004;5:119-32.

[194] Shen YQ, Hebert G, Lin LY, Luo YL, Moze E, Li KS, et al. Interleukine-1beta and interleukine-6 levels in striatum and other brain structures after MPTP treatment: influence of behavioral lateralization. *J Neuroimmunol* 2005;158:14-25.

[195] Akiyama H, McGeer PL. Microglial response to 6-hydroxydopamine-induced substantia nigra lesions. *Brain Res* 1989;489:247-53.

[196] Cicchetti F, Brownell AL, Williams K, Chen YI, Livni E, Isacson O. Neuroinflammation of the nigrostriatal pathway during progressive 6-OHDA dopamine degeneration in rats monitored by immunohistochemistry and PET imaging. *Eur J Neurosci* 2002;15:991-8.

[197] Depino AM, Earl C, Kaczmarczyk E, Ferrari C, Besedovsky H, del Rey A, et al. Microglial activation with atypical proinflammatory cytokine expression in a rat model of Parkinson's disease. *Eur J Neurosci* 2003;18:2731-42.

[198] Betarbet R, Sherer TB, MacKenzie G, Garcia-Osuna M, Panov AV, Greenamyre JT. Chronic systemic pesticide exposure reproduces features of Parkinson's disease. *Nat Neurosci* 2000;3:1301-6.

[199] Fleming SM, Zhu C, Fernagut PO, Mehta A, DiCarlo CD, Seaman RL, et al. Behavioral and immunohistochemical effects of chronic intravenous and subcutaneous infusions of varying doses of rotenone. *Exp Neurol* 2004;187:418-29.

[200] Lapointe N, St-Hilaire M, Martinoli MG, Blanchet J, Gould P, Rouillard C, et al. Rotenone induces non-specific central nervous system and systemic toxicity. *Faseb J* 2004;18:717-9.

[201] Brooks AI, Chadwick CA, Gelbard HA, Cory-Slechta DA, Federoff HJ. Paraquat elicited neurobehavioral syndrome caused by dopaminergic neuron loss. *Brain Res* 1999;823:1-10.

[202] Thiruchelvam M, Richfield EK, Baggs RB, Tank AW, Cory-Slechta DA. The nigrostriatal dopaminergic system as a preferential target of repeated exposures to combined paraquat and maneb: implications for Parkinson's disease. *J Neurosci* 2000;20:9207-14.

[203] McCormack AL, Thiruchelvam M, Manning-Bog AB, Thiffault C, Langston JW, Cory-Slechta DA, et al. Environmental risk factors and Parkinson's disease: selective degeneration of nigral dopaminergic neurons caused by the herbicide paraquat. *Neurobiol Dis* 2002;10:119-27.

[204] Manning-Bog AB, McCormack AL, Purisai MG, Bolin LM, Di Monte DA. Alpha-synuclein overexpression protects against paraquat-induced neurodegeneration. *J Neurosci* 2003;23:3095-9.

[205] McCormack AL, Atienza JG, Johnston LC, Andersen JK, Vu S, Di Monte DA. Role of oxidative stress in paraquat-induced dopaminergic cell degeneration. *J Neurochem* 2005;93:1030-7.

[206] Liou HH, Chen RC, Tsai YF, Chen WP, Chang YC, Tsai MC. Effects of paraquat on the substantia nigra of the wistar rats: neurochemical, histological, and behavioral studies. *Toxicol Appl Pharmacol* 1996;137:34-41.

[207] Wu XF, Block ML, Zhang W, Qin L, Wilson B, Zhang WQ, et al. The role of microglia in paraquat-induced dopaminergic neurotoxicity. *Antioxid Redox Signal* 2005;7:654-61.

[208] Iravani MM, Kashefi K, Mander P, Rose S, Jenner P. Involvement of inducible nitric oxide synthase in inflammation-induced dopaminergic neurodegeneration. *Neuroscience* 2002;110:49-58.

[209] Liu B, Du L, Hong JS. Naloxone protects rat dopaminergic neurons against inflammatory damage through inhibition of microglia activation and superoxide generation. *J Pharmacol Exp Ther* 2000;293:607-17.

[210] Ling Z, Gayle DA, Ma SY, Lipton JW, Tong CW, Hong JS, et al. In utero bacterial endotoxin exposure causes loss of tyrosine hydroxylase neurons in the postnatal rat midbrain. *Mov Disord* 2002;17:116-24.

[211] Gayle DA, Ling Z, Tong C, Landers T, Lipton JW, Carvey PM. Lipopolysaccharide (LPS)-induced dopamine cell loss in culture: roles of tumor necrosis factor-alpha, interleukin-1beta, and nitric oxide. *Brain Res Dev Brain Res* 2002;133:27-35.

[212] Qin L, Liu Y, Wang T, Wei SJ, Block ML, Wilson B, et al. NADPH oxidase mediates lipopolysaccharide-induced neurotoxicity and proinflammatory gene expression in activated microglia. *J Biol Chem* 2004;279:1415-21.

[213] Block ML, Wu X, Pei Z, Li G, Wang T, Qin L, et al. Nanometer size diesel exhaust particles are selectively toxic to dopaminergic neurons: the role of microglia, phagocytosis, and NADPH oxidase. *Faseb J* 2004;18:1618-20.

[214] Dehmer T, Lindenau J, Haid S, Dichgans J, Schulz JB. Deficiency of inducible nitric oxide synthase protects against MPTP toxicity in vivo. *J Neurochem* 2000;74:2213-6.

[215] Morale MC, Serra PA, Delogu MR, Migheli R, Rocchitta G, Tirolo C, et al. Glucocorticoid receptor deficiency increases vulnerability of the nigrostriatal dopaminergic system: critical role of glial nitric oxide. *Faseb J* 2004;18:164-6.

[216] Yrjanheikki J, Tikka T, Keinanen R, Goldsteins G, Chan PH, Koistinaho J. A tetracycline derivative, minocycline, reduces inflammation and protects against focal cerebral ischemia with a wide therapeutic window. *Proc Natl Acad Sci U S A* 1999;96:13496-500.

[217] Tikka TM, Koistinaho JE. Minocycline provides neuroprotection against N-methyl-D-aspartate neurotoxicity by inhibiting microglia. *J Immunol* 2001;166:7527-33.

[218] Tikka T, Fiebich BL, Goldsteins G, Keinanen R, Koistinaho J. Minocycline, a tetracycline derivative, is neuroprotective against excitotoxicity by inhibiting activation and proliferation of microglia. *J Neurosci* 2001;21:2580-8.

[219] Wu DC, Jackson-Lewis V, Vila M, Tieu K, Teismann P, Vadseth C, et al. Blockade of microglial activation is neuroprotective in the 1-methyl-4-phenyl-1,2,3,6-tetrahydropyridine mouse model of Parkinson disease. *J Neurosci* 2002;22:1763-71.

[220] Du Y, Ma Z, Lin S, Dodel RC, Gao F, Bales KR, et al. Minocycline prevents nigrostriatal dopaminergic neurodegeneration in the MPTP model of Parkinson's disease. *Proc Natl Acad Sci U S A* 2001;98:14669-74.

[221] Lin S, Zhang Y, Dodel R, Farlow MR, Paul SM, Du Y. Minocycline blocks nitric oxide-induced neurotoxicity by inhibition p38 MAP kinase in rat cerebellar granule neurons. *Neurosci Lett* 2001;315:61-4.

[222] Sanchez Mejia RO, Ona VO, Li M, Friedlander RM. Minocycline reduces traumatic brain injury-mediated caspase-1 activation, tissue damage, and neurological dysfunction. *Neurosurgery* 2001;48:1393-9.

[223] Teismann P, Ferger B. Inhibition of the cyclooxygenase isoenzymes COX-1 and COX-2 provide neuroprotection in the MPTP-mouse model of Parkinson's disease. *Synapse* 2001;39:167-74.

[224] Feng ZH, Wang TG, Li DD, Fung P, Wilson BC, Liu B, et al. Cyclooxygenase-2-deficient mice are resistant to 1-methyl-4-phenyl1, 2, 3, 6-tetrahydropyridine-induced damage of dopaminergic neurons in the substantia nigra. *Neurosci Lett* 2002;329:354-8.

[225] Feng Z, Li D, Fung PC, Pei Z, Ramsden DB, Ho SL. COX-2-deficient mice are less prone to MPTP-neurotoxicity than wild-type mice. *Neuroreport* 2003;14:1927-9.

[226] Klivenyi P, Gardian G, Calingasan NY, Yang L, Beal MF. Additive neuroprotective effects of creatine and a cyclooxygenase 2 inhibitor against dopamine depletion in the 1-methyl-4-phenyl-1,2,3,6-tetrahydropyridine (MPTP) mouse model of Parkinson's disease. *J Mol Neurosci* 2003;21:191-8.

[227] Hunot S, Vila M, Teismann P, Davis RJ, Hirsch EC, Przedborski S, et al. JNK-mediated induction of cyclooxygenase 2 is required for neurodegeneration in a mouse model of Parkinson's disease. *Proc Natl Acad Sci U S A* 2004;101:665-70.

[228] Sanchez-Pernaute R, Ferree A, Cooper O, Yu M, Brownell AL, Isacson O. Selective COX-2 inhibition prevents progressive dopamine neuron degeneration in a rat model of Parkinson's disease. *J Neuroinflammation* 2004;1:6.

[229] Carrasco E, Casper D, Werner P. Dopaminergic neurotoxicity by 6-OHDA and MPP+: differential requirement for neuronal cyclooxygenase activity. *J Neurosci Res* 2005;81:121-31.

[230] Wang T, Pei Z, Zhang W, Liu B, Langenbach R, Lee C, et al. MPP+-induced COX-2 activation and subsequent dopaminergic neurodegeneration. *Faseb J* 2005;19:1134-6.

[231] Lorenzl S, Albers DS, Narr S, Chirichigno J, Beal MF. Expression of MMP-2, MMP-9, and MMP-1 and their endogenous counterregulators TIMP-1 and TIMP-2 in postmortem brain tissue of Parkinson's disease. *Exp Neurol* 2002;178:13-20.

[232] Gu Z, Kaul M, Yan B, Kridel SJ, Cui J, Strongin A, et al. S-nitrosylation of matrix metalloproteinases: signaling pathway to neuronal cell death. *Science* 2002;297:1186-90.

[233] Rachakonda V, Pan TH, Le WD. Biomarkers of neurodegenerative disorders: how good are they? *Cell Res* 2004;14:347-58.

[234] Hayley S, Crocker SJ, Smith PD, Shree T, Jackson-Lewis V, Przedborski S, et al. Regulation of dopaminergic loss by Fas in a 1-methyl-4-phenyl-1,2,3,6-tetrahydropyridine model of Parkinson's disease. *J Neurosci* 2004;24:2045-53.

[235] Martin LJ. Neuronal cell death in nervous system development, disease, and injury (Review). *Int J Mol Med* 2001;7:455-78.

[236] Vila M, Jackson-Lewis V, Vukosavic S, Djaldetti R, Liberatore G, Offen D, et al. Bax ablation prevents dopaminergic neurodegeneration in the 1-methyl- 4-phenyl-1,2,3,6-tetrahydropyridine mouse model of Parkinson's disease. *Proc Natl Acad Sci U S A* 2001;98:2837-42.

[237] Kordower JH, Emborg ME, Bloch J, Ma SY, Chu Y, Leventhal L, et al. Neurodegeneration prevented by lentiviral vector delivery of GDNF in primate models of Parkinson's disease. *Science* 2000;290:767-73.

[238] Patel NK, Bunnage M, Plaha P, Svendsen CN, Heywood P, Gill SS. Intraputamenal infusion of glial cell line-derived neurotrophic factor in PD: a two-year outcome study. *Ann Neurol* 2005;57:298-302.

[239] Breidert T, Callebert J, Heneka MT, Landreth G, Launay JM, Hirsch EC. Protective action of the peroxisome proliferator-activated receptor-gamma agonist pioglitazone in a mouse model of Parkinson's disease. *J Neurochem* 2002;82:615-24.

[240] Angelov DN, Waibel S, Guntinas-Lichius O, Lenzen M, Neiss WF, Tomov TL, et al. Therapeutic vaccine for acute and chronic motor neuron diseases: implications for amyotrophic lateral sclerosis. *Proc Natl Acad Sci U S A* 2003;100:4790-5.

[241] Kipnis J, Mizrahi T, Hauben E, Shaked I, Shevach E, Schwartz M. Neuroprotective autoimmunity: naturally occurring CD4+CD25+ regulatory T cells suppress the ability to withstand injury to the central nervous system. *Proc Natl Acad Sci U S A* 2002;99:15620-5.

[242] Bakalash S, Kipnis J, Yoles E, Schwartz M. Resistance of retinal ganglion cells to an increase in intraocular pressure is immune-dependent. *Invest Ophthalmol Vis Sci* 2002;43:2648-53.

[243] Kipnis J, Yoles E, Porat Z, Cohen A, Mor F, Sela M, et al. T cell immunity to copolymer 1 confers neuroprotection on the damaged optic nerve: possible therapy for optic neuropathies. *Proc Natl Acad Sci U S A* 2000;97:7446-51.

[244] Arnon R, Sela M. Immunomodulation by the copolymer glatiramer acetate. *J Mol Recognit* 2003;16:412-21.

[245] Benner EJ, Mosley RL, Destache CJ, Lewis TB, Jackson-Lewis V, Gorantla S, et al. Therapeutic immunization protects dopaminergic neurons in a mouse model of Parkinson's disease. *Proc Natl Acad Sci U S A* 2004;101:9435-40.

[246] Boska MD, Lewis TB, Destache CJ, Benner EJ, Nelson JA, Uberti M, et al. Quantitative 1H magnetic resonance spectroscopic imaging determines therapeutic immunization efficacy in an animal model of Parkinson's disease. *J Neurosci* 2005;25:1691-700.

In: New Research on Parkinson's Disease
Editors: T. F. Hahn, J. Werner

ISBN: 978-1-60456-601-7
© 2008 Nova Science Publishers, Inc.

Chapter V

Frontal Lobe Mediation of the Sense of Self: Evidence from Studies of Patients with Parkinson's Disease

Patrick McNamara[*], *Raymon Durso* and *Erica Harris*

Department of Neurology (127), Boston University School of Medicine and Veterans, Administration New England Healthcare System, Boston, MA.

Abstract

Recent theoretical accounts of the brain's construction of the sense of Self have described widely distributed neural networks which participate in support of various aspects of the sense of self. In this paper, we suggest that right frontal cortex is a key node in these distributed networks which supports the sense of an enduring Self. Independent evidence suggests that patients with Parkinson's disease (PD) exhibit impairment on cognitive tasks that depend on both the right and left frontal lobes. If the sense of Self requires intact frontal function, then the sense of Self should be impaired in PD, particularly in those patients with right frontal dysfunction. In this paper, we review a series of studies we conducted to examine links between changes in the sense of Self/personality to changes in mood, neuropsychologic and dopaminergic function in PD patients. We used sentence completion tests of identity development ('self-test'), personality inventories and measures of mood, memory and neuropsychologic functioning to assess the sense of Self in PD. We found that Self and personality test responses significantly correlated with performance scores on tests of frontal function but not parietal or temporal lobe function. Patients with predominantly left-sided onset/involvement exhibited a different personality profile and performed poorly on tests of autobiographical memory recall relative to patients with right-sided onset/involvement. We conclude that a healthy autonomous sense of Self depends on intact right frontal function.

[*] Correspondence concerning this article should be addressed to Patrick McNamara, Department of Neurology (127), Boston University School of Medicine and Veterans Administration New England Healthcare System, 150 South Huntington Avenue, Boston, MA 02130 mcnamar@bu.edu, 617-232-9500 x4-5007.

Keywords: Self, ego development, Parkinson's disease, frontal lobes, executive functions, consciousness.

Author Note: This material is based upon work supported in part by the office of Research and Development, Medical Research Service, Department of Veterans Affairs.

Introduction

Throughout the history of Psychology and indeed of all the Human Sciences, the question of the nature and origins of the Self has loomed large. Study of the Self is important for the human sciences as each Self is unique and irreplaceable and thus human dignity is linked with the sense of Self we each experience. In addition, modern cognitive neuroscientific studies of the Self seem to indicate that virtually every higher cognitive function is influenced by the Self: memories are encoded more efficiently when referred to the Self, feelings and affective responses always include the Self, fundamental attributions of intentionality, agency and Mind all concern selves in interaction with other selves and so on. Finally, study of the Self is crucial for understanding many clinical disorders which involve breakdowns in the sense of Self. These disorders may involve dramatic breakdowns in the sense of Self such as schizophrenia or Alzheimer's …or more common disorders of Self such as depression or anxiety where the sense of Self is experienced as chronically under threat or oppressed etc.

The problem of the Self has been somewhat intractable to analysis because the sense of Self is so complex. The sense of Self appears to draw on several psychologic and neuropsychologic domains such as autobiographical memory, emotional and evaluative systems, agency or the sense of being the cause of some action, self-monitoring, bodily-awareness, mind-reading or covert mimicking of other's mental states, subjectivity or perspectivalness in perception, and finally, the sense of unity conferred on consciousness when it is invested with the subjective perspective [1,2,3,4]. Any account of the psychology of Self should at least be consistent with most or all of these properties.

In the absence of a theory that can account for all of the above properties of Self, we argue that carefully considering the neuropsychologic correlates of the sense of Self will help us to narrow down key aspects of the Self that might help us treat clinical disorders of Self (see also [5,6,4]). We draw on our work with patients with Parkinson's Disease (PD) to probe a neuropsychologic system that we hypothesize to be key to the sense of Self: the right frontal cortex. We will describe this system in more detail below. We first review previous work on the potential contributions of the frontal system to realization of the self experience. We then turn to a review of some of our studies with PD patients and conclude with a discussion of the implications of the PD data for theories of the neuropsychologic basis of the Self.

Frontal Lobes and Self

A number of investigators have recently suggested that the human sense of self depends crucially on prefrontal cortex [7,8,9]. A review of the behavioral effects of prefrontal leucotomies led Weingarten [10] to suggest that prefrontal lobes mediate some aspects of social sense of self and autonomy. Families of persons who sustain traumatic brain injury with orbitofrontal lesions invariably report that their relative's identity is profoundly altered, if not destroyed [11]. Similarly, when a dementing process begins to invade basal forebrain and medial frontal sites, personality changes become marked and striking. Miller et al.[12], reported that seven of 72 patients with probable frontal-temporal dementing disorders exhibited a dramatic change in self. In six of these seven patients, the selective dysfunction involved the right frontal region. In contrast, only one of the other 65 patients without selective *right* frontal dysfunction showed a change in self.

Experimental and functional imaging studies have also pointed to the frontal lobes as crucial for the sense of self. Right frontal activation has recently been associated with experience of the self itself [8]. Craik et al. showed that right frontal sites were activated whenever subjects processed or memorized materials referring to the self. Similarly, Fink et al., [13]reported selective activation of right prefrontal cortical regions in subjects engaged in recall of personal versus impersonal long term episodic memories. In a more recent functional imaging study, Kelley et al.[14] confirmed that self-referential processing could be functionally dissociated from other forms of semantic processing within the human brain. Volunteers were imaged while making judgments about trait adjectives under three experimental conditions (self-relevance, other-relevance, or case judgment). Relevance judgments, when compared to case judgments, were accompanied by activation of the left inferior frontal cortex and the anterior cingulate. A separate region of the medial prefrontal cortex was selectively engaged during self-referential processing implying that medial prefrontal sites support self-related information processing functions. In a seminal review of PET studies on episodic encoding and retrieval processes, Wheeler, Stuss and Tulving [15] (see also [16]) conclude that episodic retrieval of personal memories is associated with an increased blood flow in the right frontal cortex with no increased blood flow in the left frontal cortex; while episodic encoding is associated with the opposite pattern, i.e., increased flow in left-frontal cortex and no increased flow in right frontal cortex. They call this set of findings HERA for hemispheric encoding/retrieval asymmetry.

In summary, a number of clinical, neuroimaging and experimental studies of brain systems that contribute to the sense of self have all tended to point to the frontal lobes as key. Right frontal cortex appears to be particularly important-at least with respect to personal recall and consciousness. Because Parkinson's disease is associated with mild to severe frontal lobe dysfunction, and asymmetric PD is associated with predominantly right-sided or left-sided frontal dysfunction (depending on the patient) the question arises as to whether the sense of self would be impaired in PD, particularly in patients with left-sided onset (or right sided disease).

Parkinson's Disease (PD)

Parkinson's disease (PD) is characterized by rigidity, bradykinesia, gait disorders, and sometimes tremors. These motor symptoms initially present predominantly on one side of the body and, though poorly understood, this asymmetric disease profile may significantly influence survival rates of PD patients[17], disease severity [18,19], response profiles to levodopa [19,20], and risk for development of neuropsychiatric syndromes and dementia [19]. The prognostic utility of asymmetric disease profiles (e.g., the presence and magnitude of asymmetric disease presentation), in short, may be considerable.

The primary pathology of PD involves loss of dopaminergic cells in the substantia nigra (SN) and in the ventral tegmental area or VTA [21]. These two subcortical dopaminergic sites give rise to two projection systems important for arousal, motor, affective and cognitive functioning. The nigrostriatal system, primarily implicated in motor functions, originates in the pars compacta of the SN and terminates in the striatum. The meso-limbic-cortical system contributes to cognitive and affective functioning. It originates in the VTA and terminates in the ventral striatum, limbic sites, amygdala, frontal lobes, and some other basal forebrain areas. Dopamine levels in the ventral striatum, and frontal lobes are approximately 40% of normal [21,22]. The degree of nigro-striatal impairment correlates with degree of motor impairment while VTA-mesocortical dopaminergic impairment correlates positively with the degree of affective and intellectual impairment [23,24,25] in affected individuals. Although these dopaminergic systems are major contributors to motor and cognitive dysfunction in PD, Lewy body (LB) degeneration and Alzhemier-type changes have been noted in brainstem nuclei, including the noradrenergic locus ceruleus, the serotonergic dorsal raphe nucleus, limbic structures, cholinergic forebrain structures and in cerebral cortex [26,27].

While it is clear that the clinical manifestations of PD are influenced by multiple neurotransmitter systems, the asymmetric symptomology itself appears to be primarily determined by degeneration of dopamine neurons in the substantia nigra pars compacta and its projections to limbic and prefrontal cortex contralateral to the affected side. Animal models have shown asymmetric behavior to be associated with an imbalance of neostriatal dopamine content [28]. SPECT and PET studies in humans, furthermore, have consistently demonstrated correlations between reduced striatal and prefrontal dopaminergic activity contralateral to the clinically more affected side and the motor, mood and cognitive functions associated with that side of the brain [29,30,31].

Frontal Dysfunction in PD

Cognitive dysfunction is typically mild in *early* PD involving a generalized slowing of cognitive processing speed (bradyphrenia) and subtle deficits in so-called executive cognitive functions or ECFs [32,33,34]. ECFs refer to such functions as planning, initiation, attention, monitoring and adjustment of non-routine and goal-directed behaviors. As the disease progresses, however, these ECF deficits become more severe and deficits in selected aspects of language and visuo-spatial functions become evident as well. Relative to age-matched controls, PD patients perform abnormally on tests of planning, switching attentional sets, verbal and semantic fluency, and selected visuo-spatial tasks [35,36,37,38,39]. Longitudinal studies of cognitive change in PD have repeatedly shown that performance on verbal and semantic fluency tasks are characteristic of the preclinical phase of dementia in PD and are significant predictors of dementia in PD [35,40,38,41].

Personality Changes in PD

Many clinicians who specialize in PD have suggested that PD may be associated with a specific personality type – even before the onset of the disease. This 'parkinsonian personality' has been described as compulsive, rigid, punctilious, serious, stoic and introverted and at least one study has found evidence for just such a premorbid personality type in PD [42]. The bulk of the studies of personality in PD, however, concern personality profiles that obtain after disease onset.

Recent studies of personality in patients diagnosed with PD have found strong correlations between the personality traits of 'reduced novelty seeking' and 'increased harm avoidance' with asymmetric disease profiles. Menza and colleagues [29] reported a significant correlation in a sample of 9 PD patients between novelty seeking and 18F-dopa uptake in the left caudate only. Kaasinen et al. [30] on the other hand, reported that the novelty seeking personality trait did not significantly correlate with18F-dopa uptake in any of the brain regions studied. Instead they found a highly significant positive correlation between *right* caudate 18F-dopa uptake and the 'harm avoidance' trait in their sample of 47 PD patients. The higher the harm avoidance (pessimism, fear of uncertainty, and shyness) in Parkinson's disease, the higher the *right-sided* caudate 18F-dopa uptake. More recently, Tomer et al. [43] studied the relation of asymmetric disease profiles on personality characteristics by dividing forty PD patients into two groups according to initial asymmetry in dopamine deficit: left hemisphere, n = 22; right hemisphere, n = 18) and then assessing personality characteristics in the two groups. Tomer et al found that only patients with greater dopamine loss in the left hemisphere showed reduced novelty seeking, whereas only patients with reduced dopamine in the right hemisphere reported higher harm avoidance than matched healthy controls. They explained their findings by drawing on Davidson et al . [44] work on right vs. left frontal networks that support negative-withdrawal and positive-approach (respectively) emotional-motivational systems. Approach and avoidance reflect different patterns of dopaminergic asymmetry. Whereas reduced novelty seeking reflects deficit in the mesolimbic branch of ascending dopamine transmission in the left hemisphere, increased harm avoidance is associated with greater dopamine loss in the right striatum. Menza et al.'s finding that novelty seeking scores were correlated with [18F] dopa uptake in the left, but not right, is consistent with the Davidson et al model of left approach and right withdrawal systems. On the other hand, Kaasinen et al.'s finding of a significant correlation between [18F]dopa uptake in the right caudate and harm avoidance is difficult to explain with the Davidson model if we assume that high right caudate DA would be associated with high left hemispheric dopamine levels and therefore increased approach tendencies (rather than avoidance). Clearly, the issue of asymmetric disease and personality characteristics in PD could be considerably clarified with a prospective examination of changes in asymmetric profiles in relation to changes in personality as the disease progresses in early, mid and late stage PD patients. The asymmetric disease profile in most PD patients would also afford us the chance to evaluate whether right frontal disease has a greater impact on the sense of Self than left frontal disease as our review of the literature above would suggest. We first, however, investigated whether the sense of Self was altered in PD and whether this alteration was correlated selectively with frontal function.

Our Studies

In 1995, we [7] documented a greater variability of responses on a standard 'sense of self' test among PD patients relative to age-matched controls. Unfortunately, we did not simultaneously assess frontal functions in these patients and so could not examine the relation of this variability to frontal lobe performance. In the set of studies we describe next, we were able to explore the relation of the sense of Self in PD as measured in various ways with performance on tests of frontal function.

We tested the hypotheses that 1) sense of self would be impaired in PD and 2) this impairment would be correlated with frontal dysfunction. In the first study, we used Loevinger's et al.'s [45,46] standardized sentence completion task (see below) to explore the sense of self and standardized tests of executive function to tap frontal function. In the second study, we explored the ways in which PD patients use pragmatic aspects of language as key components of pragmatics are thought to be mediated by the right frontal cortex [47]. In the third study, we looked at personality and autobiographical memory changes in PD relative to age-matched controls. To forecast one of our major conclusions, we find that frontal dysfunction is a major correlate of change in the sense of Self in PD while other neuropsychologic systems do not correlate or correlate less strongly with change in Self in PD. Measures of right frontal cortex function, in particular, correlate with change in the sense of Self in PD.

Methods used in all of the following studies are described in detail elsewhere [48,59,50,51]. In brief, patients with PD were recruited from the outpatient Movement Disorders Clinic at the VA New England Healthcare System, Boston, MA. Patients were individually diagnosed by Dr. Raymon Durso, Director of the clinic. Most were male and right-handed. Mean years of duration of disease was typically between 12-14 years. None of these patients were demented according to clinical examinations and DSM-III criteria. All were on some form of dopaminergic medication. Patients with a history of substance abuse or head injury were excluded. Healthy age-matched control participants were recruited from the community and support staff of the same facility and the Boston area community. There were typically no significant differences in education or age between the PD patients and the controls.

In the first study to be described, we were interested in the subjective sense of Self experienced by PD patients. All participants in the study completed a battery of tests that included standardized sense of self/ego development test, three measures of prefrontal function, and one measure of temporal lobe function.

Sense of Self

Loevinger [46] pioneered the study of the sense of self by using a sentence completion procedure to gather data on the development of identity. She and her colleagues [45,46] utilized 36 sentence stems such as "The thing I like about myself is..."; "What gets me into trouble is..." "I am...", etc. After testing hundreds of subjects, Loevinger et al. devised a standardized coding system based on thousands of responses for each stem. The responses were classified into separate categories which seemed to reflect stable personality traits or modes of responding. Loevinger then noticed that these modes were characteristically associated with different age groups and so probably reflected distinct stages in the development of the sense of self or identity. Nevertheless, depending on context, adults at all ages may manifest frequent responses more characteristic of earlier stages of development. This fact makes it possible to use the Loevinger test to identify potentially maladaptive coping strategies in patients with chronic diseases.

The general picture that emerges from Loevinger's analyses of identity development might best be illustrated with a description of typical response modes associated with the "I am..." stem. Impulsive personalities (classified in Loevinger's system as I-2) do not reflect on their responses but tend to provide short, simple and uninformative responses such as "I am nice." or "I am tall." These people tend to dichotomize all events into good and evil categories and prefer not to consider the complexities of social life. They are concerned only with themselves rather than the world but do not hold considered or nuanced views of themselves. At the next stage of ego development ("delta" transitional) the individual seems to become more aware of the world around him but has no sense of the complexities of the world. He is suspicious, self-protective and opportunistic. He eschews responsibility and is pre-occupied with staying out of trouble. His humor is often hostile and rejecting.

The next (I-3) stage of development involves a broad socializing trend. The individual turns towards the world but often in a conformist way. He describes himself only in socially acceptable terms. He uses a kind of self-deprecating and ingratiating humor: e.g. "I am a big mouth". "I am a pain-in-the-butt." He uses broad, sweeping generalizations to describe others. He relies on formulaic and stereotyped responses in social interactions. His focus concerning self is concrete and oriented towards his physical appearance.

The next stage (I-3/4) involves a series of responses that are transitional between conformism and the I-4 stage: "conscientious". The I-3/4 transitional stage is characterized by self-criticism and self-consciousness. The individual's view of the world and himself is now rich and nuanced but negative reactions to self predominate. No simple straightforward responses are given to the "I am..." stem. Instead one gets responses like "I am...impossible to describe." The next stage, I-4 is dubbed "conscientious". There is a rich inner life and true conceptual complexity. The individual has a strong sense of responsibility and has developed a moral sense and standards of excellence. There is a general awareness and orientation towards long-term goals and a restlessness and impatience to reach them.

The I-4/5 transitional stage is characterized by complex responses. The individual provides nuanced descriptions of self. There is a tendency to try to justify all of one's responses. The I-5 "autonomy" stage is characterized by the ability to balance dimensions of personality that seem to be in conflict. The individual cultivates a rich array of preferences, inclinations and behaviors but may not be able to integrate, and thus be enriched by, all these options. The last stage (I-6) is characterized by "integration". Here the individual harmoniously balances opposing tendencies within himself. He enjoys a rich internal life but is oriented to the world and sees service to others as his greatest concern.

We selected 8 of Loevinger's sentence stems to use with our subjects and we used Loevinger, Wessler and Redmore's [45,46] scoring procedures to classify our subject's responses. These scoring procedures have been extensively validated by Loevinger and colleagues [45,46]. Two raters, blind to this study's hypothesis, assigned ego stage classifications to each stem completion, based on these procedures. The two raters scored the first 10 protocols by openly discussing each stem completion and assigning a stage value. After the initial ten protocols, reliability was established, and each rater scored the remaining protocols independently. If the raters had any question about the classification of an individual stem, they would refer to the Loevinger coding manual guidelines and discuss the item together thoroughly until an agreement was made as to which stage assignment would be the most accurate description as defined by Loevinger. Numerical ratings between 1 and 8 were assigned to each subject's responses to the stem completion tests, where 1=impulsive and 8=integrated.

Neuropsychologic Tests

The Animals Category Verbal Fluency Test [52] was used as a measure of semantic and verbal fluency. Participants are asked to generate as many names of animals as they can in the space of one minute. Mean number of words produced per minute is the main outcome measure. Recent reports [53,54] suggest that the two major cognitive strategies subjects employ to perform this task differentially depend on striatal-frontal and temporal lobe systems. The *clustering* strategy or the tendency to generate words within clusters or subcategories, is related to intact temporal lobe functioning; while *switching*, or the tendency to shift between clusters, is related to frontostriatal integrity. In order to directly compare measures that are linked to fronto-striatal functions with a measure of temporal lobe function, we assessed clustering and switching performance on the animals fluency task in both PD patients and Controls. We followed Troyer et al.'s [55] procedures for scoring these elements in fluency performance. If sense of self scores are more strongly correlated with prefrontal systems than with other neuropsychologic systems (such as the temporal lobe networks) then we should find stronger correlations between self and switching scores rather than self and clustering scores.

The Stroop procedure requires the subject to name the color of the ink in which a color-word is printed. Sometimes the word will name the color of the ink (the word blue in blue ink) and sometimes the word will be the name of a different color than the ink (e.g. the 'incongruent' word blue printed in green ink). The subject must ignore the word and name the color. Susceptibility to cognitive interference is calculated as a ratio of the time taken to name the colors in the incongruent condition. PET studies show that right orbitofrontal cortex is predominantly activated in normals during the interference condition [56].

In the Tower of London task disks have to be moved from a starting configuration on three sticks of equal length to a target arrangement in a minimum number of moves. Subjects are asked to rearrange the disks on the sticks so that their positions match the target array (presented as a colored drawing). The starting position, as well as number of the discs are varied so that in any particular trial the solution can only be reached following a minimum number of moves. The subject's task is to solve the problem with the minimum number of possible moves. We used 'mean time elapsed until completion of first move' (a measure of planning), 'mean time per move' (a measure of thinking and problem solving) and overall move accuracy as our outcome measures. SPECT study has demonstrated left prefrontal cortex activation in subjects attempting to plan their moves[57].

There were no significant differences between mean response levels on the Loevinger et al. sense of self stem completion test between the PD patients (M = 3.58 (.6)) and age-matched control participants (M = 3.65 (.6); t = -.275, p = .78) indicating that both groups of participants tended to emit 'conformist' responses or responses transitional to the conscientious stage (see Tables 1 and 2). There were, however, important contrasting patterns in the range of responses emitted by each group (see Table 2). While 12.84% of PD responses were classified as impulsive/self-protective, only 7.5% of control responses were so classified. On the other hand a slightly greater number (24% vs 18%) of PD responses reached the conscientious level (I-4 or above) as compared to control responses. The bulk of PD responses were classified as conformist (36%) or transitional between conformism and conscientious (28%). The corresponding percentages for controls were 41% (conformist) and 32% (transitional). No subject in any group emitted responses that were classified into the highest possible category: "integrated".

Table 1. Comparisons between PD patients and control participants on sense of self and neuropsychologic measures.

Measure	PD	Control	p
Mean SS	3.58(.60)	3.65(.60)	.78
Animals	16.0(5.3)	16.7(5.4)	.76
Clustering	1.6(1.99)	.89(.35)	.14
Switching	8.78(4.3)	8.2(3.8)	.73
Stroop	86.0(20.2)	58.6 (11.2)	.0001
ToMove acc	1.31(.37)	1.32(.29)	.90
Tower 1st	4.90(6.2)	10.1(3.9)	.027
Tower T/move	8.35(11.2)	6.44(4.2)	.59

Note. SS = sense of self test score; Animals = Verbal fluency task; Clustering = mean semantic cluster length in animals task; Switching = total switches in animals task; Stroop = interference time; Tower 1st = mean elapsed time before first move on Tower of London; Tower T/move = mean time per move on Tower of London task;
Value is the mean; value in parenthesis is the standard deviation.

Table 2. Percent of PD patients emitting given ego-level responses by stage of disease.

	Stage # 2 (n=8)	Stage # 3(n=10)
Impulsive (I-2)	7.02%	3.85%
Self Protective (delta-transitional)	12.28%	6.41%
Conformist (I-3)	28.07%	44.87%
Conformist / Conscientious (I-3/4)	24.56%	26.92%
Conscientious (I-4)	28.07%	14.10%
Conscientious/Autonomous (I-4/5)	0%	3.85%
Total	100%	100%

Interestingly, conscientious and conscientious/autonomy responses of PD patients tended to enunciate effective coping strategies. For example, in response to the stem: "When I am nervous..." a typical response was "I sit and think and appreciate the things I have." Or again in response to the stem: "When I am criticized..." response: "I try to sit back and look at the situation and find out what I did wrong," or "I try to understand it objectively, not emotionally." To complete "When I get mad", one patient stated, "I try to control myself, there are two sides to every argument." The Loevinger self-test, however, did not typically elicit examples of coping strategies from control participants. One typical response by controls to the stem "What gets me into trouble..." was: "is worrying about things." For the stem "When I get mad..." a typical response from controls was: "I tend to harbor ill-feelings for a while."

Analysis of 'sense of self' scores as a function of Hoehn-Yahr stage revealed that patients classified into Stage III emitted a greater percentage (an increase of 14%) of conformity responses as compared to stage II patients, and conversely, fewer conscientious responses (decrease of 16%) than Stage II patients (see Table 2).

With respect to tests of neuropsychologic function, we found that PD patients performed significantly more poorly than controls (see Table 1). On the Stroop interference test we found significant differences in mean interference completion times for controls (M=58.6 (11.2) secs) versus PD patients (M-PD patients = 86.0 (20.2) secs; t(25) = 4.51, p = .0001). On the Tower of London task controls were significantly slower or more deliberative in mean (planning) times for first move (M =10.1 (3.9) secs) as compared to PD patients (M-PD patients = 4.90 (6.2) secs; t(19) = -2.39, p = .027). Mean times per move, mean move accuracy and mean verbal fluency scores did not significantly differ between the two groups. We also found no significant differences between controls and patients for either switching or clustering scores. (See Table 1).

Performance on tests of executive function predicted mean self score (see Table 4), but only in the PD group. Among PD patients Stroop interference scores were strongly and inversely related to mean self score (Pearson r = -.72, p = .0001). Mean time per move on the Tower of London was also significantly related (Pearson r = -.436, p = .05) to mean self score, but again only for PD patients. Interestingly, sense of self score was strongly and positively correlated with switching (r = .66, p = .001) but not clustering (r = .16, p = .58) strategies on the category fluency task for PD patients.

Table 3. Mach subscale mean scores for PD vs. controls
(p-values are for one-sided tests).

Variable	Mean (SD)	Mean (SD)	p
Positive interpersonal Tactics	18.2 (4.0)	25.3 (2.8)	.04*
Negative Interpersonal Tactics	13.4 (5.2)	11.5 (3.2)	.12
Positive view of human nature	14.3 (1.4)	13.3 (2.8)	.30
Cynical view of human nature	21.0 (4.2)	16.8 (4.5)	.03*

* p < 0.05

Table 4. Right vs. Left sided onset: Impact on personality and memory.

	Left sided onset (N=8)	Right sided onset (N=7)	P value (Bonferroni-corrected)
Age	67.2 (10.6)	75.4 (7.4)	0.10
MMSE	24.6 (2.5)	26.7 (2.2)	0.12
DASS anxiety	5.3 (3.5)	5.2 (3.2)	0.96
DASS depression	3.8 (2.4)	5.7 (6.0)	0.52
DASS stress	4.8 (3.2)	5.4 (5.4)	0.82
TPQ novelty seeking	19.3 (5.1)	18.4 (5.7)	.74
Harm avoidance	16.3 (7.4)	(14.5 (4.3)	.53
Reward dependence	11.5 (5.3)	16.0 (5.8)	.05*
Persistence	6.0 (1.0)	4.1 (1.5)	.05*
Self-directedness	30.2 (4.9)	33.4 (3.5)	.17
Cooperativeness	32.5 (6.7)	33.8 (5.0)	.66
Self-transcendence	15.3 (6.3)	12.5 (5.5)	.30

* p < 0.05

In summary, we found that the sense of self in patients with PD was not significantly impaired relative to age-matched controls when tested with Loevinger's standardized 'sense of self' stem completion tests. This partially replicates results of McNamara et al. [7] who similarly found no mean differences in sense of self scores between PD patients and age matched controls-despite increased variability of responding among the PD patients. But we also documented a relative increase of 'conformist' responses and a decrease of 'conscientious' responses among Hoehn-Yahr Stage III patients as compared to Stage II patients. While PD patients performed more poorly than controls on tests of executive function, their 'sense of self' scores were significantly related to performance on selected measures of executive function (Stroop interference scores and time per move on the TOL) while controls' responses were not. In addition, while PD self score was strongly related to the 'switching' score (reflecting striatal-frontal function) on the fluency task, it was not significantly related to the clustering score -a measure related to temporal lobe function. We conclude that while the 'sense of self' changes as a function of disease stage in PD, the core experience of a sense of self in PD is intact when compared to age-matched controls, and may depend, in part, on frontal lobe function.

In the next study, we [51] examined the ways in which the Parkinsonian patient interacted with others in a social context. We studied how PD patients used pragmatic aspects of language included speech acts, prosody, turn-taking in conversations, topic control and coherence and so forth. There is considerable evidence for right frontal mediation of both verbal and non-verbal components of conversational topic control ('relevance'), prosody, facial expressions, and some speech act comprehension [47], though, of course, both hemispheres interact to support core aspects of language use and comprehension. We reasoned that we would be able to identify strengths and weaknesses in the sense of Self in these patients when the patient was challenged in a social context.

The challenge was merely to interact conversationally and casually for about 10-15 minutes with a partner in conversation. We could measure the extent to which the patient utilized 'pragmatic communication skills' to interact with another person. Among these skills we measured processes that could give us some clue to the Parkinsonian sense of self: to what extent did the patient appropriately use speech acts, gesture and speech to convey agreement, mood, comfort, desire, disapproval, convey requests, and so forth.

To assess conversational fluency and pragmatic competence, we presented the patient with a series of pre-scripted open-ended questions in an attempt to elicit as much casual conversation as possible. We used the Prutting and Kirchner [58] checklist of core pragmatic skills to score patient's responses as they interacted with a conversational partner. The checklist covers verbal, paralinguistic and non-verbal aspects of the patient's conversational and social skills. Appropriate and inappropriate responses were tallied and then converted to percentage outcomes scores for each of the participants. We used percentage *inappropriate* as our main pragmatic outcome measure. Prutting and Kirchner [58] show that the test protocol and scoring reaches adequate reliability and validity levels when used with brain damaged persons.

Patients with PD were significantly impaired (scored as inappropriate) on 20.4% of the items (a mean of 6 items per patient) on the Prutting and Kirchner pragmatic checklist while controls were impaired on only 3.8% of items (p = .008). The overall appropriateness score correlated with performance on Design fluency and Stroop interference tasks.

In order to estimate the clinical severity of the pragmatic disorder in PD, we also assessed the extent to which PD patients were aware of their pragmatic social communication deficits. To measure self-awareness we asked patients to rate themselves on specific pragmatic communication skills –the same skills assessed on the Prutting and Kirchner pragmatic checklist. We then asked spouses or significant others to rate patients on these same pragmatic communication skills.

Spousal-patient ratings were significantly discrepant for several pragmatic domains including speech act comprehension/production, conversational appropriateness, turn-taking, 'quantity' or conciseness and stylistics. Thus, PD patients may to some extent be unaware of their problems with social communication. This is an extremely important clinical finding as unawareness may hinder attempts to overcome social communication problems.

From the point of view of understanding the experience of Self in PD results indicate that the sense of Self is impaired in PD. To interact 'appropriately' in a social context one must be able to monitor one's responses and adjust them if they do not fit the context. Thus failures in appropriate turn taking, fluency, topic maintenance etc all indicate, at a minimum, failures in self-monitoring. These failures in 'social presence' and social interaction led us to look further into the ways in which the parkinsonian personality interacted with others in a social context.

As mentioned above, studies of personality in PD suggest that PD patients are less talkative, less flexible, more socially conformist, suspicious and cautious compared with age-matched healthy controls as well as controls with chronic disease [42]. There is some evidence that this personality profile may actually precede onset of PD signs and symptoms and thus might be predictive of PD [42] though the claim remains controversial [59].

As reviewed above, studies using the tridimensional personality questionnaire (TPQ) of Cloninger et al [60] patients with Parkinson's disease show less "novelty seeking" activity, greater harm-avoidance behavior, and less consistency in performance on "reward dependence" tasks than controls [61,62]. It has been suggested that the reduction in novelty-seeking, elevation in harm-avoidance and inconsistent findings on reward-dependence might all be related to the damage of nigro-striatal and mesocortical dopaminergic systems that occurs in association with the disorder.

These findings concerning personality profile of PD as well as our earlier cited-findings with the Loevinger stem completion tasks and the examination of social communication skills in patients with PD suggest that PD patients may utilize (unconsciously of course) the interesting behavioral strategy known as "Machivellianism". We therefore decided to more directly examine Machiavellian personality strategies in PD.

People scoring high on a Mach inventory [63] are characterized by a propensity for interpersonal manipulation, and cynicism with respect to views about human nature [64,65]. High Machs can also be charming, good leaders, and aggressive and successful salespersons. Negative traits associated with the Machiavellianism personality profile involve a diminished affect or a lack of interpersonal empathy, along with increased egocentricity or narcissism and high levels of social anxiety.

To our knowledge, no studies have yet examined Machiavellianism in patients with PD. Given that some patients with PD exhibit a shift towards socially conformist, opportunistic and suspicious responses on stem-completion tasks as PD progresses from Hoehn-Yahr Stage II to III, we hypothesized that Mach scores would be *elevated in PD* patients relative to age-matched controls and to college-age students on which the original Mach norms were developed.

We studied a group of 35 patients with PD and 20 age-matched healthy controls. We used the Mach IV scale [63] to assess Machiavellianism in PD patients and age-matched controls. This is a self-report Likert type scale, with scores ranging from 1 to 7 (where 1=I totally disagree; 4=no opinion; and 7=I totally agree), composed of 20 items, each consisting of a statement with which the respondent is to indicate his level of agreement. Following the scoring rules of Corral and Calvete [66] who based their procedures on a exhaustive factor and dimensional analyses, we extracted 4 subscales from the MACH: positive interpersonal tactics, negative interpersonal tactics, positive view of human nature and cynical view of human nature.

Once again we administered neuropsychologic tests described above (Stroop and verbal fluency) that are known to be sensitive to detection of frontal dysfunction in PD as well as tests of memory and mood.

The PD patients consistently scored higher on the 'negative' and lower on the 'positive' subscales of the Mach IV, with the differences being significant for the 'cynical views of human nature' and the 'positive interpersonal tactics' subscales (see Table 3). PD patients apparently entertain more cynical views of human nature and are less likely to endorse use of positive interpersonal tactics when interacting with others (however they are no more likely than controls to endorse negative tactics).

In PD patients, no evidence of correlation was found between the Mach subscales and any of the following variables: age, years of education, Mini-Mental State Exam (MMSE), autobiographical memory recall and any of the mood scales, (all $p > 0.25$). The positive interpersonal tactics subscale score correlated inversely with the Stroop interference score; the higher the Stroop interference score (greater frontal dysfunction) the lower the positive tactics score.

In short, in these as yet unpublished pilot studies of Machchiavellianism in PD patients, we found that patients with Parkinson's Disease reported significantly greater levels of Machiavellianism than did healthy age-matched controls.

Now why might Mach scores be elevated in patients with PD? Depressed mood due to the chronic disease obviously might contribute to enhanced cynicism in anyone –yet the MACH subscales did not correlate with any of the DASS mood scales. An alternative possibility begins with the observation that PD patients experience significant prefrontal dysfunction as the disease progresses. Prefrontal dysfunction is typically associated with decreased inhibitory control in social situations. Decreased inhibitory control in our patients was evidenced by their abnormal performance on the Stroop color-word interference test. We contend that cognitive-behavioral dis-inhibition in these PD patients explains their consistently elevated (relative to healthy controls) Mach scores.

In the final set of studies, we wish to describe here we conducted a pilot study to assess the impact of asymmetric disease on personality and autobiographical memory functions in 15 PD patients—all with mid-stage disease. To calculate presence and degree of asymmetry we followed recommendations of Uitti et al. [20]. In their study a modified UPDRS motor score was composed of UPDRS part II other than item 24 and an additional item for arm swing using the same scaling (normal _ 0, slight reduction _ 1, moderate reduction _ 2, severe reduction _ 3, marked reduction _ 4). We calculated difference scores as the absolute value of the right- minus left-sided UPDRS items 20, 21, 22, 23, 25, 26, and the additional arm swing item. On the basis of these scores, patients were classified into right vs. left onset groups.

We used the Cloninger Personality Inventory (Tri-dimensional Character Inventory; TCI; Cloniger, 1987 [60]), to assess personality changes in PD. The TCI yields three basic personality dimensions (novelty-seeking, harm avoidance and reward dependence) and 4 other sub-scale scores (persistence, self-directedness, cooperativeness and self-transcendence) that have been reliably noted to be altered in PD relatively to controls (see above).

Table 4 displays personality, mood, and Mini mental state exam scores in right-sided onset vs. left sided onset PD patients. If the sense of Self depends more heavily on right prefrontal systems, then the personality dimensions measured by the TCI should be reduced in the left-sided onset group relative to the right-sided onset group. What we found is that only some of these dimensions (reward dependence and persistence) were significantly reduced in left-sided onset patients relative to right-sided onset patients (see Table 4). Of course, these are only pilot findings based on a small number of patients, but these results are consistent with the overall hypothesis of this paper: that the right frontal cortex is especially important in mediating the sense of Self.

Summary and Discussion

We have seen that patients with PD (in mild to moderate stages of the disease) evidence a shift (relative to healthy controls) in their subjective sense of Self towards egocentric and socially conformist responses and that this shift is related to prefrontal dysfunction. The correlation with prefrontal dysfunction was selective (there was no correlation with other neuropsychologic measures). In addition, we have seen that PD patients evidence significant degrees of impairment in pragmatic communication skills, specifically those skills that have been independently linked to right prefrontal cortex. The marked inappropriateness in social communication among PD patients was once again correlated with several measures of prefrontal dysfunction. In a set of studies designed to explore changes in PD personality traits we found that PD patients evidenced an increase (relative to healthy controls) in 'Machiavellianism', a reduction in reward dependence and persistence among patients with a history of left sided onset and greater right hemisphere dysfunction. Taken together these disparate findings on personality and Self-related changes in PD all point to profound disruption in the experience of Selfhood in this disease. Although we have explored the sense of Self in PD from several directions in these sets of studies, there is still a tremendous number of questions to be answered: Are those patients with greater Self-related impairment the ones most vulnerable to neuropsychiatric and dementing illnesses? Is the profile of personality change in PD related to premorbid personality types in persons vulnerable to PD? What is the relation of Self-related impairment to the well known cognitive and affective dysfunction associated with PD? It seems reasonable to assume that Self-related impairment will predict both mood disturbance and cognitive dysfunction. Finally what is the relation of Self-related disturbance to care giver burden in PD? All of these questions must be addressed if we are to develop more effective therapeutic interventions for PD.

The above set of findings on Self-related changes in PD also point to a key network in the neural substrates of the Self experience. We consistently found that the Self –related deficits were correlated with indices of right frontal function. Our findings taken together with the findings reviewed above from clinical and neuroimaging studies of other investigators suggest that the right frontal cortex is crucial for a normal sense of Self. In support of this conlusion are the recent intriguing findings of Keenan et al. [67]. Keenan, Nelson, O'Connor and Pascual-Leone [67] presented a series of pictures to a group of patients undergoing an intracarotid amobarbital (WADA) test. The pictures represented faces generated by morphing the image of a famous person with the patient's own face, and participants were asked to remember what picture was shown during selective anaesthesia of the right and the left hemispheres. Results indicated that most patients were unable to remember seeing their own face following an inactivation of the right hemisphere, whereas anaesthesia of the left hemisphere did not interfere with recall of the "self" face. These results once again implicate right frontal cortex is support of the Self.

The right frontal cortex (both at the orbito- and dorsalateral poles) differs from its left sided counterpart in that it receives a more dense set of afferents coursing up from the neo-striatal and limbic systems and it may also receive greater innervation from serotoninergic and noradrenergic cell groups in the brain stem [68,69]. Dopaminergic cell groups which project to the right prefrontal cortex display a more enhanced response to stress than dopaminergic cell groups projecting to the left prefrontal cortex [70]. Despite these intriguing anatomical perculiarities it is not clear how they might relate to, much less support a structure as complex as that of the Self. One thing is clear: investigation of the neuropsychologic correlates of the Self has only begun, but the prospects for some substantial breakthroughs are real and inviting.

References

[1]   Metzinger, T. (2003). *Being no one: The self-model theory of subjectivity.* Cambridge: MIT Press.

[2]   Churchland, P.S. (2002). Self-representation in nervous systems. *Science, 296,* 308–310.

[3]   Gallagher, S. (2000). Philosophical conceptions of the self: Implications for cognitive science. *Trends in Cogitive Siences, 4(1),* 14–21.

[4]   Northoff, G., & Bermpohl, F. (2004). Cortical midline structures and the self. *Trends in Cognitive Sciences, 8(3),* 102-107.

[5]   LeDoux, J.E. (2002). *Synaptic self: How our brains become who we are.* New York: Viking.

[6]   Vogeley, K., & Fink, G.R. (2003). Neural correlates of the first-person perspective. *Trends Cogn Sci, 7(1),* 38–42.

[7]   McNamara, P., von Harscher, H., Scioli, T., Krueger, M., Lawson, D., & Durso, R. (1995). The sense of self after brain damage: Evidence from aphasics and individuals with Parkinson's disease. *Journal of Cognitive Rehabilitation, November/December,* 16-23.

[8]   Craik, F.I.M., Moroz, T.M., & Moscovitch, M. (1999). In search of the self: A positron emission tomography study. *Psychological Science, 10,* 129-178.

[9]   Vogeley, K., Kurthen, M., Falkai, P., & Maier, W. (1999). Essential functions of the human self model are implemented in the prefrontal cortex. *Consciousness and Cognition, 8(3),* 343-363.

[10]   Weingarten, S.M. Psychosurgery. In B.L. Miller, & J.L. Cummings (Ed.), *The human frontal lobes: Functions and disorders* (pp. 446-460). New York: Guilford Press.

[11]   Schnider, A., & Gutbrod, K. (1999). Traumatic brain injury. In B.L. Miller, & J.L. Cummings (Ed.), *The human frontal lobes: Functions and disorders* (pp. 487-508). New York: Guilford Press.

[12] Miller, B., Seeley, W.W., Mychack, P., Rosen, H.J., Mena, I., & Boone, K. (2001). Neuroanatomy of the self: Evidence from patients with frontotemporal dementia. *Neurology, 57(1),* 817-821.

[13] Fink, G.R., Markowitsch, H.J., Reinkemeier, M., Bruckbauer, T., Kessler, J., & Heiss, W.D. (1996). Cerebral representation of one's own past: Neural networks involved in autobiographical memory. *Journal of Neuroscience, 16(13),* 4275-4282.

[14] Kelley, W.M., Macrae, C.N., Wyland, C.L., Caglar, S., Inati, S., & Heatherton, T.F. (2002). Finding the self? An event-related fMRI study. *Journal of Cognitive Neuroscience, 14(5),* 785–794.

[15] Wheeler, M.A., Stuss, D.T., & Tulving, E. (1997). Toward a theory of episodic memory: The frontal lobes and autonoetic consciousness. *Psychological Bulletin, 121(3),* 331-354.

[16] Nyberg, L., McIntosh, A.R., Cabeza, R., Nilsson, L-G., Houle, S., Habib, R., & Tulving, E. (1996). Network analysis of positron emission tomography regional cerebral blood flow data: Ensemble inhibition during episodic memory retrieval. *Journal of Neuroscience, 16(11),* 3753-3759.

[17] Elbaz, A., Bower, J.H., Peterson, B.J., Maraganore, D.M., McDonnell, S.K., Ahlskog, E., Schaid, D.J., & Rocca, W.A. (2003). Survival study of Parkinson disease in Olmsted County, Minnesota. *Archives of Neurology, 60(1),* 91–96.

[18] Biary, N., & Koller, W. (1985). Handedness and essential tremor. *Archives of Neurology, 42,* 1082–1083.

[19] Direnfeld, L.K., Albert, M.L., Volicer, L., Langlais, P.J., Marquis, J., & Kaplan, E. (1984). Parkinson's disease: The possible relationship of laterality to dementia and neurochemical findings. *Archives of Neurology, 41,* 935–941.

[20] Uitti, Y., Baba, N.R., Whaley, Z.K., Wszolek, M.D., & Putzke, J.D. (2005). Parkinson's disease: Handedness predicts asymmetry. *Neurology, 64(11),* 1925–1930.

[21] Agid, Y., Javoy-Agid, M., & Ruberg, M. (1987). Biochemistry of neurotransmitters in Parkinson's disease. In C.D. Marsden, & S. Fahn (Eds.), *Movement disorders 2.* New York: Butterworth's and Co.

[22] Javoy-Agid, F., & Agid, Y. (1980). Is the mesocortical dopaminergic system involved in Parkinson's disease? *Neurology, 30,* 1326-1330.

[23] German, D., Manaye, K., Smith, W., Woodward, D., & Saper, C. (1989). Mid-brain dopaminergic cell loss in Parkinson's disease: Computer visualization. *Annals of Neurology, 26,* 507-514.

[24] Rinne, J.O., Rummukainen, J., Paljarvi, L., & Rinne, U.K. (1989). Dementia in Parkinson's disease is related to neuronal loss in the medial substantia nigra. *Annals of Neurology, 26,* 47-50.

[25] Torack, R.M., & Morris, J.C. (1988). The association of ventral tegmental area histopathology with adult dementia. *Archives of Neurology, 45(5),* 497-501.

[26] Emre, M. (2003). What causes mental dysfunction in Parkinson's disease? *Movement Disorders, 18(Suppl. 6),* 563-571.

[27] Jellinger, K.A., Seppi, K., Wenning, G.K., & Poewe, W. (2002). Impact of coexistent Alzheimer pathology on the natural history of Parkinson's disease. *Journal of Neural Transmission, 109(3),* 329-339.

[28] Glick, S.D., Ross, D.A., & Hough, L.B. (1982). Lateral asymmetry of neurotransmitters in human brain. *Brain Research, 234,* 53–63.

[29] Menza, M.A., Mark, M.H., Burn, D.J., & Brooks, D.J. (1995). Personality correlates of [18F] dopa striatal uptake: Results of positron-emission tomography in Parkinson's disease. *Journal of Neuropsychiatry & Clinical Neurosciences, 7,* 176–179.

[30] Kaasinen, V., Nurmi, E., Bergman, J., Eskola, O., Solin, O., Sonninen, P., & Rinne, J.O. (2001). Personality traits and brain dopaminergic function in Parkinson's disease. *Proceedings of the National Academy of Sciences of the USA, 98(23),* 13272-13277.

[31] Starkstein, S.E., & Merello. M. (2002). *Psychiatric and cognitive disorders in Parkinson's disease.* Cambridge: Cambridge University Press.

[32] Lange, K.W., Paul, G.M., Naumann, M., & Gsell, W. (1995). Dopaminergic effects on cognitive performance in patients with Parkinson's disease. *Journal of Neural Transmission, Supplement,, 46,* 423-432.

[33] Lees, A. J., & Smith, E. (1983). Cognitive deficits in the early stages of Parkinson's disease. *Brain, 106(Pt 2),* 257-270.

[34] Levin, B.E., Llabre, M.M., & Weiner, W.J. (1989). Cognitive impairments associated with early Parkinson's disease. *Neurology, 39(4),* 557-561.

[35] Bayles, K.A., Tomoeda, C.K., Wood, J.A., Montgomery, E.B., Jr., Cruz, R.F., Azuma, T., & McGeagh, A. (1996). Change in cognitive function in idiopathic Parkinson disease. *Archives of Neurology, 53(11),* 1140-1146.

[36] McNamara, P., & Durso, R. (2000). Language functions in Parkinson's disease: Evidence for neurochemistry of language. In L. Obler, & L.T. Conner (Eds.), Neurobehavior *of language and cognition: Studies of normal aging and brain damage* (pp. 201-212). New York: Kluwer Academic.

[37] Piccirilli, M., D'Alessandro, P., Finali, G., Piccinin, G. L., & Agostini, L. (1989). Frontal lobe dysfunction in Parkinson's disease: Prognostic value for dementia? *European Neurology, 29(2),* 71-76.

[38] Troster, A.I., & Woods, S.P. (2003). Neuropsychological aspects of Parkinson's disease and parkinsonian syndromes. In R. Pahwa, K.E. Lyons, & W.C. Koller (Eds.), *Handbook of Parkinson's disease* (pp. 127-157). New York: Dekker.

[39] Wolters, E., & Scheltens, P. (1995). *Mental dysfunction in Parkinson's disease.* The Netherlands: ICG.

[40] Caparros-Lefebvre, D., Pecheux, N., Petit, V., Duhamel, A., & Petit, H. (1995). Which factors predict cognitive decline in Parkinson's disease? *Journal of Neurology, Neurosurgery, & Psychiatry, 58(1),* 51-55.

[41] Woods, S.P., & Troster, A.I. (2003). Prodromal frontal/executive dysfunction predicts incident dementia in Parkinson's disease. *Journal of the International Neuropsychological Society, 9(1),* 17-24.

[42] Hubble, J.P., & Koller, W.C. (1995). The Parkinsonian personality. In W.J. Weiner, & A.E. Lang (Eds.), *Behavioral neurology of movement disorders* (pp. 43–48). New York: Raven Press.

[43] Tomer, R., & Aharon-Peretz, J. (2004). Novelty seeking and harm avoidance in Parkinson's disease: Effects of asymmetric dopamine deficiency. *Journal of Neurology, Neurosurgery, & Psychiatry, 75,* 972-975.

[44] Davidson, R.J. (2001). Toward a biology of personality and emotion. *Annals of the New York Academy of Sciences, 935,* 191-207.

[45] Loevinger, J., Wessler, R., & Redmore, B. (1970). *Measuring ego development.* San Francisco: Jossey-Bass.

[46] Loevinger, J. (1976). *Ego development: Conceptions and theories.* San Francisco: Jossey-Bass.

[47] Paradis, M. (1998). The other side of language. *Journal of Linguistics, 11(1-2),* 1-10.

[48] McNamara, P., Clark, J., Krueger, M., & Durso, R. (1996). Sentence comprehension and grammaticality judgments in Parkinson's disease: A comparison with Broca's aphasia. *International Journal of Neuroscience, 86,* 151-166.

[49] McNamara, P., Durso, R., Brown, A., & Lynch, A. (2003). Counterfactual cognitive deficit in persons with Parkinson's disease. *Journal of Neurology, Neurosurgery, & Psychiatry, 74(8),* 1-6.

[50] McNamara, P., Durso, R., & Brown, A. (2003). Relation of "sense Of self" to executive function performance in Parkinson's disease. *Cognitive & Behavioral Neurology, 16(3),* 139-148.

[51] McNamara, P., & Durso, R. (2003). Pragmatic communication skills in Parkinson's disease. *Brain and Language, 84,* 414-423.

[52] Lezak, N.D. (1995). *Neuropsychological assessment* (3rd ed.). New York: Oxford University Press.

[53] York, M.K., Levin, H., Grossman, R.G., Lai, E.C., & Krauss, J.K. (2003). Clustering and switching in phonemic fluency following pallidotomy for the treatment of Parkinson's disease. *Journal of Clinical & Experimental Neuropsychology, 25(1),* 110-121.

[54] Troyer, A.K., Moscovitch, M., Winocur, G., Alexander, M.P., & Stuss, D.T. (1998). Clustering and switching on verbal fluency: The effects of focal frontal- and temporal-lobe lesions. *Neuropsychologia, 36(6),* 499-504.

[55] Troyer, A.K., Moscovitch, M., & Winocur, G. (1997). Clustering and switching as two components of verbal fluency: Evidence from younger and older healthy adults. *Neuropsychology, 11(1),* 138-146.

[56] Bench, C.J., Frith, C.D., Grasby, P.M., Friston, K.J., Paulesu, E., & Frackowiak, R.S. (1993). Investigations of the functional anatomy of attention using the Stroop test. *Neuropsychologia, 31(9),* 907-922.

[57] Morris, R.G., Ahmed, S., Syed, G.M., & Toone, B.K. (1993). Neural correlates of planning ability: Frontal lobe activation during the Tower of London test. *Neuropsychologia, 31(12),* 1367-1378.

[58] Prutting, C.A., & Kirchner, D.M. (1987). A clinical appraisal of the pragmatic aspects of language. *Journal of Speech & Hearing Disorders, 52(2),* 105–119.

[59] Glosser, G., Clark, C., Freudlich, B., Kliner-Krenzel, L., Flaherty, P. & Stern, M. (1995). A controlled investigation of current and premorbid personality: Characteristics of Parkinson's disease patients. *Movement Disorders, 10,* 201–206.

[60] Cloninger, C.R. (1987). A systematic method for clinical description and classification of personality variables. *Archives of General Psychiatry, 44,* 573–588.

[61] Menza, M.A., Golbe, L.I., Cody, R.A., Forman, N.E. (1993). Dopamine-related personality traits in Parkinson's disease. *Neurology, 43,* 505–508.

[62] Fujii, C., Harada, S., Ohkoshi, N., Hayashi, A., & Yoshizawa, K. (2000). Cross-cultural traits for personality of patients with Parkinson's disease in Japan. *American Journal of Medical Genetics, 96(1),* 1–3.

[63] Christie, R., & Geis, F.L. (1970). *Studies in Machiavellianism.* New York: Academic Press.

[64] Fehr, B., Samsom, D., & Paulhus, D.L. (1992). The construct of Machiavellianism: Twenty years later. In C.D. Spielberger, & J. M. Butcher (Eds.), *Advances in personality assessment* (vol. 9). New Jersey: Lawrence Erlbaum.

[65] McHoskey, J.W., Worzel, W., & Szyarto, C. (1998). Machiavellianism and psychopathy. *Journal of Personality & Social Psychology, 74,* 192-210.

[66] Corral, S., & Calvete, E. (2000). Machiavellianism: Dimensionality of the Mach IV and its relation to self monitoring in a Spanish sample. *Spanish Journal of Psychology, 3(1),* 3-13.

[67] Keenan, J.P., Nelson, A., O'Connor, M., Pascual-Leone, A. (2001). Self-recognition and the right hemisphere. *Nature, 409(6818),* 305.

[68] Ongur, D., & Price, J.L. (2000). The organization of networks within the orbital and medial prefrontal cortex of rats, monkeys and humans. *Cerebral Cortex, 10(3),* 206–219

[69] Bruder, G.E. (2003). Frontal and parietotemporal asymmetries in depressive disorders: Behavioral electrophysiologic and neuroimaging findings. In K. Hugdahl, & R.J. Davidson (Eds.), *The asymmetrical brain* (pp. 719-742). Cambridge: MIT Press.

[70] Berridge, C.W., Espana, R.A., & Stalnaker, T.A. (2003). Stress and coping: Asymmetry of dopamine efferents within the prefrontal cortex. In K. Hugdahl, & R.J. Davidson (Eds.), *The asymmetrical brain* (pp. 69-104). Cambridge: MIT Press.

In: New Research on Parkinson's Disease
Editors: T. F. Hahn, J. Werner

ISBN: 978-1-60456-601-7
© 2008 Nova Science Publishers, Inc.

Chapter VI

New Findings about Cardiovascular Dysfunction in Parkinson's Disease

Carl-Albrecht Haensch[*]

Department of Neurology and Clinical Neurophysiology of the University of
Witten/Herdecke, HELIOS Klinikum Wuppertal; Heusnerstr. 40, D-42283
Wuppertal, Germany

Abstract

Sympathetic neurocirculatory failure in Parkinson`s disease is common. Orthostatic hypotension is the most frequent symptom. Cardiovascular disturbances have so far been met with the highest degree of clinical and scientific interest. Histological studies have proven the presence of Lewi`s bodies in sympathetic and parasympathetic neurons and also in central structures associated with the autonomic regulation.

Extrasystoles occur in normal subjects, but are more frequently seen in Parkinson patients. Heart rate variability is a useful non-invasive test to assess autonomic dysfunction in PD. It allows a differentiation of the sympathetic and parasympathetic activation, which are related to a low-frequency (0.05 - 0.15 Hz; LF) and a high-frequency (0.15-0.5Hz; HF) component of the heart rate variability (HRV) signal, respectively. The resulting LF/HF ratio is a quantitative index of the sympatho-vagal balance. The physiological function of HRV is commonly known to be to buffer changes in blood pressure. In the PD-patients group (n=107, mean age 71 years, mean PD-duration 7.0 years, Hoehn and Yahr 3.0 ± 0.9) the LF/HF ratio was lower than in the control group in rest (2.19 vs. 1.25, $p < 0.05$); in deep respiration (3.3 vs. 2.4, $p < 0.01$) and in tilt-table testing (2.6 vs 1.9, $p < 0.01$). The LF/HF ratio in tilt-table testing was significantly more reduced in PD with OH than without (2.1 vs. 1.3, $p < 0.05$). Scintigraphy with ^{123}I-Metaiodobenzylguanidine (MIBG) appears to be a highly sensitive and useful in demonstrating sympathetic postganglionic cardiac nerve disturbances. In the heart, MIBG uptake in all examined 57 Parkinson's (PD) patients was decreased (H/M-Ratio: 1.14 ± 0.16). Loss of sympathetic innervation of the heart seems to occur

---

[*] Carl-Albrecht Haensch: Email: carl-albrecht.haensch@helios-kliniken.de

independent of orthostatic hypotension and baroreflex failure in PD. We found no correlation between myocardial MIBG uptake and sympathovagal balance, blood pressure or other autonomic findings. This result could be explained by different time course of loss of intact postganglionic sympathetic cardial innervation and disturbed baroreflex response or the involvement of central autonomic pathways in PD.

The significance of the abnormalities in cardiovascular regulation among PD patients is not fully known yet. It is possible that the dysbalance of the sympathetic and parasympathetic tone is connected with heart arrhytmias. The connection between autonomic dysregulation and arrhythmia related death has recently been considered in PD. The mortality of PD patients is almost twice that for age and sex-matched healthy control groups.

Parkinson`s disease is a continuously progressive degenerative disorder of the central, peripheral and autonomic human nervous systems. Affecting an estimated 1% of the population over the age of 65 years, it causes tremor, bradykinesia, rigidity, and the loss of postural reflexes [31]. In addition to major motor symptoms, patients with Parkinson`s disease (PD) are known to suffer from disturbances of the autonomic nervous system. The most common autonomic dysfunction is orthostatic hypotension. However, symptoms of dysautonomia are variable, and include cardiovascular symptoms, gastrointestinal, urogenital, sudomotor and thermoregulatory dysfunction, pupillary abnormalities, sleep and respiratory disorders [58]. About 60-80 % of PD-patients show signs of autonomic dysfunction, some leading to severe complications such as urinary tract infections, falls and megacolon. Such nonmotor features are often not formally assessed and may be frequently misdiagnosed, so the true prevalence remains poorly defined [28, 42, 58]. Magerkurth et al. estimated that about 50% of PD patients rated the impact of the symptoms of autonomic failure on their daily lives as "a lot" or "very much" due to orthostatic dizziness, bladder dysfunction and constipation, which were more statistically significant than in age-matched controls [50]. The combined effects of aging and PD on the autonomic nervous system result in a high prevalence of orthostatic hypotension when dopamine agonists are prescribed, frequently not recognized by patients or their doctors unless systematically examined for [49]. The high prevalence of orthostatic hypotension likely contributes to the high prevalence of falls, and hip fracture, reported in these patients [48].

In addition to the dopaminergic system, the degenerative process of PD also involves noradrenergic locus coeruleus, the dorsal motor vagal nucleus and the cholinergic nucleus basalis of Meynert [40]. Lewy bodies which are eosinophilic intracytoplasmic inclusions, accompany the nerve cell loss with reactive gliosis in structures involved in autonomic regulation, are found in multiple areas of brain, spinal cord and in sympathetic and parasympathetic neurons [13, 14, 41]. Baroreceptor afferent activity, relayed and integrated in central medullary autonomic nuclei such as the nucleus tractus solitarius, increases vagal and inhibits sympathetic discharge to the heart, and inhibits vasoconstrictor discharge to resistance vessels. Because the PD process seems to involve the central nuclei as well as the peripheral autonomic ganglia and also the hypothalamus, the cardiovascular dysregulation may be of both central and peripheral origin [77]. Thus the cardiovascular autonomic control and reactivity system may be injured at multiple sites.

First Complaints, Early Diagnosis and Autonomic Disturbances

In average it takes two years to diagnose Parkinson´s disease after the onset of first complaints. Because Parkinsonism is common among elderly people and its prevalence increases markedly with age, there are important public health concerns as the worldwide life expectations grow steadily. PD belongs to the most frequent neurodegenerative illnesses and concerns up to one per cent of people older than 65 years. Although usually the onset of classic symptoms like rest tremor, bradykinesia, and rigidity allows the correct diagnosis, the early diagnosis is often difficult. Clinical signs of dysautonomia are often non-specific, and dizziness due to orthostatic hypotension may be difficult to recognize [37, 53]. The latter is important for two reasons: Recently, some drugs may have had a neuroprotective effect when given in an early state of the disease. Though there exist well-established regimes for the treatment of PD, in the beginning nonspecific symptoms can cause diagnostic mistakes. Concerning the relationship between patient and doctor, a late diagnosis often leads to a loss of confidence. Partially unnecessary and expansive investigations should be avoided.

It was the aim of our previous study based on a group of 73 patients (42 female, 31 male; mean age 69 ± 11 [39-87] years) suffering from PD to find out subjective complaints in early stages, motives for visit and the time lag from the first onset of unspecific complaints until diagnosis [35]. Clinical diagnosis of idiopathic definite PD was made according to the criteria set forth by the U.K. Parkinson's Disease Society Brain Bank [39]. The method was based on on anonymous, structured questionnaire about 26 items. We estimated the mean interval between onset of discomforts until diagnosis to be about 2 years (± 4,4 [0-20] y.). First onset of shoulder or brachial pain (72 % vs. 47%; p= 0,001), sleep disturbance (72 % vs. 47 %; p=0,001), inappetence (36% vs. 14 %; p=0,008), "internally tremblement" (81% vs., 56 %; p<0,001) and dysarthrophonia (72 % vs. 58 %; p=0,018) correlate significantly with a delayed (more than 2 years) diagnosis finding. Moreover, Parkinsonian patients (46%) often complain of psychopathological features like depression as primary symptom of PD. A variety of autonomic nervous system symptoms, such as constipation (49.3%), sexual dysfunction (28.8%), mouth dryness (58.9%), sleep disturbance (50.7%), sweating (38.4%) or inappetence (16.4%) occurs already in the first six months of clinical course.

Otherwise, most frequently (36.5%) tremors led to visits. Sleep impairment is present in about 50% of the patients. These sleep disturbances are due in part to nocturnal akinesia, painful dystonia, depression or a sleep-apnea syndrome. Among the patients with a delayed diagnosing (more than 2 years), the described vague and subtle however typical early symptoms were significantly more frequent than in those patients without a delayed diagnosing. Our results were based on retrospective questioning, which is subject to the methodical restriction of a "recall bias" (distorted memory ability illness-causes). For example, depression and cognitive impairment may influence that self-report.

It can also be assumed that our patient group was more conscious of their symptoms as they were confronted with similar questions during neurological investigation and history taking, and this may have produced a higher sensitivity.

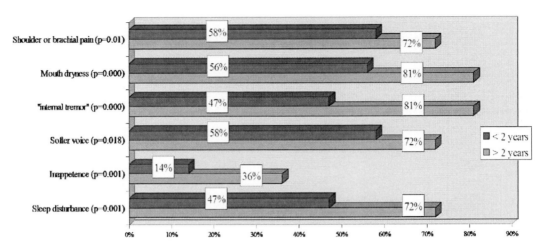

Figure 1. Preclinical and premotor complaints significantly more frequently noticed in delayed diagnosed PD.

Among the patients with a delayed diagnosing (more than two years), early symptoms were significantly more frequent (figure 1). The opportunity for diagnostic confusion is greatest early on in the clinical course, when some of the more distinctive clinical features may not have yet developed. Symptoms at the time of the first diagnosis and at the beginning of the first clinical manifestation of PD are often not identical. Those patients with subtle symptoms were diagnosed significantly later. As diagnosis can be made unchanged only clinically, physicians must be aware of this "soft" signs in early stages of PD.

Because of the therapeutic success in the beginning, PD should be diagnosed as early as possible. Diagnostic mistakes may occur early in the course of the disease. Neuroprotective therapeutic approaches can be utilized optimally only with early onset of treatment. Although the hallmark of PD is a syndrome of movement disorders, in early stages, clinical symptoms are often very subtle.

Autonomic Function Tests

The cardiovascular autonomic function tests use based on blood pressure and heart rate at rest and after various stimulations under standardized environmental conditions with a room temperature of 20° C [17, 61]. 107 PD-patients were tested (mean age 71 years, mean PD-duration 7.0 years, Hoehn and Yahr 3.0 ± 0.9). All tests were done in the morning. Finger arterial pressure was measured beat-to-beat continuously and non-invasivily using the volume clamp method with the Portapres device (TNO TPD, Amsterdam, The Netherlands). The cuff was placed on the second phalanx of the third finger. A synchronous recording of a standard 4 channel ECG, respiratory effort measured by thoracic strain gauges and the Portapres signal was performed simultaneously with the fan device (Schwarzer GmbH, Munich, Germany). The duration of recording was approximately 45 minutes. After the rest phase, a head-up tilt table, testing with a 70° upright position within 20s with an electrically driven tilt table, was performed. The Valsalva manoeuvre was performed by asking the subject to blow into a mouthpiece attached to an aneroid pressure gauge at a pressure of 40 mm Hg and to hold pressure for 15 s. A return of the cardiovascular parameters to baseline was waited for in between each test. The Valsalva ratio, the diastolic blood pressure in phase II, the latency between the minimum blood pressure in phase III of the Valsalva manoeuvre and the maximum in phase IV were qualified [16]. The response was considered to be normal if the diastolic pressure increased before the end of straining and if the systolic blood pressure during phase IV increased to a value exceeding the baseline in not more than 7 s. Orthostatic hypotension was diagnosed based on the Consensus statement on the definition of orthostatic hypotension using a decrease of at least 20 mm Hg in systolic blood pressure or at least 10 mm Hg within 3 minutes of standing [1-3, 45]. Myocardial adrenergic function was analyzed by imaging with ^{123}I-Meta-iodobenzylguanidine (MIBG) using single-photon emission computed tomography (SPECT) technique in patients with PD. MIBG is an analog of norepinephrine and a tracer for sympathetic neuron integrity and function. Cardiac MIBG uptake was assessed qualitatively for heart visualisation on planar studies by an nuclear medicine specialist, who was unaware of the autonomic function status.

Premature Ventricular Contractions

Standard cardiovascular autonomic responses to physiological stimuli have provided much evidence suggesting mild autonomic nervous system disturbances in PD [12]. The most frequent cardiac rhythm disturbances in PD are premature ventricular contractions (PVCs), often appearing as monomorphic, single PVCs, or rarely as bigeminy, trigeminy or pairs. Extrasystoles occur in normals, but are more frequently (16.25 % vs. 55 %; $Chi^2 = 19.3$, p < 0.001) seen in PD [36]. The clinical significance of the significantly higher frequency of premature ventricular contractions in PD, than in normals, is unknown. It is possible that the postganglionic sympathetic dysfunction in cardiac innervation leads to susceptibility for cardiac dysrhythmia. In the great majority of instances, sustained dysrhythmias do not arise simply in association with speeding or slowing of heart rate. Usually there are one or more premature beats as well. Recently, we described reduced baroreflex sensitivity in PD not limited to experimental reflex conditions, but causing an impaired blood pressure regulation that occuring spontaneously [36].

Heart Rate Variability

The function of Heart rate variability is commonly known to be buffer changes in blood pressure [70]. Analysis of Heart rate variability (HRV) has been used as a measure of cardiac autonomic control. It can be performed in two main ways, by statistical operations on R-R intervals (time-domain analysis) or by spectral analysis of a series of successive R-R intervals (frequency-domain analysis). It allows a differentiation of the sympathetic and parasympathetic activation, which are related to a low-frequency (LF) and a high-frequency (HF) component of the heart rate variability (HRV) signal, respectively.

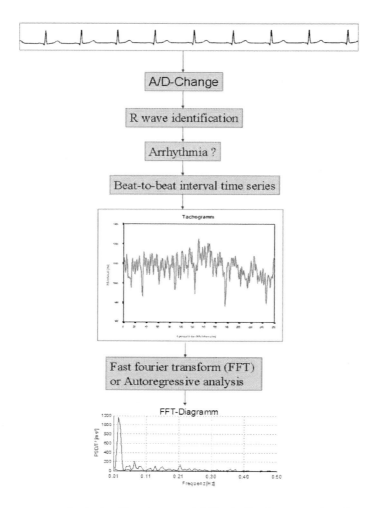

Analysis of heart rate variability in the frequency domain

Figure 2. Analysis of heart rate variability in the frequency domain.

The resulting LF/HF ratio is a quantitative index of the sympatho-vagal balance. The HF component is similar in shape and centre to the frequency of the respiratory signal and is generally considered a marker of vagal activity, although a sympathetic influence has been advocated on the basis of inconclusive studies using ß-blockers. The LF component seems to depend on more complex mechanisms. Manoeuvres enhancing the sympathetic drive or abnormal conditions associated with sympathetic hyperactivity led to a marked relative increase in the LF component. Many factors influence heart rate and explain the great variability of the parameters recorded, such as age [5, 26], drugs, breathing frequency [71], orthostatic stress [20, 21] and physical exercise [69]. The laboratory should be environment controlled, especially for temperature. International recommendations includes suggestions for the analysis of heart rate variability, blood pressure monitoring, tilt-table testing, Valsalva manoeuvre [2, 4, 6, 17, 24]. The measurement of autonomic parameters using power spectrum analysis of heart rate does not require the active participation of patients.

In the PD-patients group (n=107, mean age 71 years, mean PD-duration 7.0 years, Hoehn and Yahr 3.0 ± 0.9) the LF/HF ratio was lower than in the control group in rest (2.19 vs. 1.25, $p < 0.05$); in deep respiration (3.3 vs. 2.4, $p < 0.01$) and in tilt-table testing (2.6 vs 1.9, $p < 0.01$). The LF/HF ratio in tilt-table testing was significantly more reduced in PD with orthostatic hypotension than without (2.1 vs. 1.3, $p < 0.05$). Diminished variability of standard RR intervals and spectral measures of HR variability have been reported in PD [33, 37, 43, 44, 51, 55-57, 59, 64, 73, 74]. Cautious interpretation of heart rate variability is required regarding the neural complexity [27]. Two studies have evaluated tonic cardiovascular control patterns, reporting dysregulation both in de novo PD patients [33] and in advanced PD [51]. A previous study support the hypothesis that sympathetic and parasympathetic balance in control of heart activity are impaired in Parkinson's disease and that this dysfunction can be assessed by frequency-domain analysis of HR changes [34]. Based on clinical experience, it is assumed that autonomic dysfunction progresses along with the underlying PD, but little is known about the association between the decline of motor function and autonomic failure [47]. In accordance with a study by Haapaniemi, the size of reduction of LF/HF-ratio correlated to the UPDRS-score, might be a objective marker for disease progression in PD. However, because the association was not strong, the mechanisms causing the motor disability in PD may differ from those leading to impairment of the cardiovascular regulation [33].

The significance of the abnormalities in cardiovascular regulation among Parkinson's disease patients is not fully known yet. The conventional time and frequency domain measures of HR variability, previously proved useful in predicting cardiac arrhythmia and mortality in coronary heart disease [11, 22]. The prevailing hypothesis is that because an intact neurocardiac autonomic regulation is essential for a normal heart rate variability, a decrease of this parameter may reflect the autonomic dysfunction associated with cardiac electrical instability [10]. Adrenergic hyperactivity and/or lack of presumably protective parasympathetic tone are the suggested pathophysiological mechanisms of sudden cardiac death [67].

It is possible that the dysbalance of the sympathetic and the parasympathetic tone is connected with the arrhythmias developing in the ischemic heart muscles [70]. The connection between autonomic dysregulation and arrhythmia-related death has recently been considered in other, non-cardiovascular diseases, such as depression [32]. Analogously, we can presume a connection between the autonomic dysbalance and the high mortality among PD-patients [8, 9].

Imaging of the Autonomic Nervous System

Cardiac ^{123}I-Metaiodobenzylguanidine (MIBG) scintigraphy is a sensitive tool for detecting cardiac sympathetic denervation in PD [25]. Many recent studies have agreed on the remarkable finding that all patients with PD and orthostatic hypotension have a loss of cardiac sympathetic innervation [15, 18, 19, 30, 60, 62, 65, 66, 72]. MIBG uptake was assessed using the ratio of the heart to the upper mediastinum (H/M) according to planar scintigraphic data. In the heart, MIBG uptake in all examined 57 PD-patients was decreased (H/M-Ratio: 1.14 ± 0.16). Loss of sympathetic innervation of the heart seems to occur independent of orthostatic hypotension and baroreflex failure in PD. We found no correlation between myocardial MIBG uptake and sympathovagal balance, blood pressure or other autonomic findings. These results could be explained by different time course of loss of intact postganglionic sympathetic cardial innervation and disturbed baroreflex response or the involvement of central autonomic pathways in PD.

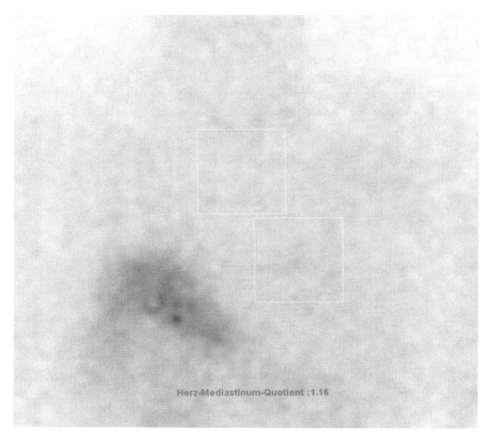

Figure 3. Decreased cardiac uptake in ^{123}I-metaiodobenzylguanidine scintigraphy in a patient with PD.

Impaired autonomic cardiovascular regulation has been associated with an increased risk of mortality both in patients with heart disease and in randomly selected general populations [33]. Sympathetic denervation leeds to denervation hypersensitivity, which is a phenomenon characterized by inadequately strong response of the denervated tissues to the physiological neurotransmitters [54]. Hypersensitivity occurs in the heart when the circulating catecholamines react with a live but sympathetically denervated myocardial tissue. The denervation hypersensitivity creates a predilection for the appearance of cardiac arrhythmias. The mortality of Parkinson's disease patients is almost twice that for age and sex-matched healthy control groups [9]. The 20-year follow-up study by Ben-Shlomo and Marmot suggested that this increased mortality is connected with an increase in heart ischemia-related deaths [8]. On the other hand Orimo et al. showed echocardiographic normal left ventricular function in 36 PD patients with myocardial sympathetic nerve damage demonstrated by ^{123}I-metaiodobenzylguanidine scintigraphy [62]. No changes in left ventricular function were observed by echocardiography studies in PD, although recently some new studies were carried out regarding valvular heart disease; associated with ergot derivative dopamine agonists therapy [7, 23, 38, 46, 63, 68, 75, 76, 78-80].

It is now clear that there is a fundamental abnormality in reflex control mechanisms like baroreceptor dysfunction in the syndrome of heart failure. Still unresolved is whether the protean abnormalities in afferent and efferent sympathetic nervous system function in heart failure are fundamental to the clinical manifestations of the syndrome or are merely epiphenomena indicative of the severity of the physiological derangement [29].

Cardiovascular dysfunction may occur in parkinsonian patients for a variety of reasons. Patients more are usually than 50 years old and on various drugs (both antiparkinsonian and for associated medical disorders), some of which may have cardiovascular effects. Autonomic failure increases with age and also is recognized in parkinsonian patients who have the disorder multiple system atrophy, in which there is substantial cardiovascular dysfunction [52]. Our results indicate that both parasympathetic and sympathetic deficits may occur in PD. Thus, recognition of cardiovascular dysfunction and its causes in parkinsonian patients is of importance in diagnosis, in determining prognosis, and finally in management.

References

(1996) Consensus statement on the definition of orthostatic hypotension, pure autonomic failure, and multiple system atrophy. *J. Neurol. Sci.* 144:218-219

(1996) Consensus statement on the definition of orthostatic hypotension, pure autonomic failure, and multiple system atrophy. The Consensus Committee of the American Autonomic Society and the American Academy of Neurology. *Neurology.* 46:1470

(1996) The definition of orthostatic hypotension, pure autonomic failure, and multiple system atrophy. *J. Auton. Nerv. Syst.* 58:123-124

(1996) Heart rate variability: standards of measurement, physiological interpretation and clinical use. Task Force of the European Society of Cardiology and the North American Society of Pacing and Electrophysiology. *Circulation.* 93:1043-1065

Agelink MW, Malessa R, Baumann B, Majewski T, Akila F, Zeit T, Ziegler D (2001) Standardized tests of heart rate variability: normal ranges obtained from 309 healthy humans, and effects of age, gender, and heart rate. *Clin. Auton. Res.* 11:99-108

Baron R (1999) Heart rate variability. *Electroencephalogr. Clin. Neurophysiol. Suppl.* 50:283-286

Baseman DG, O'Suilleabhain PE, Reimold SC, Laskar SR, Baseman JG, Dewey RB, Jr. (2004) Pergolide use in Parkinson disease is associated with cardiac valve regurgitation. *Neurology.* 63:301-304

Ben-Shlomo Y, Marmot MG (1995) Survival and cause of death in a cohort of patients with parkinsonism: possible clues to aetiology? *J. Neurol. Neurosurg. Psychiatry.* 58:293-299

Bennett DA, Beckett LA, Murray AM, Shannon KM, Goetz CG, Pilgrim DM, Evans DA (1996) Prevalence of parkinsonian signs and associated mortality in a community population of older people. *N. Engl. J. Med.* 334:71-76

Bernardi L (2000) The autonomic nervous system in heart disease. In: Appenzeller O (ed) *The autonomic nervous system.* Part II. Elsevier, Amsterdam; New York, pp 425-452

Bigger JT, Jr., Steinman RC, Rolnitzky LM, Fleiss JL, Albrecht P, Cohen RJ (1996) Power law behavior of RR-interval variability in healthy middle-aged persons, patients with recent acute myocardial infarction, and patients with heart transplants. *Circulation.* 93:2142-2151

Bolis L, Licinio J, Govoni S (2003) Handbook of the autonomic nervous system in health and disease. *Marcel Dekker,* New York

Braak H, Bohl JR, Muller CM, Rub U, de Vos RA, Del Tredici K (2006) Stanley Fahn Lecture 2005: The staging procedure for the inclusion body pathology associated with sporadic Parkinson's disease reconsidered. *Mov. Disord.* 21:2042-2051

Braak H, Ghebremedhin E, Rub U, Bratzke H, Del Tredici K (2004) Stages in the development of Parkinson's disease-related pathology. *Cell Tissue Res.* 318:121-134

Braune S (2001) The role of cardiac metaiodobenzylguanidine uptake in the differential diagnosis of parkinsonian syndromes. *Clin. Auton. Res.* 11:351-355

Braune S, Auer A, Schulte-Monting J, Schwerbrock S, Lucking CH (1996) Cardiovascular parameters: sensitivity to detect autonomic dysfunction and influence of age and sex in normal subjects. *Clin. Auton. Res.* 6:3-15

Braune S, Baron R, Low P (1999) Assessment of blood pressure regulation. Electroencephalogr *Clin. Neurophysiol. Suppl.* 50:287-291

Braune S, Reinhardt M, Bathmann J, Krause T, Lehmann M, Lucking CH (1998) Impaired cardiac uptake of meta-[123I]iodobenzylguanidine in Parkinson's disease with autonomic failure. *Acta Neurol. Scand.* 97:307-314

Braune S, Reinhardt M, Schnitzer R, Riedel A, Lucking CH (1999) Cardiac uptake of [123I]MIBG separates Parkinson's disease from multiple system atrophy. *Neurology.* 53:1020-1025

Butler GC, Yamamoto Y, Hughson RL (1994) Heart rate variability to monitor autonomic nervous system activity during orthostatic stress. *J. Clin. Pharmacol.* 34:558-562

Butler GC, Yamamoto Y, Xing HC, Northey DR, Hughson RL (1993) Heart rate variability and fractal dimension during orthostatic challenges. *J. Appl. Physiol.* 75:2602-2612

Chakko S, Mulingtapang RF, Huikuri HV, Kessler KM, Materson BJ, Myerburg RJ (1993) Alterations in heart rate variability and its circadian rhythm in hypertensive patients with left ventricular hypertrophy free of coronary artery disease. *Am. Heart J.* 126:1364-1372

Chung EJ, Yoon WT, Kim JY, Lee WY (2006) Valvular heart disease in a patient with Parkinson's disease treated with a low daily dose and a low cumulative dose of pergolide. *Mov. Disord.* 21:586-587

Claus D, Schmitz J, Nouri S (1999) Value and limits of cardiovascular autonomic function tests. *Electroencephalogr. Clin. Neurophysiol. Suppl.* 50:288-292

Courbon F, Brefel-Courbon C, Thalamas C, Alibelli MJ, Berry I, Montastruc JL, Rascol O, Senard JM (2003) Cardiac MIBG scintigraphy is a sensitive tool for detecting cardiac sympathetic denervation in Parkinson's disease. *Mov. Disord.* 18:890-897

Dawson SL, Robinson TG, Youde JH, Martin A, James MA, Weston PJ, Panerai RB, Potter JF (1999) Older subjects show no age-related decrease in cardiac baroreceptor sensitivity. *Age Ageing.* 28:347-353

Devos D, Kroumova M, Bordet R, Vodougnon H, Guieu JD, Libersa C, Destee A (2003) Heart rate variability and Parkinson's disease severity. *J. Neural. Transm.* 110:997-1011

Dewey RB, Jr. (2004) Autonomic dysfunction in Parkinson's disease. *Neurol. Clin.* 22:S127-139

Francis G, Cohn J (1999) Cardiac failure and the autonomic nervous system. In: Bannister R, Mathias CJ (eds) *Autonomic failure: a textbook of clinical disorders of the autonomic nervous system.* Oxford University Press, Oxford; New York, pp 477-486

Goldstein DS (2003) Imaging of the autonomic nervous system: focus on cardiac sympathetic innervation. *Semin. Neurol.* 23:423-433

Grubb BP, Olshansky B, Huang SK (1998) *Syncope: mechanisms and management.* Futura Pub. Co., Armonk, NY

Guinjoan SM, Bernabo JL, Cardinali DP (1995) Cardiovascular tests of autonomic function and sympathetic skin responses in patients with major depression. *J. Neurol. Neurosurg. Psychiatry.* 59:299-302

Haapaniemi TH, Pursiainen V, Korpelainen JT, Huikuri HV, Sotaniemi KA, Myllyla VV (2001) Ambulatory ECG and analysis of heart rate variability in Parkinson's disease. *J. Neurol. Neurosurg. Psychiatry.* 70:305-310

Haensch C-A, Jörg J (2001) Disturbed Sympatho-Vagal Balance in Heart Rate Variability as Marker of Progression in Parkinson's Disease. *J. Neural. Sci.* 187:133

Haensch C-A, Jörg J (1999) Preclinical symptoms in delayed diagnosed Parkinson`s disease. *J. Neural. Transm.* 106: XI

Haensch CA, Jorg J (2006) Beat-to-beat blood pressure analysis after premature ventricular contraction indicates sensitive baroreceptor dysfunction in Parkinson's disease. *Mov. Disord.* 21:486-491

Holmberg B, Kallio M, Johnels B, Elam M (2001) Cardiovascular reflex testing contributes to clinical evaluation and differential diagnosis of Parkinsonian syndromes. *Mov. Disord.* 16:217-225

Horvath J, Fross RD, Kleiner-Fisman G, Lerch R, Stalder H, Liaudat S, Raskoff WJ, Flachsbart KD, Rakowski H, Pache JC, Burkhard PR, Lang AE (2004) Severe multivalvular heart disease: a new complication of the ergot derivative dopamine agonists. *Mov. Disord.* 19:656-662

Hughes AJ, Daniel SE, Kilford L, Lees AJ (1992) Accuracy of clinical diagnosis of idiopathic Parkinson's disease: a clinico-pathological study of 100 cases. *J. Neurol. Neurosurg. Psychiatry.* 55:181-184

Jellinger K (1987) The pathology of parkinsonism. In: CD Marsden, Fahn S (eds) *Movement Disorder.* 2. Butterworths, London, pp 124-165

Jellinger KA (1991) Pathology of Parkinson's disease. Changes other than the nigrostriatal pathway. *Mol. Chem. Neuropathol.* 14:153-197

Jost WH (2003) Autonomic dysfunctions in idiopathic Parkinson's disease. *J. Neurol.* 250 Suppl 1:I28-30

Kallio M, Haapaniemi T, Turkka J, Suominen K, Tolonen U, Sotaniemi K, Heikkila VP, Myllyla V (2000) Heart rate variability in patients with untreated Parkinson's disease. *Eur. J. Neurol.* 7:667-672

Kallio M, Suominen K, Bianchi AM, Makikallio T, Haapaniemi T, Astafiev S, Sotaniemi KA, Myllya VV, Tolonen U (2002) Comparison of heart rate variability analysis methods in patients with Parkinson's disease. *Med. Biol. Eng. Comput.* 40:408-414

Kaufmann H (1996) Consensus statement on the definition of orthostatic hypotension, pure autonomic failure and multiple system atrophy. *Clin. Auton. Res.* 6:125-126

Kim JY, Chung EJ, Park SW, Lee WY (2006) Valvular heart disease in Parkinson's disease treated with ergot derivative dopamine agonists. *Mov. Disord.* 21:1261-1264

Korchounov A, Kessler KR, Yakhno NN, Damulin IV, Schipper HI (2005) Determinants of autonomic dysfunction in idiopathic Parkinson's disease. *J. Neurol.* 252:1530-1536

Kuchel GA (2004) Autonomic nervous system in old age. Karger, Basel; New York

Kujawa K, Leurgans S, Raman R, Blasucci L, Goetz CG (2000) Acute orthostatic hypotension when starting dopamine agonists in Parkinson's disease. *Arch. Neurol.* 57:1461-1463

Magerkurth C, Schnitzer R, Braune S (2005) Symptoms of autonomic failure in Parkinson's disease: prevalence and impact on daily life. *Clin. Auton. Res.* 15:76-82

Mastrocola C, Vanacore N, Giovani A, Locuratolo N, Vella C, Alessandri A, Baratta L, Tubani L, Meco G (1999) Twenty-four-hour heart rate variability to assess autonomic function in Parkinson's disease. *Acta Neurol. Scand.* 99:245-247

Mathias CJ (1998) Cardiovascular autonomic dysfunction in parkinsonian patients. *Clin. Neurosci.* 5:153-166

Mathias CJ, Mallipeddi R, Bleasdale-Barr K (1999) Symptoms associated with orthostatic hypotension in pure autonomic failure and multiple system atrophy. *J. Neurol.* 246:893-898

Matveev M, Prokopova R, Nachev C (2006) Normal and abnormal circadian characteristics in autonomic cardiac control: *new opportunities for cardiac risk prevention.* Nova Science Publishers, New York

Meco G, Pratesi L, Bonifati V (1991) Cardiovascular reflexes and autonomic dysfunction in Parkinson's disease. *J. Neurol.* 238:195-199

Mesec A, Sega S, Kiauta T (1993) The influence of the type, duration, severity and levodopa treatment of Parkinson's disease on cardiovascular autonomic responses. *Clin. Auton. Res.* 3:339-344

Mesec A, Sega S, Trost M, Pogacnik T (1999) The deterioration of cardiovascular reflexes in Parkinson's disease. *Acta Neurol. Scand.* 100:296-299

Micieli G, Tosi P, Marcheselli S, Cavallini A (2003) Autonomic dysfunction in Parkinson's disease. *Neurol. Sci. 24 Suppl.* 1:S32-34

Mihci E, Kardelen F, Dora B, Balkan S (2006) Orthostatic heart rate variability analysis in idiopathic Parkinson's disease. *Acta Neurol. Scand.* 113:288-293

Oka H, Mochio S, Yoshioka M, Morita M, Onouchi K, Inoue K (2006) Cardiovascular dysautonomia in Parkinson's disease and multiple system atrophy. *Acta Neurol. Scand.* 113:221-227

Oribe E (1999) Testing autonomic function. In: Vinken PJ, Bruyn GW, Appenzeller O (eds) *The autonomic nervous system Part I.* Elsevier, Amsterdam; New York, pp 595-648

Orimo S, Ozawa E, Nakade S, Sugimoto T, Mizusawa H (1999) (123)I-metaiodobenzylguanidine myocardial scintigraphy in Parkinson's disease. *J. Neurol. Neurosurg. Psychiatry.* 67:189-194

Peralta C, Wolf E, Alber H, Seppi K, Muller S, Bosch S, Wenning GK, Pachinger O, Poewe W (2006) Valvular heart disease in Parkinson's disease vs. controls: An echocardiographic study. *Mov. Disord.* 21:1109-1113

Pursiainen V, Haapaniemi TH, Korpelainen JT, Huikuri HV, Sotaniemi KA, Myllyla VV (2002) Circadian heart rate variability in Parkinson's disease. *J. Neurol.* 249:1535-1540

Reinhardt MJ, Jungling FD, Krause TM, Braune S (2000) Scintigraphic differentiation between two forms of primary dysautonomia early after onset of autonomic dysfunction: value of cardiac and pulmonary iodine-123 MIBG uptake. *Eur. J. Nucl. Med.* 27:595-600

Saiki S, Hirose G, Sakai K, Kataoka S, Hori A, Saiki M, Kaito M, Higashi K, Taki S, Kakeshita K, Fujino S, Miaki M (2004) Cardiac 123I-MIBG scintigraphy can assess the disease severity and phenotype of PD. *J. Neurol. Sci.* 220:105-111

Schwartz PJ, La Rovere MT, Vanoli E (1992) Autonomic nervous system and sudden cardiac death. Experimental basis and clinical observations for post-myocardial infarction risk stratification. *Circulation.* 85:I77-91

Scozzafava J, Takahashi J, Johnston W, Puttagunta L, Martin WR (2006) Valvular heart disease in pergolide-treated Parkinson's disease. *Can. J. Neurol. Sci.* 33:111-113

Stein PK, Ehsani AA, Domitrovich PP, Kleiger RE, Rottman JN (1999) Effect of exercise training on heart rate variability in healthy older adults. *Am. Heart J.* 138:567-576

Szili-Török T, Dibó G, Kardos A, Paprika D, Rudas L (1999) Abnormal cardiovascular autonomic regulation in Parkinson's disease. *Journal of Clinical and Basic Cardiology.* 2:245-247

Taylor JA, Eckberg DL (1996) Fundamental relations between short-term RR interval and arterial pressure oscillations in humans. *Circulation.* 93:1527-1532

Tipre DN, Goldstein DS (2005) Cardiac and extracardiac sympathetic denervation in Parkinson's disease with orthostatic hypotension and in pure autonomic failure. *J. Nucl. Med.* 46:1775-1781

Turkka JT (1987) Correlation of the severity of autonomic dysfunction to cardiovascular reflexes and to plasma noradrenaline levels in Parkinson's disease. *Eur. Neurol.* 26:203-210

Turkka JT, Tolonen U, Myllyla VV (1987) Cardiovascular reflexes in Parkinson's disease. *Eur. Neurol.* 26:104-112

Van Camp G, Flamez A, Cosyns B, Goldstein J, Perdaens C, Schoors D (2003) Heart valvular disease in patients with Parkinson's disease treated with high-dose pergolide. *Neurology.* 61:859-861

Van Camp G, Flamez A, Cosyns B, Weytjens C, Muyldermans L, Van Zandijcke M, De Sutter J, Santens P, Decoodt P, Moerman C, Schoors D (2004) Treatment of Parkinson's disease with pergolide and relation to restrictive valvular heart disease. *Lancet.* 363:1179-1183

Wakabayashi K, Takahashi H (1997) Neuropathology of autonomic nervous system in Parkinson's disease. *Eur. Neurol.* 38 Suppl 2:2-7

Waller EA, Kaplan J, Heckman MG (2005) Valvular heart disease in patients taking pergolide. *Mayo Clin. Proc.* 80:1016-1020

Yamamoto M, Uesugi T, Nakayama T (2006) Dopamine agonists and cardiac valvulopathy in Parkinson disease: a case-control study. *Neurology.* 67:1225-1229

Zanettini R, Antonini A, Gatto G, Gentile R, Tesei S, Pezzoli G (2007) Valvular heart disease and the use of dopamine agonists for Parkinson's disease. *N. Engl. J. Med.* 356:39-46

In: New Research on Parkinson's Disease   ISBN: 978-1-60456-601-7
Editors: T. F. Hahn, J. Werner   © 2008 Nova Science Publishers, Inc.

Chapter VII

Parkinson's Disease: A Perfect Target for Gene Therapy

Rocío García Miniet[*] *and Esteban Alberti Amador*

Neurobiology Department, International Center of Neurological Restoration,
Havana City, Cuba.

Abstract

Parkinson's disease is a neurodegenerative disorder characterized by a progressive
loss of dopaminergic neurons of the substantia nigra pars compacta, followed by
dopamine depletion in the striatum. Cellular death takes place in a well-defined group of
neurons, this fact becomes Parkinson's disease in a perfect target for the development of
gene therapy. A variety of methods have been used in order to delivery genes into the
Central Nervous System and they can be contained into two approaches. The first, *in vivo*
gene therapy, includes the delivery of a therapeutic gene directly into host cells using
viral vectors. Each one of these viral vectors has advantages and disadvantages but the
most suitable, up to date, seem to be adeno-associated viruses and lentiviruses. For
application of the second approach, *ex vivo* gene therapy, cells should be genetically
modified *in vitro* and implanted into a recipient host. A great variety of cellular sources
have been used as vehicle of gene delivery, but the ideal cells to be employed in gene
therapy seem to be stem cells due to its capacity to differentiate and generate an
unlimited number of cells. Gene therapy carried out in Parkinson's disease includes
delivery of genes encoding biosynthetic enzymes for dopamine synthesis and
neurotrophic factors. However, protective therapy using GDNF, with the aim to prevent
neuronal death, is the most promising approach. Gene therapy is a powerful tool in the
treatment of neurodegenerative disorders and it has potentiality to be applied in
Parkinson's disease.

[*] Corresponding author: Rocío García Miniet. Neurobiology Department, International Center of Neurological
Restoration, Ave 25 # 15805, Playa, CP 11 300, Havana City, Cuba

Current Surgical Strategies in Parkinson's Disease

Parkinson's disease (PD), one of the most common neurological disorders, was described in 1917 by James Parkinson [1]. The prevalence of the PD is approximately 1 % in population over 65 years old [2]. The neuropathological characteristics of the illness are the progressive loss of dopaminergic neurons of the substantia nigra pars compacta (SNpc) and presence of Lewy bodies in neuron cytoplasm [3]. Biochemically, the most relevant feature is the dopamine depletion into striatum and SNpc [4]. These damages lead to the development of several symptoms, which do not presented until approximately 80 % of dopaminergic neurons are lost [5].

Clinical manifestations of PD include the tried of muscular rigidity, resting tremor, and bradykinesia. With the disease progress others features such as postural abnormality, cognitive changes, depression, and effective disturbances are developed [6,7].

There are several risk factors for PD, however the exact etiology is unknown. It has been suggested the hypothesis of a multifactor etiology and it has been taken into account the interaction between genetic and environmental factors, as an important aspect associated with the onset of the disease [8]. Currently hypotheses including oxidative stress, mitochondrial dysfunction, excitotoxicity, and trophic factor deficit have been considered as possible mechanisms that induce nigro-striatal degeneration [9].

At the present time, dopamine precursor administration constitutes the main base of pharmacological treatment of PD. Although this treatment is generally effective in early-stage of the disease, chronic administration is often associated with severe adverse effects, especially motor response complications, limiting the use of antiparkinsonian drugs [4]. Because of oral administration of dopamine precursor results inadequate to maintain the symptom improvement of PD, it has been necessary searching other therapeutic approaches such as surgeries.

Anatomical description of the dopaminergic nigro-striatal pathway and the depletion of striatal dopamine, have been identified. These discoveries next to the existence of a well-established model which described alterations in basal ganglia (figure 1), responsible for the onset of PD, have lead to the development of several surgical strategies [10]. Surgical procedures include ablation of different nuclei of basal ganglia, deep brain stimulation and cellular transplant into the Central Nervous System (CNS).

Pallidotomy and deep brain stimulation are very used and there is a great experience in performing these kinds of surgeries. However, bilateral deep brain stimulation of the subthalamic nucleus is considered the surgical technique of election for majority of patients. It's necessary to point up that the main disadvantage of functional surgeries is that these approaches are just a symptomatic treatment but none of them are able to prevent neither cellular death nor reverse neurodegenerative process [11].

Cellular transplants attempt to restore striatal dopaminergic transmission by implantation of cells with neuronal phenotype or cells producing dopamine. Many cellular sources have been used in human: chromaffin cells [12], embryonic porcine mesencephalic tissue [13], and carotid body cells aggregated [14]. This approach brings up a clinical improvement and, in some cases, it has been possible to eliminate pharmacological treatment [11]. Recently, the first controlled transplantation study with dopamine-producing cells was carried out in human. Even though, in the complete group of transplanted patients, it was not observed a significant change in the rate of UPDRS; it was shown that dopaminergic cells grafts turned out in a clinical improvement of younger patients [15].

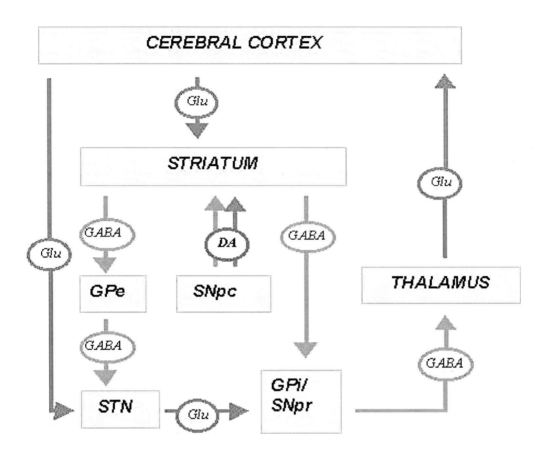

Figure 1. Model representing circuits of the basal gaglia. The degeneration of the dopaminergic nigrostriatal neurons occurring in PD with the progression of the disease induces a dopamine deficit in the striatum. Dopaminergic depletion provokes an increased and abnormally patterned output to the thalamus, which may in part be responsible for the motor disturbances of patients. Blue arrows represent projections with excitatory effect and red arrows represent projections with inhibitory effect. GABA: gabaergic projections; DA: dopaminergic projections; Glu: glutamatergic projections; SNpc: substantia nigra pars compacta; SNpr: substantia nigra pars reticularis; Gpe: external globus pallidus; Gpi: internal globus pallidus.

Another treatment strategy, which is being very explored at this moment, is the application of gene therapy in order to get an overexpression of a gene having therapeutic interesting in the injured brain. With this aim, also, exist the possibility to combine both the cellular and gene therapy to obtain cells expressing proteins in high levels.

Gene Therapy

Treating the brain is very difficult due to it is an organ with a great complexity whose characterization still remains incomplete. As well, the CNS contains a great number of neurons which establish connection among them, therefore, anything that affect the interaction among cells or the activity of them can produce serious effects in the organism functioning. The possibility to apply a pharmacological treatment in the CNS is more difficult than in systemic affections due to the presence of the cranium, the meninges, and the blood-brain barrier that partially isolate the brain. In spite of all the above-mentioned inconvenience, gene therapy constitute a promise for the future on account of this approach gives the possibility to allow a maintained delivery of a desired gene product into the brain.

The term "gene therapy" refers to the introduction of foreign genetic material into a sick host organism, using the host genetic machinery in order to produce a protein with therapeutic effect. This approach, with a great potentiality to application, includes several strategies. The first refers to the replacement of flawed genes by its functional homologues for correcting a genetic defect, this is a difficult goal because of a long-term expression genes in all affected cells is required [16]. The second includes the expression of molecules, which block synthesis or action of a protein having harmful effects, by coding an antisense mRNA [17]. The third refers to strategies in which enhanced expression of specific genes is gotten with the aim of reaching *in situ* production of therapeutic proteins by a population of cells [18]. The last approach is the most widely used in several disorders of the CNS, including PD.

Neurodegenerative disorders are targets of gene therapy in the nervous system Nevertheless, there are several reasons that become PD in the neurodegenerative disorder more sensible to gene therapy:

- Some illness such as Alzheimer's disease, Amyotrophic Lateral Sclerosis, and Leukoystrophies, affect in a global way many types of neurons. So, this element hinders the application of gene therapy due to the population of affected cells are distribute in a great part of the brain and the delivery of gene product to the whole damaged neurons group is a real problem. This trouble is not present in PD because in this case, at early states, only a well-defined and compact group of neuron is damaged, the dopaminergic cells of the SNpc. Consequently an easier strategy can be carried out because the required gene delivery is localized [19].
- In spite of its etiology has not been described, several pathological elements have been well characterized, the biochemical alteration is understood (figure 1) and it's known the genes whose manipulation produces a therapeutic benefit. This group of genes will be discussed in this review afterward.
- The existence of well-characterized animal models in PD has help to the development of several experimental strategies. Although parkinsonism is not manifested in animals in a spontaneous way, several experimental animal models of PD that have helped to study mechanisms involved in the pathogenesis of the illness and to carry out therapeutic strategies have been developed. The most used animal models of PD are probably the rat 6-hydroxydopamine (6-OHDA) lesion model. The

selective accumulation of this neurotoxin in dopaminergic neurons produces their death, maybe for oxidative stress [20]. The massive unilateral destruction of the dopaminergic neurons produces an asymmetry in the dopamine levels between injured and non-injured side. Probably, this asymmetry is responsible of the rotational behavioral observed in injured animals that is increased with the use of dopaminergic agonist [21]. The quantification of D-amphetamine and apomorfine rotations is one of the behavioral tests most widely used to evaluate the motor imbalance before and after the application of a therapeutic treatment.

In the other way, taken into account that there is not any effective treatment that stop the disease progression, the development of gene therapy as a promising strategy is welcome.

Approach of Gene Delivery to the CNS

Two general methods have been used to delivery genes into the CNS: *in vivo* gene therapy and *ex vivo* gene therapy. The selection of one of these methods is a key decision when developing a gene therapy strategy. In both cases, it's indispensable evaluate the effectiveness of gene expression in the animal models used. This evaluation is carried out by histological studies, behavioral tests, and/or determination of protein expression.

Ex Vivo Gene Therapy

Ex vivo gene therapy includes the use of cells, with neural or non-neural origin, genetically modified that are implanted in the CNS in order to act as delivery gene vehicle. The whole process of cell manipulation is carried out in vitro allowing the screening of toxicity risks associated with viral systems. The transgene expression can be monitored and its biochemical and immunological effects can be characterized. So, the principal advantage of this approach is performing a great control of gene transfer process before genetically modified cells are implanted into the brain. Also, it is possible selecting the cells able to express the trangene. Hence, an enriched cellular population is obtained and consequently a major desired protein production is achieved.

Nevertheless, ex vivo gene therapy application into the CNS is associated with several inconveniences. In some cases, these handicaps have been minimized but not completely eliminated. When cells are implanted into the brain, gene expression is generally transient and its control is not well characterized. Sometimes grafts are immunogenic and they just survive few months. Regarding the cellular source used, transplant can form tumors whose continuous growth produces the animal death. In order to obtain enough gene product expression it is essential a great quantity of cells to be grafted. This is a limitation because eventually the accessibility to the selected cellular sources is difficult or the possibility to multiply the cellular population is critic. Also, large grafts can displaces the host cerebral tissue producing variations in the brain physiology. Generally the desired protein expression is limited to the injection site, there is not diffusion of the therapeutic products and the graft effectiveness decrease. Genetic modifications of cells to be implanted into the CNS include the introduction of genes codifying just secretable proteins like neurotrophic factors and neurotransmitters because infected cells act as a genes delivery vehicle whose products can not cross the host cells membrane.

A key decision when ex vivo gene therapy is going to be developed is what cellular source should be used. Although it is very difficult that a cell population owns all necessary requirement to be implanted into the CNS, they must possess the possible major number of ideal characteristics [11,22]. These characteristics could be summarized in:

1. In order to select the cellular source it is important takes into account the possibility to culture, multiply, and modify them. With this aim cells easy of obtaining, which have the genetic information for carrying out postranscriptional modifications and for expressing the desired genetic material, are required. This aspect can limit or stimulate the use of the selected cellular cells.
2. They should be susceptible to the modification with the vector that contains the desired gene. As well, cells should own genetic characteristic allowing them surviving to the selection process used to enrich cellular population expressing the desired gene products.
3. Cells should survive long time after the transplant and this characteristic should not change with the genetic modification of cells.
4. The cellular source used should be non-oncogenic and immunologically compatible with the recipient in order to avoid rejection problems.
5. Preferably, an inexhaustible cellular source to be implanted should exist. This guarantees the total cells availability.
6. When cells are going to be implanted into the brain, it is important guaranteeing a correct integration and differentiation of these cells in order to reestablishing the normal functioning of basal ganglia circuits.

Until the moment, it has been utilized a great numbers of cells as gene delivery vehicle in PD which have some characteristics of those above-mentioned. These cellular sources include fibrablasts, astrocytes, and recently stem cells.

Genetically modified non-neural cells can be employed to gene delivery into the CNS, for instance, skin fibroblasts. These cells are easily obtainable and growth from small biopsies, so there is the possibility to be used as autologous transplant avoiding rejection problems. It have been shown that both primary fibroblasts and fibroblasts-derived cell lines can survive as intracerebral grafts for at least two months without evidence of tumorogenesis. After this time, immortalized cells occasionally show evidence of excessive growth [23]. When fibroblasts are implanted they tend to form a globular clump of cells that displaces the brain parenchyma and interrupt the normal functions of the neural tissue [24]. The disadvantages of fibroblasts are associated with their non-neural origin. These cells don't have the capacity to integrate broadly into the host brain in a functional manner after graft. For this reason, circuits may not be reformed and the regulated release of important molecules may be missing [25]. It has been developed many research using fibroblasts genetically modified with tyrosine hydroxylase (TH), the limiting enzyme in catecholamine synthesis and from these results a main conclusion is drawn [10]. Fibroblasts even when expressing active TH, can not produce dopamine due to they require an external source of the cofactor necessary for completing the first reaction in the pathway to synthesize this neurotransmitter (see the explanation later on).

Astrocytes are an important cellular source because of their neural origin. In the brain, these cells perform vital functions regarding survival and maintenance of neurons, so they are considered as a versatile platform to express molecules of therapeutic interest in the CNS [26]. Astrocytes are able to synthesize dopamine and released it into the medium [27]. For this reason and considering that these cells possess an efficient secretory system, when they are genetically modified to express TH, they can produce and release dopamine, without the necessity to add an external source of cofactors involved in the biosynthetic pathway of this neurotransmitter. Astrocytes are relatively resistant to oxidative stress, this element is important because dopamine synthesis produce reactive oxidative species [27]. The main handicap of these cells is that there is not the possibility to use them as an autologous transplant, consequently rejection problems are not avoided.

An important cellular type to the treatment of neurological disorders is the stem cells population. A stem cell is a cell from the embryo, fetus, or adult that has, under certain conditions, the capacity for self-renewal during long periods or, in the case of adult stem cells, throughout the life of the organism [28]. Of late these cells are being explored as gene delivery vehicle in specific tissues.

Bone marrow stromal cells (BMSC) is a population of adult stem cells having features that become them in an attractive cellular source to be used both in cellular and gene therapy. Human BMSC are relatively easy to isolate from small aspirates of whole bone marrow by their adherence to tissue culture surfaces [29,30]. Also, it has been shown that stromal cells, in culture, maintain the ability to differentiate in several cell lineages [29]. In addition, it is not difficult to gene-engineer them and obtain a large quantity of modified cells [31,32]. They have the ability to differentiate into tissues other than the ones from which they originated. *In vitro* studies showed that BMSC can generate non-mesenchymal cell types including myocytes, hepatocytes, microglia, and even neuronal cells [33,34]. There are evidences that BMSC injected into the lateral ventricles of neonatal mice can migrate throughout the forebrain and cerebellum, and they can differenciate into astrocytes and cells with neural phenotype [35]. In a similar study, it was confirmed that direct infusion of human BMSC into rat striatum give rise to astrocytes [36]. It has been demonstrated their ability to produce and secrete neurotrophic factors such as IGF-1 [37], NGF [38], BDNF [39], and GDNF [40]. It is an important feature to the treatment of PD because of these proteins are able to protect and rescue dopaminergic neurons [41] also, GDNF is the protein with the strongest trophic effect over dopaminergic neurons.

With the use of BMSC in gene therapy approach, implanted cells have a dual role. First, they behave like pumps delivering genes of interesting that act upon host cells. On the other hand, these cells when are implanted have the potentiality to migrate and differentiate into neuronal phenotypes. Hence, theoretically, combination of both properties gives rise the possibility that BMSC could re-establish the interactions cell-cell into the brain and get the delivery of the desired gene in a great area of the brain.

In Vivo Gene Therapy

In vivo gene therapy involves the introduction of interest gene in a non-viral or viral vector and the direct treatment of the brain with this expression system. Non-viral vectors include cationic liposomes, naked DNA and, DNA-proteins complex. On the other hand, viral vectors get from viruses that are engineered to prevent the infective destruction in target tissues. Although non-viral vectors are considered safer than viral vectors, they are less efficient because they achieved very low levels of transgenes expression. For this reason, the use of non-viral vectors in animal models on CNS disorders is more limited. Contrarily, viral vectors are widely used in neurological diseases due to they generally reach high transgenes expression in a great number of target cells.

One of the advantages of in vivo gene therapy is that viral systems are small molecules, which do not interrupt the normal brain architecture, contrarily to what happen when cellular grafts are used. Viral vector systems are applied in situ to host cells, over which therapeutic gene products should act. That is why, this approach is not only restricted to the expression of secretable proteins acting upon the cellular surface but it can be used to express intracellular proteins such as enzymes, transporters, and receptors [22]. Nervous cells are the best equipped to produce desired CNS gene products because they have the genetic information for producing and secreting neurotransmitters, the ability to carry out transcriptional modifications of these gene products, and they possess the adequate cofactors [42].

On the other hand, it has been exposed that generally modified host cells are very close to injection site or in the tissue surface acquiring a restricted distribupion [16]. This situation provokes a therapeutic limited effect bounded to a small number of cells. This problem can be minimized using multiple inoculations in several transplant sites allowing a greater number of infected cells and a more efficient gene product delivery. Viral vectors application results in functional modifications of infected cells and the evaluation of these modifications is very difficult when the infected cells are the host one. Hence, a clinical application of the in vivo gene therapy should be preceded of an intense study in animal model that undertakes the determination of transgenes expression levels and the possibility of forming tumors. Nevertheless, the major inconveniences include the safety of using viral vector systems. It is known that these vectors cause toxicity and inflammatory respond in the host tissue.

Viral Vectors Used for Ex Vivo and In Vivo Gene Therapy

Viruses are obligate intra-cellular parasites designed through the course of evolution to infect cells. Generally they are very efficient at transfecting their own DNA into the host cell. When genes needed for viral genome replication are substituted with genes of therapeutic interest, recombinant viral vectors are obtained and they maintain the ability to transduce cells. With this aim, removed genes, which are necessary for replication, are provided in trans, either integrated into the genome of the packaging cell line or on a plasmid.

Even though it has been explored many viruses as vectors for gene therapy, those described later on are the most broadly used for transgenes delivery in the CNS. Each of them have advantageous and disadvantageous, and although there is no consensus regarding the ideal vector system, the most suitable, up to date, seem to be adeno-associated viruses and lentiviruses.

Adenovirus Vectors

The adenovirus (Ad) is a double-stranded DNA virus, which in its wild type form, causes acute upper respiratory tract. The adenoviral long genome (36 kb) is well-characterized. It is constituted by early (E1-E4) and late (L1-L5) expression genes codifying for structural and non-structural proteins; two inverted terminal repeat (ITR), one of them is necessary for the initiation of viral DNA replication; and an DNA packaging signal [43].

First generation of recombinant adenoviruses has been widely described. These vectors are made replication-defective through deletions in the E1 region including E1A and E1B genes. Using cell lines expressing E1 region genes in *trans*, it can be possible to produce preparation of recombinant viral particles with high titer, (10^8-10^{12} IU/ml) [43-46]. Ad vectors infect a broad range of cellular type, dividing and non-dividing cells, with high efficiency both *in vitro* and *in vivo* [47]. The main limitation of this generation of adenovirus is that they express residual viral genes producing a strong immune response. This has been associate with the decrease in the duration of transgen expression observed in many studies using recombinant adenovirus [48,49]. In addition, higher titers of recombinant Ad vectors (> 5 x 10^7 IU) resulted in cellular toxicity with both gliosis and vascular inflammatory responses [50]. Also, if the animal has been previously exposed to adenovirus, which is the cases in most of the humans, infected cells are quickly eliminated by an specific anti-adenovirus immune response [51]. Another inconvenience of these vectors is that they are present as an episomal DNA and it is not ideal for obtaining long-term expression of the transgenes. In the other hand, these vectors only allow accommodate insert of up to approximately 8 kb [42]. Nevertheless, this is not a problem for PD because of the majority of therapeutic interest genes for this disorder do not exceed this size.

Recently, it has been developed high capacity Ad vectors, also named "gutless" Ad vectors. In these new adenoviral constructions almost all viral genes are deleted and only ITRs and packing signal remain [52]. For obtaining recombinant viral particles it is necessary the presence of a helper virus providing, in *trans*, required genes for replication, packaging, and encapsidation. These new generation adenoviral vectors allow insert sequences of foreign DNA of approximately 28 kb [47]. Studies carried out *in vivo* using "gutless" adenoviral vectors have shown high levels of transgenes expression with very low toxicity [51]. Nevertheless, it is necessary to improve technical aspects in order to obtain viral preparations with higher titers and lower contamination with helper virus [47].

Adeno-Associated Virus Vectors

Adeno-associated virus (AAV) is a small, single-stranded DNA parvovirus, non-pathogenic to human. Six AAVs (AAV-1 to 6) have been isolated from primates, and their genome has been studied. The most known is the AAV-2 and it is very used for the development of gene therapy vectors [53]. The AAV-2 genome contains two open reading frames (ORF) flanked by two ITRs that are indispensable for packaging of viral DNA and act as the replication origin. One of the ORFs, encodes a set of four non structural Rep proteins, which are essential for AAV genome replication. The other ORF encodes a group of proteins participating in viral encapsidation, they are VP1, VP2, and VP3 [54].

The production of recombinant AAV include the transfection with a plasmid containing a sequences encoding the therapeutic gene flanking by the AVV ITRs and other one providing in *trans* the Rep and VP proteins. The co-transfection is carried out along with a helper virus that contains adenoviral gene products necessary for carry out helper functions [55]. It has been developed protocols which do not use helper virus but a helper plasmid, so the contamination with adenovirus is avoided and the preparation of recombinant AAV is safer [50,56].

AVV have the ability to integrate its DNA into a specific locus of the host genome, which is chromosome 19 in humans, allowing prolonged transgene expression. Nevertheless, a large amount of AAV vectors remains episomal [50,57]. AAV can infect a wide range of dividing and quiescent cells. A further and main advantage of the use of recombinant vectors is that they have minimal viral sequences. Thus their *in vivo* administration, apparently, does not produce a serious immune response nor toxicity [47].

However, AAV present two disadvantages. The total length of AAV genome is relatively small, for this reason the insert cannot greatly exceed 5 kb [58,59], although as we previously mention, generally this is not a disadvantage in the case of the EP. In the other hand, the obtaining of high titers is cumbersome, although with new procedures it has been possible to obtain titers of 10^9 IU/ml [58].

Recently, the US Food and Drug Administration (FDA) approved a clinical trial for the application of AAV in humans. The treatment was designed to delivery a recombinant AAV containing glutamic acid decarboxylase (GAD) gene, the key enzyme in the synthesis of GABA, into the subthalamic nucleus in order to ameliorate Parkinson's symptoms [60].

Herpes Virus Vectors

Herpes simple virus type I (HSV-1) is an enveloped double strand DNA virus containing a large genome (~ 150 kb). Two approach for using HSV-1 as gene delivery vector have been developed, they are named amplicon and recombinant systems.

The amplicon system contains the foreign gene and a fraction of the complete HSV-1 genome including the origin of DNA replication and a cleavage/packaging signal. This segment is repeated several times until the size of the total HSV-1 genome is generated [50]. When the amplicon is transfected into a cell line containing a helper virus (a temperature sensitive mutant) that provide *in trans* necessary proteins for viral replication and packaging, the repeated sequences of the HSV-1 are replicated, cleaved into 150 kb units, and package into an HSV-1 virion particle. As result, several copies of the interest gene are delivery in a cell, amplifying the signal [50,61].

Recombinant system, are made replication deficient by deletion of one or some essential genes from the HSV-1 genome. Therefore, replication mutants are only able to replicate in certain cell lines that supply cellular proteins to complement the missing gene products. Gene of interest is inserted into the viral genome and homologous recombination occurs. In turn, recombinant viruses containing the foreign gene are obtained [62].

The attractive features of these vectors include the ability to establish latency in neurons, it can infect dividing and non dividing cells, and it is possible to obtain viral stocks of high titers (10^8 –10^9 UI/ml) [63]. Due to the large genome of the virus, HSV-1 vectors allow accommodate large inserts or more than one transgenes (30-40 kb). Besides, insertional mutagenesis is not a trouble for these vectors because HSV genome remains as an episomal element [64].

However, the use of HSV-1 vectors is associated with inflammation, immune response, and toxicity. There is the possibility that HSV-1 vectors revert to wild-type virus by recombination producing encephalitis. In some studies, it has been reported that 10-20 % of animals treated with an HSV-1 vector died, probably due to the above-mentioned reason [50,65]. These elements limit the use of HSV-1 vectors to treat neurodegenerative disorders in humans.

Retroviral Vectors

Retrovirus is an enveloped virus whose genome is represented by a single stranded RNA molecule. After infection, the viral genome is reverse transcribed into double stranded DNA, which integrates into the host genome and is expressed as proteins. The viral genes are replaced with the transgene of interest and expressed on plasmids in the packaging cell line. The viral genome is approximately 10kb, so the accommodation capacity of the inserted gene is ~7.5 kb [66].

Retroviruses integration requires that target cells are dividing. Thus, these viral vectors are ideal for ex vivo approach but they do not allow the direct transfer of transgene into non-dividing CNS cells. It is not easy to obtain stock viral preparation of recombinant retroviruses at high titers, usually titers produced are in the range between 10^4-10^6 IU/ml [26,31,42]. The possibility of reversion to the wild type virus by homologous recombination exists. Retroviruses do not stay episomal but the viral vector is integrated into the chromosome at random. Although this ability is ideal for the long-term expression of the transgene, it could produce insertional mutagenesis and cause cancer by disrupting a tumour suppresser gene. The use of retroviruses in a clinical trials was applied to 11 chlidren treated for X-linked severe combined immunodeficiency. Three years later, two children developed leukaemia, probably due to the retroviral vector insertional mutagenesis [67]. For this reason, the FDA suspended all gene therapy studies using retroviral vectors.

Lentivirus Vectors

Lentiviruses are a subclass of retroviruses, able to infect both proliferating and non-proliferating cells, including neurons and stem cells. It has been developed two classes of lentiviruses, HIV-1 and HIV-2 lentiviral vectors. However, HIV-2 has more advantages than HIV-1 for human gene therapy because generally is less pathogenic [68]. Lentiviral vectors integrate into the host genome of their targets and a long-term expression of the transgene is achieved (until 8 months). The gene expression observed in this study occurred without evidence of significant toxicity [69]. Besides, it can be possible to obtain high titers of viral preparation of ~ 10^8 IU/ml [70]. These characteristics of the lentiviral vectors make them in one of the most attractive vectors for application of gene therapy, although more studies regarding safety of these vectors are necessary before use them in a clinical trials.

Gene of Therapeutic Interesting in Parkinson's Disease

As etiology of Parkinson's disease is unknown, current strategies carried out regarding the delivered genes for the treatment of PD are based in the elements of the illness that have been described. Dysfunctions of the motor responses due to alteration of the basal ganglia functioning are the result of the striatal dopamine deficit, so the first approach leads to the dopamine replacement by expression of enzymes participating in the biosynthetic pathway of this neurotransmitter. In contrast, the decrease of the secreted dopamine levels in the putamen is a direct consequence of the progressive loss of the substantia nigra dopaminergic neurons. Thus, considering that one of the elements theoretically implicated in the cellular death, occurring in neurodegenerative disorders, involves the deficit of neurotrophic factors; the second approach include the delivery of gene encoding these proteins.

Dopamine Replacement

The first step in the synthesis of dopamine takes places from L-tyrosine, an essential amino acid that is present in all cells of the organism. L-tyrosine hydroxylation to produce L-DOPA is carried out by tyrosine hydroxylase (TH). This enzyme, which is limiting of this biosynthetic pathway, requires the presence of three cofactors: tetrahydrobiopterin (BH_4), oxygen, and iron. The second reaction, the L-DOPA decarboxylation to produce dopamine, is catalyzed by the Aromatic-L-Amino-Acid Decarboxylase (AADC) that uses pyridoxal phophate as cofactor. In the other hand, BH_4 is synthesized from GTP in several enzymatic reactions. The GTP cyclohydrolase I (GTPCH I) catalyzes the first step in this sequence of reactions and it is the limiting enzyme in the synthesis of BH_4 (figure 2).

With the aim to increase dopamine levels into the striatum in animal models of PD several studies have been carried out. They include the introduction of TH cDNA into a viral vector and delivery of the construction encoding this enzyme into the CNS, both directly or by means of cells. It has been used astrocytes genetically modified to produce the TH gene under the control of an astrocytes-specific promoter derived from the glial fibrillary acidic protein (GFAP) gene. The use of this promoter offers several advantages, it has a built-in regulatory system that increase its transcripcional activity in responds to reactive gliosis, which take place when a brain injury is produced [71], and in responds to intracellular signals (i.e, variations of cAMP levels) [27]. So, the activity of the GFAP promoter increases due to the progression of the illness. In all these studies a significant recovery of the function was observed since in treated animals a reduction of about 50 % in the turning behavior occurring in response to apomorphine was detected.

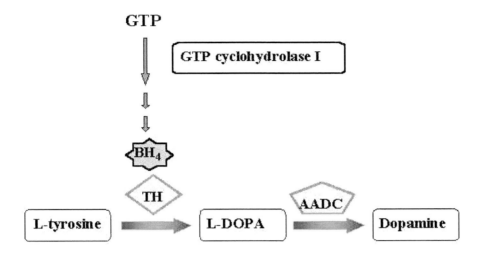

Figure 2. Schematic representation of the dopamine synthesis. The limiting enzyme, TH, requires BH_4 as cofactor for carry out the L-tyrosine hydroxylation.

In vivo TH transfer using adenovirus as alternative to the treatment of PD was evaluated [72]. All animals received the same quantity of recombinant adenoviral particles but experimental groups differed in the number of injection sites and the location of viral vector dispersion. The treatment with adenovirus expressing TH resulted in behavioral recovery in 6-OHDA-lesioned rats. Nevertheless, it was observed that animals receiving multi-site steriotactic injections showed highly significant behavioral recovery, major number of TH-immunoreactive cells, and consequently, major TH expression in the striatum that those receiving single-site injection. Moreover, it was concluded that subregional effects of TH expression might be important to obtain a reduction in turning behavior.

Many cells used as gene delivery vehicle do not synthesize BH_4. In addition, endogenous levels of this cofactor in the denervated striatum are insufficient to support TH activity. Thus, exogenous BH_4 infusion is necessary to obtain a good recovery when TH transfer is applied. It has been demonstrated that BH_4 penetrates poorly into the nervous system [73]. For that reason, gene transfer of GTPCH I may be an option for support TH activity [24]. Several studies, *in vivo* [74] and *ex vivo* [24,75], have concluded that the expression of both TH and GTPCH I is required for the production of L-DOPA since BH_4 has an important role in the biochemical restoration of animal models of PD.

Although patients of PD suffer a significant loss of dopaminergic neurons, which are the principal source of AADC, L-DOPA is transformed in dopamine into the brain of these patients. The source and site of the remainder AADC in dopamine depleted animals is unknown because there is not any significant non-enzymatic L-DOPA decarboxylation *in vivo* [42]. As the importance of the AADC supply is not clear, some studies including expression of this enzyme, in order to evaluate its role in the dopamine production, have been carried out.

At the present time, L-DOPA administration together with carbidopa, the peripheral inhibitor of the AADC, is the pharmacological treatment most widely used in patients of PD. This approach is beneficial in early stages of the disease but with the progression of the illness AADC levels decrease and the treatment effectiveness declines. With the aim to resolve this trouble, *in vivo* AADC gene transfer using an AAV vector together with systemic administration of L-DOPA was carried out [76]. It was detected a more efficient dopamine production from L-DOPA by restoration of AADC levels into the striatum. Therefore, using this strategy it is possible reduce the dose of L-DOPA / carbidopa with a better clinical response and fewer side effects.

Considering that endogenous AADC activity in the striatum of animal models of PD is low, cotransduction of rat model striatal cells using two separate AAVs expresing TH or AADC was performed. Cotransduction with these two recombinant AAV vectors resulted in a more efficient dopamine production and a better behavioral recovery in lesioned rats compared with AAV expresing TH alone. It was concluded that the decrease of endogenous decarboxylase levels in the striatum limits the therapeutic effects of the TH gene transfer alone [77]. Taking into account these results, the effects of triple-transduction with AAV expressing TH, AADC, and GTPCH I upon biochemical and behavioral improvement compared with double-transduction with AAV expresing TH and AADC was evaluated [78]. A more remarkable decrease in turning behavior was observed in triple-transduced rats than double transduced ones. The major dopamine levels was detected in animals receiving a triple transduction, this result was in correspondence with the behavioral improvement observed in this group of animals. This study showed than TH as well as AADC and GTPCH I are key enzymes necessary for reaching an efficient production of dopamine.

Protective and Restorative Therapy

Neurotrophic factors are small proteins with capacity to promote sprouting of surviving neurons. These proteins are able to maintain neuronal cultures *in vitro* and protect neurons, *in vitro* and *in vivo*, of toxic damage. It has been widely describe the role of neurotrophic factors in the protection of dopaminergic neurons that are lost during PD progression and most of the research has focused on Glial Cell Line-derived Neurotrophic Factor (GDNF).

GDNF gene transfer induces a therapeutic benefit in 6-OHDA-lesioned rats and MPTP-treated monkeys. This effect is achieved due to neuroprotective and neurorestorative ability of GDNF. The *in vivo* transduction of lentivirus vector expressing GDNF, into the striatum of MPTP lesioned mice and into the substantia nigra of MPTP treated monkeys, prevented loss of TH positive cells observed in animal models of PD [69,79]. Similar protection of dopaminergic neurons against 6-OHDA-induced degeneration was obtained with a recombinant AVV expressing GDNF delivered in either substantia nigra or striatum [55]. Nevertheless, the rescue of dopaminergic cells was most pronounced in animals receiving injection in the substantia nigra. The injection of recombinant AAV in the striatum produced an incomplete protection of nigral dopaminergic neurons, maybe because a greater spread of GDNF throughout this region may be required to obtain a complete protection.

Recently, the first study demonstrating that BMSCs has ability for acting as gene delivery vehicle to achieve neuroprotection was carried out [31]. BMSCs were genetically modified with a retroviral vector expressing GDNF and they were injected in the tail vein of MPTP-lesioned mice. Although GDNF secreted by modified cells has very poor penetration across the blood brain barrier, these authors reported a clear protective effect of nigral neurons and their striatal terminals. They consider that this effect could be intensified using brain-specific promoters to regulate the transgene expression.

The application of a neuroprotective strategy in human is not a practical approach since clinical symptoms of PD begin to show up when more than 80 % of dopaminergic neurons have died. Hence, an ideal therapy could allow slowing down the death of the remainder healthy neurons and rescuing damaged neurons from dying [5]. For this reason, the evaluation of neurorestorative effect of GDNF using viral vectors has been performed in several studies.

It have been reported that the treatment with GDNF, *ex vivo* [80] and *in vivo* [69,80], produce an increase in the number of TH-immunoreactive cells. This effect could be explained because GDNF may induce plasticity in the dopamine-depleted brain of animal treated by converting striatal neurons to dopaminergic cells [80]. Nevertheless, it has been demonstrated that intrastiatal but not intranigral treatment of the brain induces functional regeneration in the damaged nigroestriatal system [55]. In other studies, furthermore, when GDNF is delivery in the substantia nigra it is possible generate enhancement of dopaminergic activity in the ventral tegmental area and induce other symptoms [81]. That is to say the ideal site of vector administration should be taken into account and more profound researches will be needed for determining it.

In this respect, the advantages of the gene transfer of GDNF as a neuroprotective and neurorestaurative factor is clear. This approach rather than symtomatic therapy is a strategy preventing degeneration of lost neurons and restoring functions of dopaminergic nigrostriatal cells. However, although a great advance has been reached in this field, some research should be carried out before clinical application of this approach [82].

Conclusions

Gene therapy is a promising approach for the treatment of PD in the future. However, some limitations should be resolve such as long-term expression of transgenes and regulation of this expression. Up to day, the most suitable viral vectors seem to be adeno-associated viruses and lentiviruses. The benefits of each one should be compared in order to establish the better vector for the application in humans. The delivery of GDNF in early-stage of PD, when patient have a relatively large number of remaining dopaminergic neurons yet, is emerging as an attractive strategy for clinical application of gene therapy. The combination of cellular and gene therapy may be favorable because the advantages of the cellular source used are profitable. The ideal cells to use as gene delivery vehicle are stem cells with the ability to differentiate to dopaminergic phenotype and susceptible to viral modification. By all means, the future development of different strategies of gene therapy in human as a treatment for PD requires the efforts of many researches but it is an optimistic hope.

References

[1]   Parkinson J. *An essay on the shaking palsy*. [London: Whittingham and Rowland for Sherwood, Neely, and Jones]. 1817.

[2]   Fernandez-Espejo E, El Banoua F, Caraballo I, Galán B, Flores JA: Trasplante de células naturales "dopaminotróficas": nuevo concepto terapéutico antiparkinsoniano. *Rev Neurol* 2003, 36:540-544.

[3]   Hurelbrink CB, Barker RA: Prospects for the treatment of Parkinson's disease using neurotrophic factors. *Expert Opinion Pharmacotherapy* 2001, 2:1531-1543.

[4]   Djaldetti R, Melamed E: New therapies for Parkinson's disease. *J Neurol* 2001, 248:357-362.

[5]   Bohn MC, Kozlowski DA, Connor B: Glial cell line-derived neurotrophic factor (GDNF) as a defensive molecule for neurodegenerative disease: a tribute to the studies of Antonia Vernadakis on neuronal-glial interactions. *Int J Devl Neuroscience* 2000, 18:679-684.

[6]   Linazasoro G: Complicaciones no motoras en la Enfermedad de Parkinson. In *Tratado sobre la Enfermedad de Parkinson*. Edited by Obeso JA, Tolosa ES, Grandas FJ. Edición en CD-ROM. Laboratorios DU PONT Pharma y Ediciones Doyma S.L.; 2000:353-364.

[7]   Aarsland D, Andersen K, Larsen JP, Lolk A, Kragh-Sorensen P: Prevalence and characteristics of dementia in Parkinson disease: an 8-year prospective study. *Arc Neurol* 2003, 60:387-392.

[8]   Allam MF, del Castillo AS, Navajas RFC: Factores de riesgo de la Enfermedad de Parkinson. *Rev Neurol* 2003, 36:749-755.

[9]   Ferrer I: Muerte neuronal. *Neurología* 2003, 18(Supl 1):62-68.

[10]   Segovia J: Gene therapy for Parkinson's disease. Current status and Future Potential. *Am J Pharmacogenomics* 2002, 2:135-146.

[11]   Linazasoro G: Células madre: ¿solución a la problemática actual de los trasplantes en la enfermedad de Parkinson? *Neurología* 2003, 18:29-52.

[12]   Drucker-Colín R, Verdugo-Díaz L, Morgado-Valle C, Solís-Maldonado G, Ondarza R, Boll C, Miranda G, Jack-Wang G, Volkow N: Transplant of cultured neuron-like differentiated chromaffin cells in a Parkinson's disease patient. A preliminary report. *Arch Med Res* 1999, 30:33-39.

[13]   Schumacher JM, Ellias SA, Palmer EP, Kott HS, Dinsmore J, Dempsey PK, et al.: Transplantation of embryonic porcine mesencephalic tissue in patients with Parkinson's disease. *Neurology* 2000, 54:1042-1049.

[14]   Mínguez A, López J, Arjona V, Montoro R, Escamilla F, Ortega A, et al: Trasplante de agregados celulares de cuerpo carotídeo en pacientes con Enfermedad de Parkinson. *Neurología* 2000, 15:580.

[15]   Freed CR, Greene PE, Breeze RE, Tsai W, DuMouchel W, Kao R, et al: Transplantation of embryonic dopamine neurons for severe Parkinson's disease. *N Eng J Med* 2001, 344:710-719.

[16]   Tinsley R, Eriksson P: Use of gene therapy in central nervous system repair. *Acta Neurol Scand* 2004, 109:1-8.

[17] Benítez JA, Segovia J: Gene therapy targeting in the central nervous system. *Current Gene Therapy* 2003, 3:127-145.

[18] González M, González ME: La terapia génica para el sistema nervioso: una tendencia en la neurología moderna. *Rev Neuro* 1998, 27:625-630.

[19] Bohn MC: Parkinson's disease: a neurodegenerative disease particularly amenable to gene therapy. *Mol Ther* 2001, 1:494-496.

[20] Venero JL, Revuelta M, Cano J, Machado A: Time courses changes in the dopaminergic nigrostriatal system following transection of the medial forebrain bundle: detection of oxidatively modified proteins in substantia nigra. *J.Neurochem* 1997, 68:2458-2468.

[21] Pavón N, Vidal L, Alvarez P, Blanco L, Torres A, Rodríguez A, Macías R: Evaluación conductual del modelo de lesión unilateral en ratas con 6-hidroxidopamina. Correlación entre las rotaciones inducidas por d-anfetamina, apomorfina y la prueba de habilidades manuales. *Rev Neurol* 1998, 26:915-918.

[22] Kang UJ, Frim DM: Gene therapy for arkinson's disease: review and update. *Exp.Opin.Invest.Drugs* 1999, 8:-1.

[23] Gage F, Fisher L, Jinnah H, Rosenberg M, Tuszynski M, Friedmann T: Grafting genetically modified cells to the brain. *Prog Brain Res* 1990, 82:1-10.

[24] Bencsics C, Wachtel SR, Milstien S, Hatakeyama K, Becker JB, Kang UJ: Double transduction with GTP cyclohydrolase I and tyrosine hydroxylaseis necessary for spontaneous synthesis of L-Dopa by primary fibroblasts. *J.Neurosc.* 1996, 16:4449-4456.

[25] Snyder EY, Wolf JH: Central nervous system cell transplantation: a novel therapy for storage diseases? *Curr.Opin.Neurol.* 1996, 9:126136.

[26] Cortez N, Trejo F, Vergara P, Segovia J: Primary astrocytes retrovirally transduced with a tyrosine ydroxylase transgene driven by a glial-specific promoter elicit behavioural recovery in experimental parkinsonism. *J.Neurosc.Res.* 2000, 9:39-46.

[27] Segovia J, Vergara P, Brenner M: Astrocyte-specific expression of tyrosine hydroxylase after intracerebral gene transfer induces behavioral recovery in experimental Parkinsonism. *Gene Ther* 1998, 5:1650-1655.

[28] Kirschstein R, Shirboll LR. *Stem Cells: scientific progress and future research directions. Rebuilding the nervous system with stem cells.* 77-85. 2001. National Institute of Health.

[29] Prockop DJ, Sekiya I, Colter DC: Isolation and characterization of rapidly self-renewing stem cells from cultures of human marrow stromal cells. *Cytotherapy* 2001, 3:393-396.

[30] Shih H, Nien Ch, Shie H, Hung L, Hsiao M, Wai L: Isolation and characterization of size-sieved stem cells from human bone marrow. *Stem cells* 2002, 20:249-258.

[31] Park KW, Eglitis MA, Mouradian MM: Protection of nigral neurons by GDNF-engineered marrow cell transplantation. *Neurosci Res* 2001, 40:315-323.

[32] Prockop D, Azizi S, Phinney D, Kopen G, Schwarz E: Potential use of marrow stromal cells as therapeutic vectors for diseases of the central nervous system. *Prog Brain Res* 2000, 128:293-297.

[33] Sanchez-Ramos J, Song S, Cardoso-Pelaez F, Hazzi C, Stedeford T, Willing A, Freeman TB, Saporta S, Janssen W, Patel N, Cooper DR, Sanberg PR: Adult bone marrow stromal cells differentiate into neural cells in vitro. *Exp Neurol* 2000, 164:247-256.

[34] Woodbury D, Schwarz EJ, Prockop DJ, Black IB: Adult rat and human bone marrow stromal cells differentiate into neurons. *J Neurosci Res* 2000, 61:364-370.

[35] Kopen GC, Prockop DJ, Phinney DG: Marrow stromal cells migrate throughout forebrain and cerebellum, and they differentiate into astrocytes after injection into neonatal mouse brains. *Proc.Natl.Acad.Sci.USA* 1999, 96:10711-10716.

[36] Azizi S, Strokes D, Augelli BJ, DiGirolamo C, Prockop DJ: Engrafment and migration of bone marrow stromal cells implanted in the brains of albino rats - similarities to astrocyte grafts. *Proc.Natl.Acad.Sci.USA* 1998, 95:3908-3913.

[37] Grellier P, Yee D, Gonzalez M, Abboud SL: Characterization of insulin-like growth factor binding proteins (IGFBP) and regulation of IGFBP-4 in bone marrow stromal cells. *Br J Haematol* 1995, 90:249-257.

[38] Auffrey I, Chevalier S, Froger J, Izac B, Vainchenker W, Gascan H, Coulombel L: Nerve growth factor is involved in the supportive effect by bone marrow-derived stromal cells of the factor-dependent human cell line UT-7. *Blood* 1996, 88:1608-1618.

[39] Dormady SP, Bashayan O, Dougherty R, Zhang XM, Basch RS: Inmortalized multipotential mesenchymal cells and the haematopoietic microenvironment. *J Haematother Stem Cell Res* 2001, 10:125-140.

[40] García R, Aguiar J, Alberti E, Dde la Cuétar K, Pavon N: Bone marrow stromal cells produce nerve growth factor and glial cell line-derived neurotrophic factors. *BBRC* 2004, 316:753-754.

[41] Kordower J: In vivo gene delivery of Glial Cell Line-Derived Neurotrophic Factor for Parkinson's disease. *Ann Neurol* 2003, 53(Suppl 3):S120-S134.

[42] Kang UJ: Potential of gene therapy for Parkinson's disease: neurobiologic issues and new developments in gene transfer methodologies. *Mov.Disord.* 1998, 13 (Suppl 1):59-72.

[43] Castro M, Hurtado A, Umana P, Smith JR, Zermansky A, Abordo E, Löwenstein P: Regulatable and cell-type specific transgene expression in glial cells: prospects for gene therapy for neurological disorders. *Prog Brain Res* 2001, 132:655-681.

[44] Breakefield X: Gene delivery into the brain using virus vectors. *Nat Genet* 1993, 3:187-189.

[45] Gerdes C, Castro M, Löwenstein P: Strong promoters are the key to highly efficient, noninflammatory and noncytotoxic adenoviral-mediated transgene delivery into the brain *in vivo*. *Mol Ther* 2000, 2:330-338.

[46] Hida H, Hashimoto M, Fujimoto I, Nakajima K, Shimano Y, Nagatsu T, Mikoshiba K, Nishino H: Dopa-producing astrocytes generated by adenoviral transduction of human tyrosine hydroxylase gene: in vitro study and transplantation to hemiparkinsonian model rats. *Neurosci Res* 1999, 35:101-112.

[47] Castro M, David A, Hurtado A, Suwelack D, Millan E, Verakis T, Xiong WD, Yuan XP, Löwenstein P: Gene therapy for Parkinson's disease: recent achievements and remaining challenges. *Histol Histopathol* 2001, 16:1225-1238.

[48] Byrnes AP, MacLaren RE, Charlton HM: Immunological instability of persistent adenovirus vectors in the brain: peripheral exposure to vector leads to renewed inflammation, reduced gene expression, and demyelination. *J Neurosc* 1996, 16:3045-3055.

[49] Yang Y, Nunes FA, Berensi K, Furth EE, Gönczöl E, Wilson JM: Cellular immunity to viral antigens limits E1-deleted adenoviruses for gene therapy. *Proc Natl Acad Sci USA* 1994, 91:4407-4411.

[50] Freese A, Stern M, Kaplitt M, O'Connor WM, Abbey M, O'Connor MJ, During MJ: Prospects for gene therapy in Parkinson's disease. *Mov Disord* 1996, 11:469-488.

[51] Thomas C, Schiedner G, Kochanek S, Castro M, Löwenstein P: Peripheral infection with adenovirus causes unexpected long-term brain inflammation in animals injected intracranially with first-generation, but not with high-capacity, adenovirus vectors: toward realistic long-term neurological gene therapy for chronic diseases. *Proc Natl Acad Sci USA* 2000, 97:7482-7487.

[52] Chen H, Mack LM, Kelly R, Ontell M, Kochanek S, Clemens PR: Persistence in muscle of an adenoviral vector that lacks all viral genes. *Proc Natl Acad Sci USA* 1997, 94:1645-1650.

[53] Muramatsu S, Wang L, Ikeguchi K, Fujimoto K, Nakano I, Ozawa K: Recombinant adeno-associated viral vectors bring gene therapy for Parkinson's disease closer to reality. *J Neurol* 2002, 249 (Suppl 2):36-40.

[54] Srivastava A, Lusby EW, Berns KI: Nucleotide sequence and organization of the adeno-associated virus 2 genome. *J Virol* 1983, 45:555-564.

[55] Kirik D, Rosenblad C, Bjorklund A, Mandel R: Long-term rAAV-mediated gene transfer of GDNF in the rat Parkinson's Model: Intrastriatal but not intranigral transduction promotes functional regeneration in the lesioned nigrostriatal system. *J Neurosci* 2000, 20:4686-4700.

[56] Xiao X, Li J, Samulski RJ: Production of high-titer recombinant adeno-associated virus vectors in the absence of helper adenovirus. *J Virol* 1998, 72:2224-2232.

[57] Lu Y: Recombinant adeno-associated virus as delivery for gene therapy - A review. *Stem Cells and Development* 2004, 13:133-145.

[58] Rabinowitz JE, Samulski RJ: Adeno-associated virus expression systems for gene transfer. *Curr Opin Biotech* 1999, 9:470-475.

[59] Smith AE: Viral vectors in gene therapy. *Annu Rev Microbiol* 1995, 49:807-838.

[60] Oransky I: Gene therapy trial for Parkinson's disease begins. *Lancet* 2003, 362:712.

[61] Spaete RR, Frenkel N: The herpes simplex virus amplicon: a new eucaryotic defective virus cloning-amplifying vector. *Cell* 1982, 30:295-304.

[62] Latchman D: Gene therapy with herpes simplex virus vectors: progress and prospects for clinical neurosciences. *The Neuroscientist* 2001, 7:537.

[63] Latchman D, Coffin R: Viral vectors in the treatment of Parkinson's disease. *Mov Disord* 2000, 15:9-17.

[64] Fink D, Glorioso J, Mata M: Therapeutic gene transfer with herpes-based vectors: studies in Parkinson's disease and motor nerve regeneration. *Exp Neurol* 2003, 184 (Suppl 1):S19-S24.

[65] Kucharczuk JC, Randazzo B, Chang MY, Amin KM, Elshami AA, Sterman DH, Rizk NP, Molnar-Kimber KL, Brown SM, MacLean AR, Litzky LA, Fraser NW, Albelda SM, Kaiser LR: Use of a replication-restricted herpes virus to treat experimental human malignant mesothelioma. *Cancer Research* 1997, 57:466-471.

[66] Verma I, Somia N: Gene therapy - promises, problems and prospects. *Nature* 1997, 389:239-242.

[67] Hacein-Bey-Abina S, von Kalle C, Schmidt M, Le Deist F, Wulffraat N, McIntyre E, Radford I, Villeval JL, Fraser CC, Cavazzana-Calvo M, Fischer A: A serious adverse event after successful gene therapy for X-linked severe combined immunodeficiency. *N Eng J Med* 2003, 348:255-256.

[68] D'Costa J, Harvey-White J, Qasba P, Limaye A, KAneski C, Davis-Warren A, Brady R, Bankiewicz K, Major E, Arya S: HIV-2 derived lentiviral vectors: gdene transfer in Parkinson's and Fabry disease models in vitro. *J Med Virol* 2003, 71:173-182.

[69] Kordower J, Emborg M, Bloch J, Ma S, Chu Y, Leventhal L, McBride J, Chen EY, Palfi S, Zion B, Brown WD, Holden JE, Pyzalski R, Taylor M, Carvey P, Ling Z, Trono D, Hantraye P, Déglon N, Aebischer P: Neurodegeneration prevented by lentiviral vector delivery of GDNF in primate models of Parkinson's Disease. *Science* 2000, 290:661-888.

[70] Hottinger A, Azzouz M, Déglon N, Aebischer P, Zurn A: Complete and long-term rescue of lesioned adult motoneurons by lentiviral-mediated expression of glial cell line-derived neurotrophic factor in the facial nucleus. *J Neurosc* 2000, 20:5587-5593.

[71] Tacconi MT: Neuronal death: is there a role for astrocytes? *Neurochem Res* 1998, 23:759-765.

[72] Leone P, McPhee SW, Janson CG, Davidson BL, Freese A, During MJ: Multi-site partitioned delivery of human tyrosine hydroxylase gene with phenotypic recovery in Parkinsonian rats. *NeuroReport* 2000, 11:1145-1151.

[73] Levine RA, Zoephel GP, Niederwieser A, Curtius HC: Entrance of tetrahydrobiopterin derivatives in brain after peripheral administration: effect on biogenic amine metabolism. *J Pharmacol Exp Ther* 1987, 242:514-522.

[74] Mandel R, Rendahl KG, Spratt SK, Snyder RO, Cohen LK, Leff SE: Characterization of intrastriatal recombinant adeno-associated virus-mediated gene transfer of human tyrosine hydroxylase and human GTP-cyclohydrolase I in rat model of Parkinson's disease. *J Neurosc* 1998, 18:4271-4284.

[75] Leff SE, Rendahl KG, Spratt SK, Kang UJ, Mandel R: In vivo L-DOPA production by genetically modified primary ratfibroblast of gliosarcoma cell grafts via coexpression of GTP cyclohydrolase I with tyrosine hydroxylase. *Exp Neurol* 1998, 151:249-264.

[76] Bankiewicz K, Eberling JL, Kohutnicka M, Jagust W, Pivirotto P, Bringas J, Cunningham J, Budinger TF, Harvey-White J: Convection-enhanced delivery of AAV vector in parkinsonian monkeys; *in vivo* detection of gene expression and restoration of dopaminergic function using pro-drug approach. *Exp Neurol* 2000, 164:2-14.

[77] Fan DS, Ogawa M, Fujimoto I, Ikeguchi K, Ogasawara Y, Urabe M, Nishizawa M, Nakano I, Yoshida M, Nagatsu I, Ichinose H, Nagatsu T, Kurtzman G, Ozawa K: Behavioral recovery in 6-hydroxydopamine-lesioned rats by cotransduction of striatum

with tyrosine hydroxylase and aromatic L-amino acid decarboxylase genes using two separate adeno-associated virus vectors. *Human Gene Therapy* 1998, 9:2527-2535.

[78] Shen Y, Muramatsu S, Ikeguchi K, Fujimoto I, Fan DS, Ogawa M, Mizukami H, Urabe M, Kume A, Nagatsu I, Urano F, Suzuki T, Ichinose H, Nagatsu T, Monahan J, Nakano I, Ozawa K: Triple transduction with adeno-associated virus vectors expressing tyrosine hydroxylase, aromatic-L-amino-acid decarboxylase, and GTP cyclohydrolase I for gene therapy of Parkinson's disease. *Human Gene Therapy* 2000, 11:1509-1519.

[79] Bensadoun JC, Déglon N, Tseng JL, Ridet JL, Zurn A, Aebischer P: Lentiviral vectors as gene delivery system in the mouse midbrain: cellular and behavioural improvements in a 6-OHDA model of Parkinson's disease using GDNF. *Exp Neurol* 2000, 164:15-24.

[80] Palfi S, Leventhal L, Chu Y, Ma S, Emborg M, Bakay R, Néglon D, Hantraye P, Aebischer P, Kordower J: Lentivirally delivered glial cell line-derived neurotrophic factor increases the number of striatal dopaminergic neurons in primate models of nigrostriatal degeneration. *J Neurosci* 2002, 22:4942-4954.

[81] Hurelbrink CB, Barker RA: The potential of GDNF as a treatment for Parkinson's disease. *Exp Neurol* 2004, 185:1-6.

[82] Kordower J: In vivo gene delivery of glial cell line-derived neurotrophic factor for Parkinson' disease. *Ann Neurol* 2003, 53 (suppl 3):S120-S134.

In: New Research on Parkinson's Disease
Editors: T. F. Hahn, J. Werner

ISBN: 978-1-60456-601-7
© 2008 Nova Science Publishers, Inc.

Chapter VIII

Manganese-Induced Parkinsonism, Parkinson's Disease and Welding

Chin-Chang Huang and *Nai-Shin Chu*
Department of Neurology, Chang Gung Memorial Hospital,
Taipei, College of Medicine, Chang Gung University, Taiwan

Abstract

Excessive manganese exposure may induce a neurological syndrome similar to Parkinson's disease (PD), called manganism. However, close observation of manganism patients reveals a clinical disease entity different from PD, not only in the clinical manifestation and therapeutic response, but also in the neuroimaging studies, such as magnetic resonance images (MRI), positron emission tomography (PET), and dopamine transporter images (DAT), and in the neuropathological findings. The differences in the clinical manifestations between manganism and PD include in the former less-frequent resting tremor, more frequent dystonia, gait en bloc, and a wide-based and characteristic cock-walk gait. In PD, a persistent focal asymmetry is noted, whereas in manganism there is a high degree of symmetry. However, a unilateral cock-walk gait and asymmetric dystonia are also found in chronic manganism. Therefore, symmetry is not a good differential clue between manganism and PD. A failure to achieve a sustained therapeutic response is noted in manganism. Neuroimaging studies may distinguish manganism from PD. The findings in manganism are hyperintensity in the basal ganglia on T1-weighted MRI scans, and normal 6-fluorodopa PET and DAT scans. Neuropathologically, PD is associated with neuronal loss in the substantia nigra pars compacta and locus ceruleus, and the presence of Lewy bodies, whereas in manganism, gliosis mainly is limited to the globus pallidum and substantia nigra pars reticularis, with an absence of Lewy bodies. Furthermore, manganism has a clinical course different from PD; in long-term follow-up, manganism patients show a prominent deterioration in the parkinsonian symptoms in the initial 5-10 years, followed by a plateau in the following 10 years.

---

* Correspondence: Chin-Chang Huang, MD; Department of Neurology, Chang Gung Memorial Hospital; 199, Tun Hwa North Road; Taipei, Taiwan; Tel: 886-3-3282200 Ext. 8413; Fax: 886-3-3287226

In the most recent few years, the possible potential risk of inhaling welding fumes to accelerate the onset of PD or induce PD has been raised. Previous studies have not provided adequate evidence to support the relationship between welding and PD because of a lack of exposure data and selection bias with the patients. However, welding fumes may contain various neurotoxic substances in addition to manganese such as iron which may increase oxidative stress. Further investigation is warranted.

Introduction

1. Background

Manganese (Mn) is the twelfth most abundant element and the fourth most widely used metal in the world. It was first found by the Swedish chemist Scheele in 1771, and named from the Latin word for magnetism, *magnes*. It is widely distributed in soils, rock, water, food, living plants and animals. Pyrolusite (MnO_2), rhodochrosite ($MnCO_3$) and rhodanate (Manganese silicate) are the most common forms in Mn-rich ores, and annually an estimated 8 million tons of manganese are extracted from open pits and shallow mines. Manganese is frequently found in nature in 11 oxidative states, including Mn^{+2}, Mn^{+3}, Mn^{+4}, and Mn^{+7}. $MnCl_2$, $MnNO_3$, $MnSO_4$ and Mn acetate are usually water soluble, while Mn_3O_4 and MnO_2 are insoluble in aqueous solution. Mn_2O_3 is the most common form of air pollution. [1-5] The Mn^{+3} ion is relatively unstable in the environment. In biological systems, the Mn^{+2} ion is similar to Mg^{+2}, while the Mn^{+3} ion acts interchangeably with Fe^{+3}.

Manganese compounds are commonly used in the production of ferromanganese alloys and other industrial products, such as dry-cell batteries, paints, glazes, and electronic parts, and chemicals for coloring glasses and tiles. [6-11] Another important application for Mn is methylcyclopentadienyl manganese tricarbonyl (MMT), an organometallic compound used in low concentrations as an octane improver and antiknock agent in unleaded gasoline in some countries such as Canada and the U.S.A.. [12-14] In addition, potassium permanganate is used as a powerful oxidizing agent in purifying drinking water, treating waste water, and removing waste odor, and as an agricultural fungicidal and bactericidal agent. [6-8] Mn is also a natural component of most foods, particularly of nuts, grains, and tea, and an essential trace element in the metabolism of humans.

Excessive exposure to Mn, mainly via occupational inhalation, may cause primarily central nervous system symptoms known as manganism. Manganese poisoning was first reported in a manganese ore-crushing plant in France. [15] Subsequently, many cases of chronic Mn poisoning were reported in industrial workers at dry-cell battery factories, [16] and among smelters [17] and welders. [18] Health risks as a result of exposure to Mn have also been found in agricultural workers who were exposed to organic Mn-containing pesticides, such as Mn ethylene-bis-dithiocarbamate (Maneb). [19] Mn is also found in the street drug called 'Bazooka', a cocaine-based drug contaminated with manganese carbonate. [20] In addition, a significant concern has been raised about airborne Mn exposure from the fuel additive MMT. [21,22] Mn has been used as a contrast agent in medical diagnostics, although there have been no reported cases of Mn intoxication. However, some cases have also been reported in patients receiving long-term parenteral nutrition [23] or in those ingesting contaminated water. [24]

2. Essentiality and Deficiency of Manganese

Manganese is an essential trace element in the animals and humans and is a potent electron-withdrawing agent particularly necessary for ubiquitous enzymatic reactions such as synthesis of lipids, proteins, and carbohydrates. [25] The adequate daily intake levels for manganese are 2.3 mg for men and 1.8 mg for women. Manganese deficiency may result in impairment of growth, skeletal defects, altered lipid and carbohydrate metabolism, and may even cause an increased prevalence of seizures during infancy. [26]

Kinetics of Manganese

1. Absorption of Manganese

A. Respiratory Absorption
Absorption of manganese via inhalation is strongly dependent on the form and size of the manganese compounds. Manganese particles > 15μm in diameter do not reach the alveoli and are eliminated from the lung and reflex into the gastrointestinal tract; particles smaller than 5um can be deposited in the distal tributaries of the lung. Most manganese particles deposited in the lung can be found in the feces within 4 days of exposure. [7] Particles 1μm or less are small enough to be deposited in the lung alveoli where clearance mechanisms are slower than for trachea-bronchial clearance. [14,27] The particle size of Mn_3O_4, the major oxide produced upon combustion of MMT, is about 0.1 to 0.4μm, small enough to reach the lung alveoli easily. [28] It is believed that respiratory absorption is more likely to lead to toxic concentration in the brain in occupational exposure.

B. Gastrointestinal Absorption
The high amount of manganese in the ordinary diet constitutes the major route of exposure for most people. Absorption via the gastrointestinal route is usually lower than that via the inhalation route. In the normal adult, absorption of radio-labeled $MnCl_2$ via the oral route was 3% of the ingested dose and remained constant as through increased loads of manganese up to 5000μg/m^3 from occupational exposure in manganese miners. [29] Low iron status may result in an increased absorption of manganese. Individuals with anemia absorbed about twice as much manganese as normal individuals. High calcium levels also reduce the absorption of manganese in humans. [30]

C. Nasal Absorption and Skin Absorption
There is no evidence to support significant nasal or skin absorption of inorganic manganese either into the bloodstream or into the subfrontal cortex through the olfactory apparatus. [7] Although transit through the olfactory route to the brain in rats, mice, and pike

has been proved, it is considered that anatomical differences make this an unlikely significant route in humans. [3, 31-33] However, MMT may enter by skin absorption. [34]

2. Tissue Distribution

A. Respiratory Exposure

Under normal circumstances, manganese is preferentially bound to transferrin and albumin. [35] Immediately following inhalation of 1,800μg/m^3 Mn$_3$O$_4$ for 2 hours, tissue distribution is highest in the lungs, followed by the liver, kidney and spleen. [36] Two days later, the lung manganese level may fall to normal, while the kidney and spleen levels are still elevated 60% above controls. The relative uptake in the brain is independent of the inhaled concentration and did does exceed 1% of lung deposition. The gastrointestinal tract and liver can remove a significant portion of absorbed manganese after inhalation intake. Iron deficiency can increase by approximately two times the retention of manganese in the brain stem, basal ganglia, and medulla of rats. [14]

B. Gastrointestinal Exposure

In human adults, whole body retention of an orally ingested dose was about 1.6% after 10 days and 0.2% after 50 days. [29] In rats, whole body retention of a single ingested dose at day 19 was 3%. Manganese content was highest in the liver, kidney and hair. Within the brain, manganese accumulates primarily in the globus pallidus (GP) and substantia nigra pars reticularis (SNr). Accumulation also occurs in the striatum, pineal gland, and olfactory bulb. MnO$_2$ can cause a significant decrease of dopamine and norepinephrine in the corpus striatum, hypothalamus, and midbrain in mouse. [14, 37]

3. Clearance of Manganese

A. Respiratory Exposure

Highly variable rates of clearance of manganese from the lung have been reported after inhalation exposure. Clearance half-time (T$_{1/2}$) is about 68 days for MnO$_2$ particles of 0.9μm diameter in humans. [38] Lung clearance appears to be inversely dependent on concentration. Differing particle sizes may explain the differences in clearance rates. Small particle sizes are likely to clear more slowly than larger particle sizes due to phagocytosis of the particles by alveolar macrophages, and translocation into the pulmonary tissue. A major clearance mechanism for respiratory exposure is the translocation of particles deposited in the respiratory tract via ciliary action, and swallowing to the gastrointestinal tract. Clearance of manganese from the brain is extremely slow with a half-time of 223-267 days for monkeys given ultra-low concentrations of MnCl$_2$. [39] After injection of radioactive [54]Mn in humans, clearance half-times for the head are 54 days in normal individuals, 37 days in manganese miners, and 62 days in symptomatic Mn-exposed miners. [29]

B. Gastrointestinal Exposure

After ingesting manganese in the diet, whole-body clearance was usually biphasic, with clearance half-times of 13 and 34 days for the fast and slow components. [40] The rate of clearance of manganese differs in various tissues, from a few hours in blood to months or even years in the brain. [39]

4. Effect of Valence State of Manganese

Both the valence state and the solubility may influence the disposition of manganese. After administration by various routes, Mn^{+2} is very rapidly cleared from the blood and efficiently excreted in bile. Mn^{+3} had a slower elimination rate than Mn^{+2} in cows and pigs. [41] A hypothesis was proposed for the differential distribution of the different valence states of manganese: manganese, usually Mn^{+2}, is absorbed from the gastrointestinal tract; in the plasma, a portion is bound to α_2-macroglobulin, while a small portion is oxidized to Mn^{+3} via ceruloplasmin and is circulated to the tissues; Mn-transferrin may cross the blood-brain barrier via an active transfer mechanism, then release manganese. [42]

Sources of Mn Exposure

1. Occupational Exposure

Occupational sources of exposure to manganese-containing dusts or fumes include:

- Mining,
- Sorting and milling ore
- Refining ore
- Production, crushing or milling ferromanganese alloys
- Production of carbon and high-temperature steel

Manufacture of dry-cell batteries, glasses, porcelains, vanishes, ceramics, fireworks, matches, fertilizer, fungicide, disinfectants, water purifiers, and preservatives for fruit and flowers.

2. Non-Occupational Exposure

Exposure may result from the ingestion of drinking water contaminated by natural sources or buried waste such as batteries. Manganese intoxication has also been reported in long-term parenteral nutrition, and ingestion of potassium permanganate and the street drug "Bazooka."

Human Manganism

1. History of Manganese Neurotoxicity

Chronic manganese poisoning was first recognized in 1837 by Couper who reported 5 patients in a manganese ore-crushing plant with whispered speech, hyper-salivation, limb tremor, a bent posture and muscle weakness. [15] The observations were ignored until Embden (1901) [43] and von Jaksch (1907) [44] reported a peculiar "cock-walk gait" in manganese intoxication. In 1919, Edsall et al. [45] established a relationship among the epidemiological, clinical and pathological effects of Mn on the CNS. In 1927, Ashizawa [46] reported the medial segment of the GP was more vulnerable to the manganese intoxication. Manganese neurotoxicity was subsequently reported in miners, [47] industrial workers such as smelters, [48, 49] welders, [50, 51] and manufacturing dry- cell battery workers. [16] In 1988, Ferraz et al. [19] reported CNS toxicity after exposure to the agriculture fungicide Maneb. Manganese toxicity can also occur in patients following ingestion of potassium permanganate [52] and receiving long-term total parental nutrition. [23]

2. Clinical Manifestations

The symptomatic onset of Mn toxicity may be delayed for up to 6 months or several years after exposure. The onset is always insidious. The clinical features include psychiatric features, Parkinsonism, and dystonia. [53-59] Patients usually have a prodrome consisting of psychiatric symptoms such as irritability, emotional lability, illusion and hallucinations, or even frank psychoses, referred to as "manganese madness." The bradykinetic-rigid parkinsonian syndrome is prominent and is characterized by diminished blinking, masked face, impaired dexterity, postural instability, bradykinesia, rigidity, micrographia, and speech disturbances such as monotonous speech and hypophonia. Dystonia consists of facial grimacing, hand dystonia and/or plantar flexion of the foot. [59]

The most characteristic clinical feature is "cock-walk gait", consisting of a high-stepping gait, strutting on the toes with flexed elbows, and an erect spine. (figure 1). [60] This peculiar walking difficulty can be unilateral or bilateral, is considered a form of dystonia, and generally becomes prominent after walking a short distance. Tremor is less prominent, usually rapid and low-amplitude, tending to be postural, and not resting. The tremor may involve the hands and sometimes the tongue.

3. Tissue Mn Concentration

Manganese concentrations are usually high in the blood and urine in manganism patients, indicating a recent exposure to manganese. Mn concentrations of scalp hair and pubic hair, are usually much higher, even up to one hundred times the normal levels, indicating a more chronic exposure. [17] However high concentrations of manganese in the tissues represent manganese exposure rather than chronic manganism. Field or environmental studies usually reveal an increased manganese concentration in the air above the threshold limited value of 5 mg/m^3. [59]

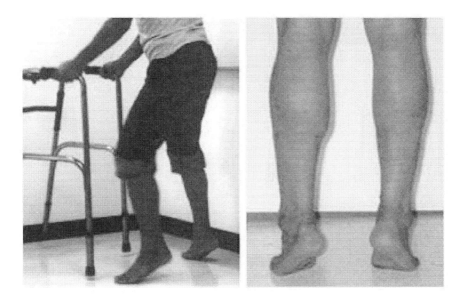

Figure 1. Cock-walk gait with a high-stepping gait, strutting on the toes in a patient with chronic manganese intoxication.

4. Neurobehavior Studies

Psychomotor disturbances usually occur in early-stage of manganism patients, particularly the Chilian miners, and are referred to as locura manganica or manganese psychosis [61]. Frequently, nervousness, irritability, emotional instability, hallucination and compulsive acts result in arguments and friction among the miners, occasionally approaching violence. However, these abnormal violent behaviors are not commonly found in industrial workers.

The early symptoms may be reversible and the earliest signs of chronic Mn intoxication in industrial workers are subtle, including fatigue, irritability, sleep disturbance, anxiety, depression, confusion, and impaired vision. [62-64] Onset can be insidious or gradual, and the illness can develop after weeks, months, or years of exposure. Neuropsychological tests may detect deficits, particularly in mood disturbance, sexual dysfunction, and memory and intellectual impairment. In the study by Hua and Huang, [65] comprehensive examinations of neurobehavioral functions were performed in two groups of workers with chronic exposure to manganese and two control groups. Impaired general intelligence, visuoperceptive impairment and defective manual dexterity, and a slowdown in the response speed were noted in manganism patients. A cross-sectional study was conducted in 1987 by Roles et al. [66] on 141 manganese-exposed workers in a manganese salt and oxide plant. Manganese exposed workers performed more poorly in visual reaction time, eye-hand co-ordination and steadiness. In 1992, the same researchers conducted a cross-sectional study on 92 Belgian workers in a battery factory with exposure to MnO_2, who were supposed to have subtle preclinical signs and were matched to a control group of 101 workers from a nearby polymer processing plant. [67] The geometric mean for "respirable" dust (particles of 5 μm mass diameter) was 215 μg/m^3, and was 948 μg/m^3 for total manganese dust (particles up to 35-45 μm). Eye-hand coordination was significantly worse in 21/92 Mn-exposed workers (23%), compared to 5/101 (5%) of the non-exposed group. The manganese-exposed workers also performed the hand steadiness test and visual reaction time less satisfactorily than the control workers. Poorer performance in all three tests was significantly increased in the highest exposure group, and a dose-response trend was evident for hand steadiness. In addition, recent studies revealed a higher prevalence of neuropsychological dysfunction in manganese-exposed welders than in unexposed controls. [68] The manganese-exposed welders performed poorly on tests measuring both verbal and visuomotor speed of information processing, sustained concentration, motor skills and working memory. [64, 68, 69]

5. Autonomic Study

Autonomic dysfunctions such as sialorrhea, seborrhea, profuse sweating, diminished libido and impotence have been reported in manganism, [1, 8, 16, 57] but their frequencies varied considerably. The autonomic function was studied using the sympathetic skin response (SSR) and RR interval variation (RRIV) in manganism patients, and compared with stage-matched PD patients and age-matched normal controls. [70] Autonomic symptoms were less common in manganism than in PD. In SSR, the latency was prolonged in PD and manganism, while the amplitude was reduced only in PD. The RRIV was decreased in PD and manganism, but the reduction in RRIV was more severe in PD than in manganism. The data indicated that autonomic disturbance may occur in manganism, but is less frequent and less severe when compared with PD.

6. Long-Term Follow-up Studies

Neurological deficits tend to become established within 1-2 years after chronic manganese intoxication. Therefore neurological deficits may remain stationary, [47] improve [54, 71, 72] or continue to progress [58, 73, 74] even after cessation of manganese exposure. There have been very few long-term follow-up studies in previous chronic manganese intoxication patients. Longitudinal follow-up studies were conducted by Huang et al. [75-77] every 5 years for 20 years following cessation of manganese exposure. The studies revealed that the parkinsonian symptoms showed a prominent progression in gait disturbances, such as freezing during turning (gait en bloc) and walking backward with retropulsion 5 years later. Slight deterioration was also found in writing (micrographia), stability, posture, speed and rigidity. Ten years later, the deterioration was still observed, particularly in the gait, rigidity, speed of foot tapping, and writing, although the concentrations of Mn in the blood, urine, scalp hair and public hair had returned to normal and the follow-up brain MRI did not show high signal intensity in the T1-weighted images. [76] The serial scores measured by the

King's College Hospital Rating Scale for Parkinson's disease showed a rapid progression in the initial 10 years, followed by a plateau in the following 10 years (figure 2). [77] Figure 3 shows the changes of micrographia during the 20-year follow-up period. These data infer that the causal event of manganese intoxication may destroy some cells and damage others, and that the damaged cells may undergo death after a long latency, which is limited to 10 years.

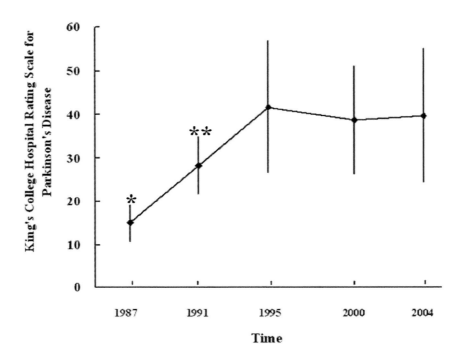

Figure 2. The long-term clinical course study showing a rapid deterioration in the initial 10 years, followed by a plateau in the following 10 years. The serial scores measured with the King's College Hospital Rating Scale for Parkinson's Disease. (*p<0.0001, the score in 1987 vs. the scores in 1991, 1995, 2000, and 2004; and **p<0.001, the score in 1991 vs. the scores in 1995, 2000, and 2004).

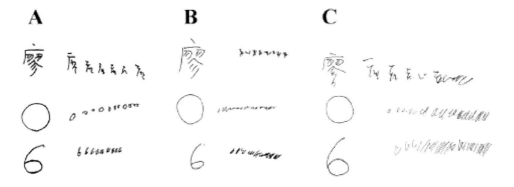

Figure 3. Serial hand writings in a patient with chronic manganese intoxication revealed micrographia (A) and a deterioration 5-10 years later (B) and then a stationary status 20 years later (C) after cessation of Mn exposure.

7. Treatment of Manganism

Previous studies revealed inconsistent results, in open trials after administering various dosages of levodopa. [55, 58] Some patients had a marked to total reduction of rigidity, improvement of postural reflexes and gait, and correction of bradykinesia; some patients had a limited response and the others had a poor response. [1, 57, 78] Huang et al. [17] also reported that manganism patients had an initial response to levodopa in an open trial, but this benefit was not sustained. A double-blind, short-term, placebo-controlled, cross-over study of levodopa was subsequently conducted and showed that parkinsonism and dystonia failed to respond to the treatment. [79] Other antiparkinsonian drugs such as bromocriptine, selegiline, amantadine and trihexylphenidyl were also ineffective (unpublished observation).

Previous chelation therapy with $CaNa_2EDTA$ showed that the Mn excretion in urine was increased and the Mn concentration in blood was decreased. [17, 80] However the manganism patients only showed transient improvement of postural stability, speech and retropulsion, or did not improve at all. [17] 5-Hydroxytryptophan (5-HTP) has been reported to be effective in some patients with hypokinetic and hypotonic features, or with abnormalities of gait and postural reflexes. [57, 78] In addition, para-amino-salicylic acid (PAS) therapy has been reported to be effective in a few patients, but the therapeutic response should be further investigated. [81, 82]

Neuroimaging Studies

1. Brain Magnetic Resonance Images (MRI)

Mn has a paramagnetic quality and a shortening of proton T1-relaxation time with MRI. Therefore manganese can be seen in the basal ganglia in experimental poisoning of non-human primates. [83] Subsequently, high signal intensities were found symmetrically in the GP and midbrain, particularly SNr on T1-weighted brain MRI in manganism patients. [84, 85] Signals in the brain MRI are commonly increased, with a frequency of 41.6% in Mn-exposed workers. [86] However, the hyperintensity lesions may resolve 6 months to 1 year after cessation of Mn exposure, indicating Mn can be cleaned out within a period of 1 year. [87] A similar MRI pattern has also been observed in patients with liver cirrhosis and a portal systemic shunt. [88-90] Many manganese-exposed workers have no clinical symptoms, but may have hyperintensities in the brain MRI. Increased signal intensities on a T1-weighted image may only reflect exposure to Mn or an accumulation of Mn. Therefore, the phenomenon does not necessarily represent manganism. [87] The pallidum index (PI) was defined as the ratio of the signal intensity of GP to frontal subcortical white matter multiplied by 100. [91] In Mn-exposed workers, blood Mn concentrations were highly correlated with PI. The Mn-exposed workers also had higher PI than the non-exposed workers. [91,92]

2. Brain Positron Emission Tomography (PET) Study

Brain PET with 6-fluorodopa (6F-Dopa) can be used to study the integrity of the nigrostriatal dopaminergic projection. [93-95] 6F-Dopa PET has been employed in manganism patients and revealed a normal 6F-Dopa uptake. [96] These findings suggest that in manganism patients, damage may occur in the pathways postsynaptic to the nigrostriatal system, probably involving the striatum or pallidal neurons. In addition, brain PET scanning with fluorodeoxyglucose showed a decreased cortical glucose metabolism indicating damage to the function of glucose metabolism. Raclopride is a PET marker for dopamine D_2 receptors. [97] In early untreated PD, the uptake of raclopride is increased, indicating an upregulation of the dopamine receptors. In advanced PD patients with levodopa therapy, the uptake of raclopride is reduced. [98] Brain PET with presynaptic and postsynaptic dopaminergic function were measured with 6F-Dopa and [^{11}C]raclopride (RAC) in a follow-up study on these manganism patients, and revealed a normal influx constants (Ki) of 6F-Dopa in the caudate and putamen. [99] However, the RAC binding was mildly reduced in the caudate, and normal in the putamen. The data again indicate that nigrostriatal dopaminergic pathway lesions were not primarily responsible for chronic Mn-induced parkinsonism.

3. Brain Single Photon Emission Computed Tomography (SPECT) Study

Dopamine transporter (DAT) SPECT is easily accessible and less expensive than 6F-Dopa. [100] Various ligands binding to DAT, such as [^{123}I]-β-CIT, [^{123}I]-fluoropropyl-CIT, and ^{99m}Tc-TRODAT-1, can be used in SPECT studies. [101-103] ^{99m}Tc-TRODAT-1 is a cocaine analogue that can bind to the DAT site, reflecting the function of presynaptic dopaminergic terminals. [104,105] Brain ^{99m}Tc-TRODAT-1 SPECT was performed on manganism patients, and showed only a slight decrease in the putamen. (figure 4) [106] The DAT results could clearly differentiate between manganism and PD.

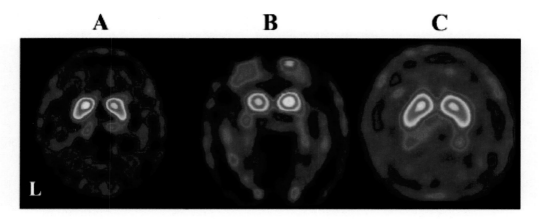

Figure 4. Brain DAT-SPECT with ^{99m}Tc-TRODAT-1 revealed a nearly normal uptake in a manganism patient (A), compared with a decrease in uptake in the corpus striatum, particularly in the left side of a PD patient (B), and a normal uptake in a healthy subject (C). (L=left).

Pathological Findings

There have been only a few pathological studies on patients or experimental animals with chronic manganese intoxication. [39,107-110] Degeneration of the basal ganglion is primarily confined to the medial segment of the GP and SNr. The putamen and the caudate are affected to a lesser degree, while the substantia nigra pars compacta (SNc) is only rarely involved. Other areas of the brain, including the cerebral cortex, thalamus, subthalamus, hypothalamus, and red nucleus may be inconsistently involved.

Experimental studies with rhesus monkeys were conducted after IV injections of manganese chloride for 2-3 months at 1-week intervals. [111] These monkeys developed a parkinsonian syndrome characterized by bradykinesia, rigidity, and facial dystonia, but no tremor, and did not respond to levodopa. Autopsy demonstrated that gliosis was confined to the GP and the SNr. Mineral deposits in the perivascular region were found in the GP and SNr. The mineral deposits were comprised of iron and aluminum. These studies demonstrated that manganese primarily damages the GP and SNr, and to a relative extent, spares the nigrostriatal dopaminergic system. [111,112] In PD and 1-methyl-4-phenyl-1,2,3,6-tetrahydropyridine (MPTP)-induced parkinsonism, the primary lesion is localized to the SNc. The results suggest that Mn-induced parkinsonism can be differentiated from PD and MPTP-induced parkinsonism. The accumulation of iron and aluminum may induce oxidants that contribute to the damage of the GP and SNr.

Non-Wilsonian Hepatolenticular Degeneration in Patients with Liver Failure

Several reports have revealed that liver cirrhosis can be associated with bilateral hyperintense lesions in the GP on brain T1-weighted MRI images- a pattern similar to that seen with manganese accumulation (figure 5). [88-90] Approximately 98% of dietary manganese is excreted from the liver, so accumulation of manganese can occur in patients with liver failure or with a portal-system shunt. The plasma manganese levels are increased in patients with liver failure, and a correlation is also found between plasma manganese levels and the severity of hyperintensity changes on T1WI. [89] Surveys of patients with chronic liver failure suggested that 20-50% of these patients have moderate to severe parkinsonian symptoms including gait disturbance, speech impairment, bradykinesia, rigidity, relative absence of resting tremor, dystonia, and a poor response to levodopa. [113] However, not all patients with MRI changes had parkinsonian features. Therefore the manganese related alteration on MRI may represent a threshold or a biological marker for manganese exposure.

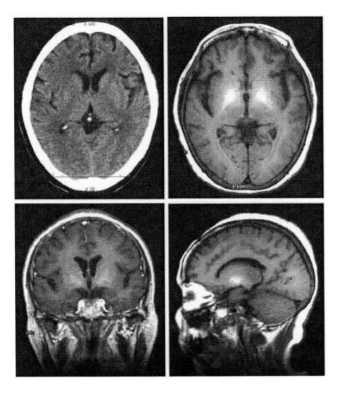

Figure 5. Brain CT scan and MRI scan of a patient with hepatic encephalopathy (a 64-year-old woman had chronic liver cirrhosis due to hepatitis B infection). The brain CT scan is normal and MRI shows an increased signal intensity indicating an accumulation of Mn in the globus pallidium.

Differential Diagnosis between Manganism and PD

Manganism is a clinically distinct disease entity from PD, and this can be differentiated based on their clinical manifestations, long-term course, and pharmacological, neuroimaging and neuropathological features. [114, 115] Similarities of clinical manifestations between manganism and PD include the presence of bradykinesia, rigidity, masked face, micrographia, monotonous speech and loss of postural reflex. Manganism differs from PD in its less-frequent resting tremor, more frequent dystonia, easy in falling backward, and a characteristic cock-walk gait. [114-116] A failure to achieve a sustained therapeutic response is noted in patients with manganism. [79] In contrast, PD patients can respond well to levodopa. [114] The pattern of focal asymmetry has been investigated during the course of PD, and revealed a persistent asymmetry. [117, 118] In manganism, a high degree of symmetry was suggested to be a differential clue between PD and manganism. [115, 116] However, an asymmetrical cock gait and asymmetrical dystonia were reported in chronic manganism. [119] The asymmetricity was noted in the early stage of manganism, and persisted during the long-term follow-up, very similar to that found in PD. [76, 100] PD patients may deteriorate continuously while manganism patients may show a rapid progression in the initial 5-10 years, followed by a plateau in the following 10 years. [77] Neuroimaging procedures including MRI, PET, and DAT-SPECT, have been used to distinguish manganism from PD. [87] Manganism is generally associated with hyperintense abnormalities in the GP, striatum, and SNr bilaterally on MRI, whereas the MRI is normal in PD patients. PET or DAT-SPECT can provide a means of discrimination between PD and manganism. [96, 99, 106] In PD, there is a reduced uptake of 6F-Dopa in the striatum, whereas PET or DAT-SPECT is generally normal or minimally abnormal in manganism. Pathologically, PD is associated with neuronal loss in the locus ceruleus, nucleus basalis of Meynert, and dorsal motor nucleus of the vagus, as well as loss of dopaminergic neurons within the SNc, whereas in manganism, neuronal loss is limited to the SNr and the medial segment of the GP, which is linked to the degeneration of GABAminergic neurons within the GP in pathways postsynaptic to the nigrostriatal system. In addition, the presence of Lewy bodies in the SN and other regions of the brain has been noted in PD, but not in manganism. [115,116]

Neuroimaging is very important in the differential diagnosis of parkinsonism, particularly in PD patients with an incidental exposure to Mn. When patients have high T1 signals on the brain MRI, with a Mn exposure history, and the brain PET or DAT-SPECT shows a prominently decreased uptake, the patients can be considered as PD with coincidental Mn exposure. [87] Table 1 shows the differences between chronic manganism and PD.

Welding, Manganism, and PD

Chronic occupational exposure to high concentrations of Mn dust and fumes in mining and some industrial settings is associated with an increased risk of "manganism." Based on the above findings, typical manganism is different from PD.

However, in recent years, questions have been raised regarding a possible causal association between neurological effects and welding. [51, 69, 120-122] Although the evidence to support the existence of such a relationship is not sufficient, welding has been suspected to be a risk factor for PD, particularly in a recent court decision which concluded that a former welder developed PD as a result of exposure to Mn in welding fumes. [123] Subsequently, many lawsuits have been filed in the United States. The Bureau of Labor Statistics reported that at least 361,970 persons are identified as having a primary occupation involving welding, cutting and soldering in the United States. [124]

1. Welding Fume Composition

A mixture of metal oxides is observed during welding processes. The welding fume is the vaporized metal that may react with air to form particles that are usually respirable in size. The individual primary particles generated during welding are in the nano-size range (about 0.01-0.10 μm) and then quickly accumulate together to form larger particles with a diameter in the range of 0.1-0.6 μm. [125] Mild and low alloy steel electrodes are comprised of mostly iron with varying amounts of manganese, whereas stainless steel electrodes contain other metals such as chromium and nickel, in addition to iron and manganese, and trace amounts of metals including zinc, aluminum, cadmium, copper, lead, silicon, magnesium, calcium and tin. [126]

Table 1. Differences between manganism and Parkinson's disease

Features	Manganism	Parkinson's disease
Clinical		
Symmetricity	Asymmetry or symmetry	Asymmetry
Tremor	Less frequent, rapid postural,	Usually frequent, resting,
Dystonia	Usually prominent in face	Sometimes
Gait disturbance	More frequent, cock-walk gait,	Festinating gait, Small-step
Long term course	Rapid deterioration in the initial	Continuous deterioration
Therapeutic response		
to levodopa	No response	Excellent response
to other	No response	Good response
Autonomic involvement	Less common	More common
Brain images		
MRI (T1-weighted	Hyperintensity in the GP in	Normal
PET with 6F-Dopa scan	Normal	Markedly decreased
PET with RAC	Mildly reduced	Increased initially, but
DAT-SPECT	Normal or mildly decreased	Markedly decreased
Pathologic findings	Degeneration in the GP and	Loss of neurons in the SNc,

MRI: mangnetic resonance images, PET: positron emission tomography, RAC: raclopride, DAT-SPECT: dopamine transporter-single photon emission computed tomography, GP: globus pallidus, SNr: substantia nigra pars reticularis, SNc: substantia nigra pars compacta, LC: locus ceruleus.

2. Manganese in Welding Fumes

Manganese is an essential ingredient in the welding of steel because Mn can increase hardness and strength. The amount of manganese in a welding rod ranges from 1% to 20% of the metal. Most welders are exposed to mixed metal fumes that contain less than 5% of manganese. However some welders may be exposed to 10-20% of manganese. Mn^{+2} and Mn^{+3} are the most probable oxidation states of manganese in welding fumes. [127]

3. Absorption of Welding Fumes

The potential health impact of inhaling welding fumes is dependent on the sites of deposition in the respiratory tract. The majority of inhaled welding particles would deposit in the alveolar or pulmonary regions of the respiratory tracts. [125] Welding particles that deposit in the trachea-bronchial regions are most likely to have a short half-time in the respiratory tracts due to removal by the mucociliary escalator, and are removed to the pharynx. Because of the fast elimination time of the particles from the body by this process, and the insoluble nature of most welding particles, it is unlikely that manganese associated with welding fumes would be reabsorbed back into the body via the gastrointestinal tract. Also the inhaled particles that reach the alveolar regions are most likely to be engulfed by alveolar macrophages. [128] The retention half-time of non-toxic, solid particles in the alveolar regions has been estimated to be up to 700 days in humans. [129] It appears that significant amounts of particles and associated metals can persist in the lungs, and thus potentially enter the pulmonary circulation for extended periods of time.

Welding particles that deposit in the nasal/head airway region may reach the brain via olfactory transport- a potential route of delivery as manganese travels from the nose to the brain. [31, 32] During olfactory transport, the blood-brain barrier is bypassed and the inhaled chemicals are conveyed along cell processes to synaptic junctions with neurons of the olfactory bulb. Recent studies have showed that inhaled nano-size radio-labeled carbon particles were rapidly transported by olfactory uptake and accumulated in the olfactory bulb in rats. [33]

Approximately 80% of the manganese in the plasma is bound to β_1-globulin, albumin and transferrin. [130] Due to the chemical similarities between Mn and Fe, these metals can compete for binding in the circulation and at the blood-brain barrier. A significant decrease of the uptake of Mn has been shown due to plasma iron overload, while iron deficiency has been associated with increased concentrations of manganese in the brain. [131]

4. Occupational Exposure Limits for Manganese

From 1988 to 1994, the American Conference of Governmental Industrial Hygienist (ACGIH) Threshold Limit Value-Time Weighted Average (TLV-TWA) was 5mg/m^3 for manganese dust and compounds in the breathing zone of welders during the welding of iron, mild steel, and aluminum. [132] In 1995, the TLV-TWA was drastically decreased to 0.2 mg/m^3 manganese for elemental and inorganic compounds, including total welding fumes. [133] In early 2002, The ACGIH published draft documentation for a new TLV for manganese and its inorganic compound recommending from 0.2mg/m^3 to 0.03mg/m^3. However the new recommendation was withdrawn and the TLV for manganese has remained 0.2 mg/m^3. [134]

In 2005, the US Occupational Safety and Health Administration (OSHA) set a permissible exposure limit (PEL) for total welding fumes at 5mg/m^3 as an 8h-TWA. [135] The National Institute of Occupational Safety and Health (NIOSH) has also established a recommended exposure limit (REL) at 1mg/m^3 as a 10h-TWA and short-term exposure limit

(STEL) at $3mg/m^3$ as a 15-min average for manganese compounds and fumes. (NIOSH, 2005) [136]

Workplace manganese levels have been measured in welding fumes that exceeded the NIOSH REL and original ACGIH TLV-TWA. Approximately 19% of welders were exposed to levels of iron that exceeded the original ACGIH TLV-TWA of $5mg/m^3$, and 68% of the welders were exposed to levels of manganese that exceeded the ACGIH-TWA of $0.2mg/m^3$. The personal exposures to Mn ranged from 0.01 to $4.93mg/m^3$. [137]

5. Clinical Studies of Manganism in Welders

In 2001, Racette et al. [120] described a potential relationship between PD and welding. They examined 15 welders treated in their Parkinson's clinic. These patients had typical clinical features of PD with good responses to levodopa and abnormal 6F-Dopa PET studies. In addition, their patients had developed the disease around age 45, on average 15 years earlier than controls. Therefore, they speculated that manganese exposure from the welding fumes might be a risk factor or could accelerate the onset of PD. In 2005, Racette et al. [122] again conducted a study to estimate the prevalence of parkinsonism in 1423 welders from Alabama, and concluded that the estimated prevalence of Parkinsonism was higher in the male welders compared to the general population of male residents from a county in Mississippi. However, the reports failed to show adequate exposure data, including air monitoring in the work place and evidence of exposure in the welders by measuring Mn in the blood, urine and hair. Neuroimaging studies, including MRI, and DAT-SPECT, were not reported. Therefore, whether those patients had an exposure to high concentrations of Mn remained uncertain.

In 2004, Koller et al. [138] also described a group of welders as having "manganese-induced parkinsonism," based on the presence of parkinsonian signs, a history of exposure to manganese in welding rods and lack of response to levodopa. The parkinsonian signs of these patients were not necessarily indicative of manganism, particularly in the presence of resting tremor and the absence of dystonia in most patients. At least some of those patients might have had PD or other types of parkinsonism instead of manganism. In addition, there was an obvious selection bias as the welders were recruited due to civil and workman's compensation litigation. The validity of the diagnosis of manganese-induced parkinsonism and the lack of qualifications of the diagnosing physicians were also questioned. [138, 139]

In 1999, Kim et al. [91] also described two cases of manganese workers who developed a PD syndrome with typical imaging changes. At first, they argued that these patients had PD with incidental exposure to manganese, but subsequently they raised the possibility that manganese might have been a risk factor for the development of PD, [140] and finally they concluded that these cases simply had idiopathic PD with incidental exposure to manganese. [87]

6. Problems of other Welder Studies

The health effects associated with welding fume inhalation have been evaluated, but are often difficult to assess due to differences in worker populations and industrial work area ventilation, welding processes, and the materials used. In addition, large-scale epidemiological studies addressing the association of welding fume inhalation with neurological disease are currently lacking. A few studies of welders have indicated that welding fume inhalation may increase subclinical neurological effects, but most of these studies have no workplace exposure data, little information on exposure to other neurotoxic substances, and small exposure population. [51, 64, 68, 69, 121] Aside from manganese exposure, other risk factors such as liver impairment, carbon monoxide poisoning, organic solvent exposure and iron accumulation that may induce parkinsonism were not mentioned. [4, 5]

Based on there above data, there is no adequate evidence to support the association between welding fume exposure, and the development of PD [142]. However, the absence of a finding of relationship does not prove the absence of relationship. There are some reasons to believe that welding fumes may have different neurotoxic effects, since these welding fumes may include manganese as well as other heavy metals such as iron. [143] Iron may increase oxidative stress through the formation of free radicals and through its effects on mitochondrial function. [144] Iron may also promote aggregation of α-synuclein [145] and provoke neuroinflammation. [146]

Conclusion

Chronic manganese poisoning can induce parkinsonism after absorption through the body circulation and transport to the CNS. Typically, manganese-induced parkinsonism differs from idiopathic PD by clinical features, therapeutic responses, neuroimaging studies, including MRI, 6F-Dopa PET, and DAT-SPECT, and neuropathological studies. In the long-term follow-up studies, PD usually presents with a continuous deterioration, while manganism presents with a rapid progression in the initial 5-10 years, followed by a plateau in the following 10 years. It has also been hypothesized that manganese-containing welding fumes may pose a hazard of inducing neurotoxicity. A rush to such a conclusion is not warranted, and some matters of risk assessment require further investigations by larger studies conducted by neurologists, toxicologists, epidemiologists, industrial hygienists, and other specialists.

References

[1] Mena, I. (1979). Manganese poisoning. In: P.J. Vinken, G.W. Bruyn, (Eds.), *Handbook of Clinical Neurology.* vol. 36. pp. 217-37, Amsterdam: Elsevier/ North Hollard.

[2]   Feldman, R.G. (1994). Manganese. In: P.J. Vinken, G.W. Bruyn, (Eds.), *Handbook of Clinical Neurology.* vol. 64. Intoxication of the Nervous System. Pt 1. F.A. de. Wolff, (ed.) pp. 303-22, Amsterdam: Elsevier Science BV.

[3]   McMillan G. (2005). Is electric arc welding linked to manganism or Parkinson's disease? *Toxical Rev.* 24:237-57.

[4]   Antonini, J.M., Santamaria, A.B., Jenkins, N.T., Albini, E., and Lucchini, R. (2006). Fate of manganese associated with the inhalation of welding fumes: potential neurological effects. *NeuroToxicology.* 27: 304-10.

[5]   Finley, B.L., and Santamaria, A.B. (2005). Current evidence and research needs regarding the risk of manganese-induced neurological effects in welders. *NeuroToxicology.* 26: 285-9.

[6]   Chu, N.S., Huang, C.C., and Calne, D.B. (2000). Manganese. In: P.S. Spencer, H.H. Schaumburg, (Eds.), *Clinical and Experimental Neurotoxicology.* 2nd ed. pp.752-5, Tokyo: Springer Science and Business Media.

[7]   Chu, N.S., Hochberg, F.H., Calne, D.B., and Olanow, C.W. (1995). Neurotoxicology of manganese. In: L.W. Chang, R.S. Dyer, (Eds.), *Handbook of Neurotoxicology.* 1st ed. pp. 91-103, New York: Marcel Dekker Inc.

[8]   Chu, N.S., Huang, C.C., Lu, C.S., and Calne, D.B.(1995). Dystonia caused by toxins. In: J.K.C. Tsui, D.B. Calne, (Eds.), *Handbook of Dystonia.* Vol. 39. 1st ed. pp. 241-65, New York, Basel, Hong. Kong: Marcel Dekker Inc.

[9]   Feldman, R.G. (1999). Manganese. *Occupational and Environmental Neurotoxicology.* 1st ed. pp. 168-88, New York: Lippincott-Raven Press.

[10]   Saric, M. (1986). Managanese. In: I. Friberg, G.I. Nordberg, V. Vouk, (Eds.), *Handbook of Toxicology of Metals.* 1st ed. pp. 354-70 Amsterdam: Elsevier.

[11]   Cersosimo, M.G., and Koller, W.C. (2006). The diagnosis of manganese-induced parkinsonism. *NeuroToxicology.* 27: 340-6.

[12]   Lynam, D.R., Pfeifer, G.D., Fort, B.F., Ter Hear, G.L., and Hollrah, D.P. (1994). Atmospheric exposure to manganese from use of methylcyclopentadienyl manganese tricarbonyl (MMT) performance additive. *Sci. Total Environ.* 146: 103-9.

[13]   Cooper, W.C. (1984). The health implications of increased manganese in the environment resulting form the combustion of fuel additives: a review of the literature. *J. Toxicol. Environ. Health.* 14: 23-46.

[14]   Good, G., and Egyed, M. (1994). Risk assessment for the combustion products of methylcyclopentadienyl manganese tricarbonyl (MMT) in gasoline. Environmental Health Directorate. *Health Canada.* pp1-110.

[15]   Couper, J. (1837). On the effects of black oxide of manganese when inhaled into the lungs. *Br. Ann. Med. Pharmacol.* 1: 41-2.

[16]   Emara, A.M., and El-Ghawabi, S.H., Madkour, O.I., El-Samra, G.H. (1971). Chronic manganese poisoning in the dry battery industry. *Br. J. Ind. Med.* 28: 78-82.

[17]   Huang, C.C., Chu, N.S., Lu, C.S., Wang, J.D., Tsai, J.L., Wolters, E.C., and Calne, D.B. (1989). Chronic manganese intoxication. *Arch. Neurol.* 46: 1104-6.

[18]   Ono, K., Komai, K., Yamada, M. (2002). Myoclonic involuntary movement associated with chronic manganese poisoning. *J. Neurol. Sci.* 199: 93-6.

[19] Ferraz, H.B., Bertolucci, P.H.F., Pereria, J.S., Lima, J.G.C., and Andrade, L.A.F. (1988). Chronic exposure to the fungicide Maneb may produce symptoms and signs of CNS manganese intoxication. *Neurology.* 38: 550-3.

[20] Ensing, J.G. (1985). Bazooka: cocaine-base and manganese carbonate. *J. Anal. Toxicol.* 9: 45-6.

[21] Lynam, D.R., Roos, J.W., Pfeifer, G.D., Fort, B.F., and Pullin, T.G. (1999). Environmental effects and exposures to manganese from use of methylcyclopentadienyl manganese tricarbonyl (MMT) in gasoline. *NeuroToxicology.* 20: 145-50.

[22] Hudnell, H.K. (1999). Effects from environmental Mn exposures: a review of the evidence from non-occupational exposure studies. *NeuroToxicology.* 20: 379-97.

[23] Ejima, A., Imamura, T., Nakamura, S., Saito, H., Matsumoto, K., and Momono, S. (1992). Manganese intoxication during total parenteral nutrition. *Lancet.* 339: 426.

[24] Kondakis, X.G., Makris, N., Leotsinidis, M., Prinou, M., and Papapetropoulos, T. (1989). Possible health effects of high manganese concentration in drinking water. *Arch. Environ. Health.* 44: 175-8.

[25] Aggett, P.G. (1985). Physiology and metabolism and essential trace elements: an outline. *Clin. Endocrinal. Metab.* 14: 513-43.

[26] Dobson, A.W., Erikson, K.M., and Aschner, M. (2004). Manganese neurotoxicity. *Ann. NY Acad. Sci.* 1012:115-28.

[27] Oberdorster, G., Obedorster, J., and Lehnert, B. (1994). Particulate air pollution: animal toxicology. Unpublished report prepared under contact for Health Canada. Environmental Health Directorate

[28] Ter Haar, G.L., Griffing, M.E., Brandt, M., Oberding, D.G., and Kepron, M. (1975). Methlcylopentadienyl manganse tricarbonyl as an anti-knock: composition and fate of manganese exhaust products. *J. Air Pollut. Contr. Assoc.* 25: 858-60.

[29] Mena, I. (1980). Manganese. Metals in the Environment. 1st ed. pp199-220. In: H.A. Waldron (Ed.), London, New York, Toronto: Academic Press.

[30] Pavidsson, L., Cederblad, A., Lonnerdal, B., and Sandstrom, B. (1985). Manganese absorption from human milk, cow's milk and infant formulas in humans. *Am. J. Dis. Child.* 143; 823-7.

[31] Tjalve, H., and Henriksson, J. (1999). Uptake of metals in the brain via olfactory pathways. *NeuroToxicology.* 20: 181-95.

[32] Tjalve, H., Mejare, C., and Borg-Neczak, K. (1995). Uptake and transport of manganese in primary and secondary neurons in pike. *Pharmacol. Toxicol.* 77:3-31.

[33] Tjalve, H., Henriksson, J., and Tallkvist, J. (1996). Uptake of manganese and cadmium from the nasal mucosa into the central nervous system via olfactory pathway in rats. *Pharmacol. Toxicol.* 79: 347-56.

[34] Arkhipova, O., Tolgskaya, M., and Kochetkova, T. (1996). Toxic properties of manganese cyclopentadienyl tricarbonyl antiknock substance. *US. SR Lit. Air Pollut. Relate Dis.* 12: 85-9.

[35] Scheuhammer, A., and Cherian, M. (1985). Binding of manganese in human and rat plasma. *Biochim. Biophys. Acta.* 840: 163-9.

[36] Adkons, B., Luginbuhl, G.H., and Gardner, D.E. (1980). Acute exposure of laboratory mice to manganese oxide. *Am. Ind. Hyg. Assoc.* 11:494-500.

[37] Komura, J., and Sakamoto, M. (1992). Effect of manganese forms on biogenic amines in the brain and behavioral alterations in the mouse: long-term oral administration of several manganese compounds. *Environ. Res.* 57; 34-44.

[38] Morrow, P.; Gibb, F.R., and Gazioglu, K.(1967). The clearance of dust from the lower respiratory tract. An experimental study. In: *Inhaled particles and vapours. II. Proceedings of an international symposium* pp.351-9. C.N.Davis (Ed.). Oxford. New York: Pergamon Pres.

[39] Newland, M.C., Cox, C., Hamada, R., Oberdorster, G., and Weiss, B. (1987). The clearance of manganese chloride in the primate. *Fund Appl. Toxicol.* 9:314-28.

[40] Sandstrom, B., Davidsson, L., Cedarblad, R., Eriksson, R., and Lonnerdal, B. (1986). Manganese absorption and metabolism in man. *Acta Pharmacol. Toxicol.* 59: 60-2.

[41] Gibbons, R.A., Dixon, S.N., Hallis, A.M., Russel, A.M., Sansom, B.F., and Symonds, H.W. (1976). Manganese metabolism in cows and goats. *Biochim. Biophys. Acta.* 444:1-10.

[42] Aschner, M., and Aschner, J.L. (1991). Manganese neurotoxicity: cellular effects and blood-brain barrier transport. *Neurosci. Behavior Rev.* 15:333-40.

[43] Embden, H. (1901). Zur Kentniss dre metallischen nervengifte. *Deutsch Med. Wochenschr.* 27: 795-6.

[44] Von Jaksch, R. (1907). Ueber Mangantoxikosen und manganophobie. *Muench. Med. Wochenschr.* 20: 969-72.

[45] Edsall, D.L., Wilbur, F.P., and Drinker, C.K. (1919) The occurrence, course and prevention of chronic manganese poisoning. *Ind. Hyg.* 1: 183-93.

[46] Ashizawa, R. (1927). Uber einen sektionsfall von chronischer manganvergiftung. *Jpn. J. Med. Sci. Trans. Intern. Med. Pediatr. Psychiat.* 1: 173-91.

[47] Rodier, J. (1955). Manganese poisoning in Moroccan miners. *Br. J. Ind. Med.* 12: 21-35.

[48] Flinn, R.H., Neal, P.A., and Fulton, W.B. (1941). Industrial manganese poisoning. *J. Ind. Hyg. Toxicol.* 23: 374-87.

[49] Smyth, L.T., Ruhf, R.C., Whitman, N.E., and Dugan, T. (1973). Clinical manganism and exposure to manganese in the production and processing of ferromanganese alloy. *J. Occup. Med.* 15: 101-9.

[50] Wang, D., Zhou, W., Wang, S., and Zheng, W. (1998). Occupational exposure to manganese in welders and associated neurodegenerative diseases in China. *Toxicologist.* 42: 24-30.

[51] Sadek, A.H., Rauch, R., and Schulz, P.E. (2003). Parkinsonism due to manganism in a welder. *Int. J. Toxicol.* 22: 393-401.

[52] Holzgraefe, M., Poser, W., Kijewski, H., and Beuche, W. (1986). Chronic enteral poisoning caused by potassium permanganate: a case report. *Clin. Toxicol.* 235-44.

[53] Canavan, M.M., Cobb, S., and Drinker, C.K. (1934). Chronic manganese poisoning. *Psychiatry.* 32: 501-12.

[54] Mena, I., Marin, O., Fuenzalida, S., and Cotzias, G.C. (1967). Chronic manganese poisoning. Clinical picture and manganese turnover. *Neurology.* 17: 128-36.

[55] Mena, I., Court, J., Fuenzalida, S., Papavasiliou, P.S., and Cotzias, G.C. (1970). Modification of chronic manganese poisoning. Treatment with L-dopa or 5-OH tryptophane. *N. Engl. J. Med.* 282: 5-10.

[56] Cotzias, G.C., Horiuchi, K., Fuenzalids, S., and Mena, I. (1968). Chronic manganese poisoning: clearance of tissue manganese concentrations with persistence of the neurological picture. *Neurology.* 18: 376-82.

[57] Cook, D.G., Fahn, S., and Brait, K.A. (1974). Chronic manganese intoxication. *Arch. Neurol.* 30: 59- 64.

[58] Rosenstock, H.A., Simons, D.G., and Meyer, J.S. (1971). Chronic manganism: neurologic and laboratory studies during treatment with levodopa. *JAMA.* 217: 1354-8.

[59] Wang, J.D., Huang, C.C., Huang, Y.H., Chiang, J.R., Lin, J.M., and Chen, J.S. (1989) Manganese induced parkinsonism: an outbreak due to unrepaired ventilation control system in a ferromanganese smelter. *Br. J. Ind. Med.* 46: 856-9.

[60] Huang, C.C., Chu, N.S., Lu, C.S., and Calne, D.B. (1997) Cock gait in manganese intoxication. *Mov. Disord.* 1997; 12: 807-8.

[61] Schuler, P., Oyanguren, H., Maturana, V., Cruz, E., Plaza, V., Schmidt, E., and Haddad, R. (1957). Manganese poisoning. Environmental and medical study at a Chilean mine. *Industr. Med. Surg.* 26: 167-73.

[62] Bowler, R.M., Mergler, D., Sassine, M.P., Larribe, F., and Hudnell, K. (1999). Neuropsychiatric effects of manganese on mood. *NeuroToxicology.* 20: 367-78.

[63] Pettersen, R., Ellingsen, D.G., Hetland, S.M., and Thomassenn, Y. (2004). Neuropsychological function in manganese alloy plant workers. *Int. Arch. Occup. Environ. Health.* 77: 277-87.

[64] Bowler, R.M., Gysens, S., Diamond, E., Booty, A., Hartney, C., and Roels, H.A. (2003). Neuropsychological sequelae of exposure to welding fumes in a group of occupationally exposed men. *Int. J. Hyg. Environ. Health.* 206: 517-29.

[65] Hua, M.S., and Huang, C.C. (1991). Chronic occupational exposure to manganese and neurobehavioral function. *J. Clin. Exp. Neuropsychol.* 13: 497-507.

[66] Roels, H., Lauwerys, R., and Genet, P. (1989). Relationship between external and internal parameters of exposure to manganese in workers from a manganese oxide and salt producing plant. *Am. J. Ind. Med.* 2: 297-305.

[67] Roels, H.A., Ghyselen, P., Buchet, J.P., Cenlemans, E., and Lauwerys, R.R. (1992). Assessment of the permissible exposure level to manganese in workers exposed to manganese dioxide dust. *Br. J. Ind. Med.* 49: 25-34.

[68] Bowler, R.M., Gysens, S., Diamond, E., Nakagawa, S., Drezgie, M., and Roels, H.A. (2006). Manganese exposure: neuropsychological and neurological symptoms and effects in welders. *NeuroToxicology.* 27: 315-26.

[69] Bowler, R.M., Koller, W., and Schulz, P.E. (2006). Parkinsonism due to manganism in a welder: neurological and neuropsychological sequelae. *NeuroToxicology.* 27:327-32.

[70] Chu, N.S., Huang, C.C., and Calne, D.B. (1996). Sympathetic skin response and RR interval variation in manganism and a comparison with Parkinson's disease. *Parkinsonism Relat. Disord.* 2: 23-8.

[71] Mena, I., Horiuchi, K., Berke, K., and Cotzia, G. (1969). Chronic manganese poisoning: individual susceptibility and absorption of iron. *Neurology.* 19: 1000-6.

[72] Smyth, L.T., Ruhf, R.C., Whitman, N.E. and Dugan, T. (1973) Clinical manganism and exposure to manganese in the production and processing of ferromanganese alloy. *J. Occup. Med.* 15:101-9.

[73] Penalver, R. (1955). Manganese poisoning. *The 1954 Ramazzini Oration. Ind. Med. Surg.* 24: 1-7.

[74] Tanaka, S., and Lieben, J. (1969). Manganese poisoning and exposure in Pennsylviania. *Arch. Environ. Health.* 19: 674-84.

[75] Huang, C.C., Lu, C.S., Chu, N.S., Hochberg, F., Lilienfeld, D., Olanow, W., and Calne, D.B. (1993) Progression after chronic manganese exposure. *Neurology.* 43: 1479-83.

[76] Huang, C.C., Chu, N.S., Lu, C.S., Chen, R.S., and Calne, D.B. (1998). Long-term progression in chronic manganism: ten years of follow-up. *Neurology.* 50: 698-700.

[77] Huang, C.C., Chen, N.S., Lu, C.S., Chen, R.S., Schulzer, M., and Calne, D.B. (2007). The natural history of neurological manganism over 18 years. *Parkinsonism Relat. Disord.* (in press).

[78] Greenhouse, A.H. (1971). Manganese intoxication in the United States. *Trans. Ann. Neurol. Associ.* 96: 248-9.

[79] Lu, C.S., Huang, C.C., Chu, N.S., and Calne, D.B. (1994). Levodopa failure in chronic manganism. *Neurology.* 44: 1600-2.

[80] Crossgroue, J., and Zheng, W. (2004). Manganese toxicity upon overexposure. *NMR. Biomed.* 17: 543-53.

[81] Ky, S., Deng, H., and Hu, W. (1992). A report of two cases of chronic serious manganese poisoning treated with sodium para-amino-salicylic acid. *Br. J. Ind. Med.* 49: 66-9.

[82] Jiang, Y.M., Mo, X.A., Du, F.Q., Fu, X., Zhu, X.Y., Gao, H.Y., Xie, J.W., Liao, F.L., Pira, E., and Zheng, W. (2006). Effective treatment of manganese-induced occupational parkinsonism with p-aminosalicylic acid: a case of 17-year follow-up study. *J. Occup. Environ. Med.* 48: 644-9.

[83] Newland, M.C., Ceckler, T.L., Kordower, J.H., and Weiss, B. (1989). Visualizing manganese in the primate basal ganglia with magnetic resonance imaging. *Exp. Neurol.* 106: 251-8.

[84] Nelson, K., Golnick, J., Korn, T., and Angle, C. (1993). Manganese encephalopathy: utility of early magnetic resonance imaging. *Br. J. Ind. Med.* 50: 510-3.

[85] Josephs, K.A., Ahlskog, E., Klos, K.J., Kumar, N., Fealey, R.D., Trenerry, M.R., and Cowl, C.T. (2005). Neurologic manifestations in welders with pallidal MRI T1 hyperintensity. *Neurology.* 64: 2033-9.

[86] Kim, Y., Kim, K.S., Yang, J.S., Park, I.J., Kim, E., Jin, Y., Kwon, K.R., Chang, K.H., Kim, J.W., Park, S.H., Lim, H.S., Cheong, H.K., Shin, Y.C., Park, J., and Moon, Y. (1999). Increase in signal intensities on T1-weighted magnetic resonance images in asymptomatic manganese-exposed workers. *NeuroToxicology.* 20: 901-8.

[87] Kim, Y. (2006). Neuroimaging in manganism. *NeuroToxicology.* 27: 369-72.

[88] Hauser, R.A., Zesiewicz, T.A., Rosemurgy, A.S., and Martinez, C., Olanow CW. (1994). Manganese intoxication and chronic liver failure. *Ann. Neurol.* 1994; 36: 871-5.

[89]   Hauser, R.A., Zesiewicz, T.A., Martinez, C., Rosemurgy, A.S., and Olanow, C.W. (1996). Blood manganese correlates with brain magnetic resonance imaging changes in patients with liver disease. *Can. J. Neurol. Sci.* 1996; 23: 95-8.

[90]   Krieger, D., Krieger, S., Jansen, O., Gass, P., Theilmann, L., and Lichtnecker, H. (1995). Manganese and chronic hepatic encephalopathy. *Lancet.* 346:270-4.

[91]   Kim, Y., Kim, J.W., Ito, K., Lim, H.S., Cheong, H.K., Kim, J.Y., Shin, Y.C., Kim, K.S., and Moon, Y. (1999). Idiopathic parkinsonism with superimposed manganese exposure: utility of positron emission tomography. *NeuroToxicology.* 20: 249-52.

[92]   Kim, E., Kim, Y., Cheong, H.K., Cho, S., Shin, Y.C., Sakong, J., Kim, K.S., Yang, J.S., Jin, Y.W., and Kang, S.K. (2005). Pallidal index on MRI as a target organ dose of manganese: structural equation model analysis. *NeuroToxicology.* 26: 351-9.

[93]   Morrish, P.K., Sawle, G.V., and Brooks, D.J. (1995). Clinical and [^{18} F] dopa PET findings in early Parkinson's disease. *J. Neurol. Neurosurg. Psychiatry.* 59: 597-600.

[94]   Calne, D.B., and Langston, J.W. (1983). Etiology of Parkinson's disease. *Lancet.* 2: 1457-9.

[95]   Snow, B.J., Tooyama, I., McGeer, E.G., Yamada, T., Calne, D.B., Takahashi, H., and Kimura, H. (1993). Human positron emission tomographic [^{18}F] fluorodopa studies correlate with dopamine cell counts and levels. *Ann. Neurol.* 34: 324-30.

[96]   Wolters, E., Huang, C.C., Clark, C., Peppard, R.F., Okada, J., Chu, N.S., Adam, M.J., Ruth, T.J., Li, D., and Calne, D.B. (1989). Positron emission tomography in manganese intoxication. *Ann. Neurol.* 26: 647-51.

[97]   Brooks, D.J., Ibanez, V., Sawle, G.V., Playford, E.D., Quinn, N., Mathias, C.J., Lees, A.J., Marsden, C.D., Bannister, R., and Frackowiak, R.S. (1992). Striatal D2 receptor status in patients with Parkinson's disease, striatonigral degeneration and progressive supranuclear palsy, measured with ^{11}C-raclopride and positron emission tomography. *Ann. Neurol.* 31: 184-92.

[98]   Rinne, U.K., Laihinen, A., Rinne, J.O., Nagren, K., Bergman, J., Ruotsalainen, V. (1990). Positron emission tomography demonstrates dopamine D2-receptor supersenitivity in the striatum of patients with early Parkinson's disease. *Mov. Disord.* 5: 55-9.

[99]   Shinotoh, H., Snow, B.J., Chu, N.S., Huang, C.C., Lu, C.S., Lee, C., Takahashi, H., Calne, D.B. (1997). Presynaptic and postsynaptic striatal dopaminergic function in patients with manganese intoxication: a positron emission tomography study. *Neurology.* 48: 1053-6.

[100] Huang, C.C., Yen, T.C., Weng, Y.H., and Lu, C.S. (2002). Normal dopamine transporter binding in dopa responsive dystonia. *J. Neurol.* 249: 1016-20.

[101] Kung, H.F., Kim, H.J., Kung, M.R., Meegalla, S.K., Plossl, K., and Lec, H.K. (1996). Imaging of dopamine transporters in humans with technetium^{99m} Tc-TRODAT-1. *Eur. J. Nucl. Med.* 23: 1527-30.

[102] Jeon, B., Jeong, J.M., Park, S.S., Kim, J.M., Chang, Y.S., Song, H.C., Kim, K.M., Yoon, K.Y., Lee, M.C., and Lee, S.B. (1998). Dopamine transporter density measured by [^{123} I]-β-CIT single photon emission computed tomography is normal in dopa-responsive dystonia. *Ann. Neurol.* 43: 782-800.

[103] Nurmi, E., Ruottinen, H.M., Kaasinen, V., Bergman, J., Haaparanta, M., Solin, O., and Rinne, J.O. (2000). Progression in Parkinson's disease: a positron emission tomography study with a dopamine transporter ligand [^{18}F] CFT. *Ann. Neurol.* 47: 804-8.

[104] Meegalla, S.K., Plossl, K., Kung, M.P., Stevenson, D.A., Mu, M., Kushner, S., Liable-Sands, L.M., Rheingold, A.L., and Kung, H.F. (1998). Specificity of diastereomers of [^{99m} Tc] TRODAT-1 as dopamine transporter imaging agents. *J. Nucl. Med.* 41: 428-36.

[105] Mozley, P.D., Schneider, J.S., Acton, P.D., Plossl, K., Stern, M.B., Siderowf, A., Leopold, N.A., Li, P.Y., Alavi, A., and Kung, H.F. (2000). Binding of [^{99m} Tc]-TRODAT-1 to dopamine transporter in patients with Parkinson's disease and in healthy volunteers. *J. Nucl. Med.* 41: 584-9.

[106] Huang, C.C., Weng, Y.H., Lu, C.S., Chu, N.S., and Yen, T.C. (2003). Dopamine transporter binding in chronic manganese intoxication. J. Neurol. 250: 1335-9.

[107] Yamada, M., Ohno, S., Okayasu, I., Okeda, R., Hatakeyama, S., Watanabe, H., Ushio, K., and Tsukagoshi, H. (1986). Chronic manganese poisoning: a neuropathological study with determination of manganese distribution in the brain. *Acta Neuropathol.* (Berlin) 70: 273-8.

[108] Neff, N.H., Barrett, R.E., and Costa, E. (1969). Selective depletion of caudate nucleus dopamine and serotonin during chronic manganese dioxide administration to squirrel monkeys. *Experientia.* 25: 1140-1

[109] Brouillet, E.P., Shinobu, L., McGarvey, U., Hochberg, F., and Beal, M.F. (1993). Manganese injection into the rat striatum produces excitotoxic lesions by impairing energy metabolism. *Exp. Neurol.* 120: 89-94.

[110] Spadoni, F., Stefani, A., Morello, M., Lavaroni, F., Giacomini, P., and Sancesario, G. (2000). Selective vulnerability of pallidal neurons in the early phases of manganese intoxication. *Exp. Brain Res.* 135: 544-51.

[111] Olanow, C.W., Good, P.F., Shinotoh, H., Hewitt, K.A., Vingerhoets, F., Snow, B.J., and Beal, M.F. (1996). Calne DB, Perl DP. Manganese intoxication in the rhesus monkey: a clinical, imaging, pathologic, and biochemical study. *Neurology.* 46: 492-8.

[112] Pal, P.K., Samii, A., and Calne, D.B. (1990). Manganese neurotoxicity: a review of clinical features, imaging and pathology. *NeuroToxicology.* 20: 227-38.

[113] Burkhard, P.R., Delavelle, J.Y., Dupasquier, R., and Spahr, L. (2003) Chronic Parkinsonism associated with cirrhosis: a distinct subset of acquired hepatocerebral degeneration. *Arch. Neurol.* 60:521-8.

[114] Calne, D.B., Chu, N.S., Huang, C.C., Lu, C.S., and Olanow, W. (1994). Manganism and idiopathic parkinsonism: similarities and differences. *Neurology.* 44: 1583-6.

[115] Olanow, C.W. (2004). Manganese-induced parkinsonism and Parkinson's disease. *Ann. NY Acad. Sci.* 1012: 209-23.

[116] Jankovic, J. (2005). Searching for a relationship between manganese and welding and Parkinson's disease. *Neurology.* 64: 2021-8.

[117] Lee, C.S., Schulzer, M., Mak, E.K., Snow, B.J., Taui, J.K., Calne, S., and Calne, DB. (1994). Clinical observations on the rate of progression of idiopathic parkinsonism. *Brain.* 117: 501-7.

[118] Lee, C.S., Schulzer, M., Mak, E.K., Hammerstad, J.P., Calne, S., and Calne, D.B. (1995). Patterns of asymmetry do not change over the course of idiopathic parkinsonism: implication for pathogenesis. *Neurology.* 45: 435-9.

[119] Abd-El Naby, S., and Hassanein, M. (1965). Neuropsychiatric manifestation of chronic manganese poisoning. *J. Neurol. Neurosurg. Psychiatry.* 28: 282-8.

[120] Racette, B.A., McGee-Minnich, L., Moerlein, S.M., Mink, J.W., Videen, T.O., and Perlmutter, J.S. (2001). Welding-related parkinsonism: clinical features, treatment, and pathophysiology. *Neurology.* 56: 8-13.

[121] Racette, B.A., Antenor, J.A., McGee-Minnich, L., Moerlein, S.M., Videen, T.O., Kotagal, V., and Perlmutter, J.S. (2005). [^{18} F] FDOPA PET and clinical features in parkinsonism due to manganism. *Mov. Disord.* 20: 492-6.

[122] Racette, B.A., Tabbal, S.D., Jennings, D., Good, L., Perlmutter, J.S., and Evanoff, B. (2005). Prevalence of parkinsonism and relationship to exposure in a large sample of Alabama welders. *Neurology.* 64: 230-5.

[123] Kaiser, J. (2003). State court to rule on manganese fume claims. *Science.* 300: 927.

[124] Bureau of Labor Statistics. Welders, cutters, solderers and brazers. In : Occupation Employment Statistics: Occupational Employment and Wages, 2002. US Department of Labor. Accessed 01/28/2004; available at http://www.bls.gw/oes/2002/oes51421.htm.

[125] Zimmer, A.T., and Biswas, P. (2001). Characterization of theaerosals resulting form arc welding processes. *J. Aerosol. Sci.* 32: 993-1008.

[126] Beckett, W.S. (1996). Welding. In Harber, P., Schenker, M.B., Balmes, J.R. (Eds). *Occupational and environmental respiratory disease.* pp. 704-17. St. Louis. MO: Mosby-Year Book Inc.

[127] Harris, M.K. (2002). Welding health and safety: A field guide for DEHS professionals. Fairfax, VA: American Industional Hygiene Association Press.

[128] McClellan, R.O. (2000). Particle interactions with the respiratory tract. In: C. Lenfant, C. (Ed.) *Particle-Lung Interactions.* pp3-76. New York: Marcel Dekker Inc.

[129] Oberdorster G. (2004). Kinnetics of inhaled ultrafine particles in the organism. In: Heinrich U, (Ed.) *Effects of air contaminants on the respiratory tract-Inter pretations from molecular to meta analysis* pp.122-43. Hannover: Fraunhofer IRB verlag.

[130] Aschner, M. (2006). Manganese: brain transport and emerging research needs. *Environ. Health Perspect.* 108 (Suppl.3): 429-32.

[131] Achner, M., and Aschner, J.L. (1990). Manganese transport across the blood –brain barrier: relationship to iron homeostasis. *Brain Res. Bull.* 24:857-860.

[132] American Conference of Governmental Industrial Hygienists (ACGIH). (1994) Threshold limit values for chemical substances in the work environment adopted by ACGIH. Cincinnati, Ohio: ACGIH.

[133] ACGIH. Manganese and inorganic compounds. In: Documentation of the Threshold Limits Values for Chemical Substances. 7th ed; Vol 3, Cincinnati, OH, American Conference of Governmental Industrial Hygienists, 2001.

[134] ACGIH. TLVs and BEIs. Threshold limit values for 4 chemical substances and physical agents and biological exposure indices. Cincinnati, OH, American Conference of Governmental Industrial Hygienists 2005, pp19.

[135] OSHA. US Department of Lebor Occupational Safety and Health Administration. Manganese compound 2007-1-30 http://www.osha.gov/dts/sltc/methods/partial/pv2004/2004.html

[136] NIOSH. Welding fumes. In NIOSH Pocket Guide to Chemical Hazards. U.S. Department of Heath and Human Services. Public Health Service, Centers of Disease Control and Prevention, National Institute for Occapational Safety and Health, Cincinnati, OH, NIOSH.

[137] Korczynski, R.E. (2002). Occupational health concerns in the welding industry. *Appl. Occup. Environ. Hyg.* 15: 936-45.

[138] Koller, W.C., Lyons, K.E., and Truly, W. (2004). Effect of levodopa treatment for parkinsonism in welders. *Neurology.* 62:730-3.

[139] Chu, N.S. (2004). Effect of levodopa treatment for parkinsonism in welders: a double-blind study. *Neurology.* 63:1541.

[140] Koller, W.C., and Lyons, K.E. (2004). Effect of levodopa treatment for parkinsonism in welders: a double-blind study. *Neurology.* 63:1541.

[141] Kim, Y., Kim, J.M., Kim, J.W., Yoo, C.I., Lee, C.R., Lee, J.H., Kim, H.K., Yang, S.O., Chung, H.K., Lee, D.S., and Jeon, B. (2002). Dopamine transporter density is decreased in parkinsonian patients with a history of manganese exposure: what does it mean? *Mov. Disord.* 17: 568-75.

[142] Antonini, J.M., Santamaria, A.B., Jenkins, N.T., Albini, E., and Lucchini, R. (2006). Fate of manganese associated with the inhalation of welding fumes: potential neurological effects. *NeuroToxicology.* 27: 304-10.

[143] Kieburtz, K., and Kurlan, R. (2005). Welding and Parkinson disease. Is there a bond ? *Neurology.* 64: 2001-3.

[144] Berg, D., Gerlach, M., Youdim, M.B., Double, K.L., Zecca, L., Riederer, P., and Becker, G. (2001). Brain iron pathways and their relevance to Parkinson's disease. J. Neuroche. 79:225-36.

[145] Wolozin, B., and Golts, N. (2002). Iron and Parkinson's disease. *Neuroscientist.* 8: 22-32.

[146] McGeer, P.L., Itagaki, S., Boyes, B.E., and McGeer, E.G. (1998). Reactive microglia are positive for HLA-DR in the substantia nigra of Parkinson's and Alzheimer's disease brains. *Neurology.* 38: 1285-91.

In: New Research on Parkinson's Disease
Editors: T. F. Hahn, J. Werner

ISBN: 978-1-60456-601-7
© 2008 Nova Science Publishers, Inc.

Chapter IX

Cognitive Disorders in Parkinson's Disease

Claudio da Cunha
Laboratory of Physiology and Pharmacology of CNS,
Department of Pharmacology,
Federal University of Paraná,
81.531-990- Curitiba,
PR, Brazil.

Introduction

At the beginning of the nineteenth century, when James Parkinson published the book entitled "Essay on the Shaking Palsy", life expectation was no longer than 45 years old. The "shaking palsy", later named Parkinson's disease by Charcot, affects mainly aged people. Nowadays, 0.3 % of the whole population and 1% of the population over 60 years old have Parkinson's disease. This percentage increases with age. Besides, now in the beginning of the XXI century, life expectancy is near 80 years old. Therefore, there are much more parkinsonian patients nowadays than two centuries ago. Hence, one can ask – is it a great advantage to live more if it means an increased probability to suffer of diseases like this?

At least, a century ago one could say that the Parkinson's disease caused only motor disabilities like bradykinesia/hypokinesia, muscular rigidity and resting tremor, but preserved cognitive functions. Unfortunately more recent studies showed that that is not the truth. A famous James Parkinson's contemporary affected by this disease, Wilhem von Humboldt, a writer and educational reformer, had already reported to be deeply impaired in a motor skill closely related to the expression of cognition – writing. Micrographia was later added to the list of symptoms observed in Parkinson's disease. In one of his famous letters, Humboldt wrote that at least his mental life had not been affected at all. He was probably referring to his capacity of consciously storing and recalling events and concepts. This kind of memory, called declarative or explicit, is indeed mostly preserved in many parkinsonian patients.

However, near one-third of the Parkinson's disease patients are not as lucky as Humboldt and become demented, a condition in which declarative memory is deeply affected. Besides, other kinds of cognitive impairments that are not so easily noticed may have been neglected by Humboldt and his relatives. Recent studies have shown that other types of learning and non-declarative (implicit) memories that are usually stored and recalled unconsciously, are more commonly affected in Parkinson's disease. Motor skills, such as the writing skill mentioned above, is an example of non-declarative memory affected by Parkinson's disease. Since many skills are closely related to motor functions, people use to see them as part of the motor disabilities of the disease. But, it must not be forgotten that skills are acquired by learning and are, therefore, cognitive in nature. Furthermore, the learning of more clearly cognitive skills, like reading mirrored image words, is also affected in this disease. Besides, other types of non-declarative memories are also impaired in non-demented Parkinson's disease patients. Forming a habit is a clear example. Habits are usually formed unconsciously by the repetitive association of a stimulus with a reinforced response. After learned, the response will be automatically triggered by the associated stimulus. Many of our daily jobs, like driving a car, turning right or left to go from home to work and even remembering that 2 X 2 = 4, are done automatically by habit. Working memory, especially visuospatial working memory, has also been reported to be impaired in Parkinson's disease. Besides those mnemonic functions, executive functions, such as attention shifting, planning, and task management are also impaired, even in non-demented Parkinson's disease patients. In the next sections of this article we will detail convincing evidence showing that these cognitive functions are impaired in Parkinson's disease.

Hence, although Humboldt and other Parkinson's disease patients thought that they had preserved their cognitive functions, careful studies have not confirmed this belief. Therefore, the question of whether it is worth living for a longer time, being thus more susceptible to this kind of disease, can be reformulated as a new question – What can we do to treat the cognitive impairments of Parkinson's disease? The prime task of the scientist is to understand why Parkinson's disease affects these specific cognitive functions. In the next part of this article we will report what scientists have already discovered about it and how this knowledge has been used to treat the cognitive functions of Parkinson's disease.

Patophysiology

The neurodegenerative processes that lead to sporadic Parkinson's disease begin many years before the appearance of the characteristic somatomotor symptoms. It seems that the pathological process start with the formation of Lewy bodies and Lewy neurites in the anterior olfactory structures as well as in regions of the medulla oblongata and pontine tegmentum, including the noradrenergic neurons of the locus coeruleus and the serotonergic neurons of the caudal raphe nuclei (stages 1-2). Later, the cholinergic nucleus basalis of Meynert also becomes affected (stage 3). By the time somatomotor disabilities are evident (stage 4 and beyond), there is considerable loss of dopaminergic neurons in the substantia nigra pars compacta (SNpc). Cortical Lewy bodies and Lewy neurites occur initially in the temporal mesocortex (stage 4) and, thereafter, in the neocortex (stages 5-6) (Figure 9.1).

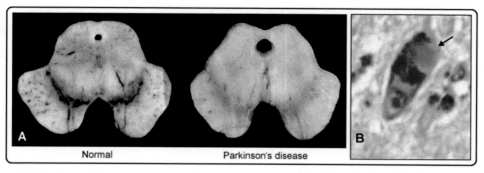

Figure 9.1. The loss of the neuromelanin-pigmented neurons of the SNpc in the midbrain (A), and the occurrence of intracellular proteinaceous inclusions known as Lewy bodies, revealed here by a hematoxinin-eosin staining (B), are the main hallmarks of Parkinson's disease.

Lewy bodies are intracitoplasmatic incrustations composed mainly by the proteins α-synuclein and ubiquitin. Many studies suggest that the death of dopamine cells in Parkinson's disease is linked to protein aggregation and dysfunction of the ubiquitin proteasome pathway. An altered form of the α-synuclein gene has been found in a case of family inherited Parkinson's disease with early onset. However, this abnormal gene was not found in most cases of the so called idiopathic Parkinson's disease that affects aged people. In these cases, no apparent genetic pattern of inheritance was found. Since the polymerization of this protein, as well as many neurotoxins that cause Parkinsonism, produce free radical species, they are often pointed as the trigger of the neurodegenerative process that leads to the disease. The inhibition of the mitochondrial complex I, oxidative stress, and inflammation have also been pointed as important steps leading to neurodegeneration (Figure 9.2). Indeed, the midbrain dopamine cells are among the most vulnerable cells to degenerative processes in the brain. However, the primary event that starts the neurodegeneration cascade and how to stop the disease progression are not precisely known.

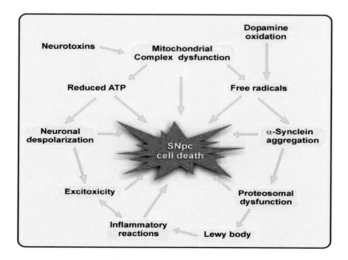

Figure 9.2. Multifactorial causes for substantia nigra pars compacta (SNpc) neurodegeneration in Parkinson's disease.

As important as knowing the cause of Parkinson's disease is to know the normal function of the brain components affected by this disease. Dopaminergic neurons of the SNpc modulate a brain system called basal ganglia. Basal ganglia are composed by the caudate nucleus and putamen (altogether called striatum), globus pallidus and the subthalamic nucleus (Figure 9.3). Neurons from all parts of the neocortex project to the striatum. Striatal neurons in turn project to the globus pallidus or to the substantia nigra pars reticulata (SNpr) that projects to the ventrolateral thalamus that in turn projects back to the frontal cortex, as can be seen in the schedule presented in Figure 9.4. Therefore, the activity of sensorial and motor parts of the cortex affects the activity of the basal ganglia that in turn modulate the activity of motor and cognitive parts of the frontal cortex. The positive modulation exerted by the glutamate thalamic neurons upon the frontal cortex is under inhibitory control of GABAergic neurons of the globus pallidus and the SNpr. This inhibition can be either blocked by a direct pathway or increased by an indirect pathway of neurons that arise in the striatum   (Figure 9.5). Midbrain dopamine neurons play a dual modulation on the activity of these striatal neurons. Acting on D1-like or D2-like dopamine receptors, the dopamine released by these neurons activates the direct pathway and inhibits the indirect pathway respectively. Both actions result in a positive modulation of the motor and cognitive functions of the frontal cortex. By this view, it is clear that the loss of midbrain dopamine neurons that occurs in Parkinson's disease results in impairments of both motor and cognitive functions.

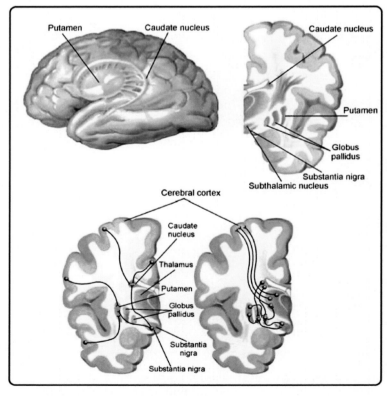

Figure 9.3. Extrinsic and intrinsic connections of the basal ganglia.

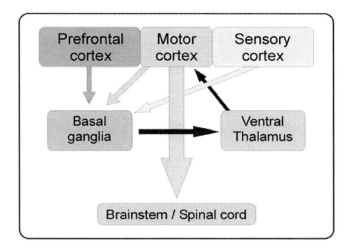

Figure 9.4. Motor loop through the basal ganglia.

How does the decrease of dopamine concentration in the striatum, and its consequent decrease in the positive modulation exerted by the basal ganglia loop upon the frontal cortex, cause the cognitive impairments observed in Parkinson's disease? Let us start by the motor skills and habit learning. Primary motor cortex, supplementary motor area and somatosensory cortex neurons directly control the firing of spinal motor neurons leading to consciously willed movements. Motor programs are the orchestrated sequences of commands to functional groups of muscles that govern movements at or around the joints. Where are these motor programs encoded and stored? The striatum is in a strategic position to participate in the encoding of such motor programs that will constitute the framework of the motor skills and habits. The ability to perform a skill demands a coordinated activity of muscle groups from different parts of the body, and the continuous integration of information about the contraction state of these muscles, and of the visual follow-up of the movement in order to make fine adjustments for proper movements. Habit learning consists in increasing the probability that a sensorial stimulus triggers a motor program designed for a particular behavioral response. As mentioned above, both sensory and motor regions of the entire cortex project to the striatum. The sensorial perception of the body in terms of tactile discrimination of shape and texture of the stimuli, response to deep stimuli, and response to muscle efferents are topographically organized in the primary somatosensory area of the cortex (SI, subdivided in anatomically distinct areas designated 1, 2, 3a and 3b). The primary motor cortex (MI) also presents a somatotopic organization. Inputs from regions of MI and SI that represent the same body parts, send projections to the same region within the striatum. This convergence is observed even for the SI regions presenting distinct somatosensory submodalities of the same body parts. However, while the cortical regions form a single and continuous representation of the entire body, the representation of these areas of the body in the striatum is broken in a mosaic and is redundant. That is, each part of the body is represented by multiple striatal unities called matrisomes. After these somato-sensory-motor inputs are processed in the striatum, the multiple matrisomes representing the same body parts send overlapping projections to the globus pallidus. There, in the globus pallidus, the unique and continuous representation of the body is restored (see Figure 9.6). Primary cortex regions for other sensorial modalities, i.e., vision, hearing and smell, also send projections to the striatum. Notice that the multiple mosaics representation of sensorial and motor information in the striatum allows the association of different stimuli with the activation of sequences of movement involving different parts of the body. The capacity of the dopamine neurons to either inhibit or stimulate the basal-cortical output and to induce firing dependent plasticity in the cortico-striatal synapses enables this system to form experience driven stimulus-response programs that are the basis of skills and habit learning.

Working memory and executive functions dependent on the activity of prefrontal cortex are also affected in Parkinson's disease. There are loops integrating the dorsolateral and the orbitofrontal areas of the prefrontal cortex with the basal ganglia. Many studies have shown increased activity of these cortical regions and the dorsolateral striatum, when subjects are performing spatial working memory tasks. The concept of working memory involves the integration and maintenance of information for its prospective use when selecting the appropriate behavior. This process could involve the transformation of sensory cues in a code response. The prefrontal cortex is in the top hierarchy of the sensorial and motor systems. In the same way as the striatum, it can receive information from all sensory modalities and control the motor output. While doing this, it works in consonance with basal ganglia loops (Figure 9.4). These cortico-basal loops can run parallel subroutines that are unconsciously operated while the prefrontal cortex is involved in solving conscious demands for the ongoing behavior. Like the striatum, the prefrontal cortex is also modulated by dopamine neurons arising in the midbrain. Therefore, it is easy to understand how the depletion of dopamine that occur in Parkinson's disease in these brain regions, can affect working memory. In the same way, attention and other executive functions of the prefrontal cortex will be affected by the dopamine depletion in the striatum and prefrontal cortex.

Cognitive Disabilities

Besides the characteristic motor symptoms, subtle cognitive impairments can be observed even in early phases of Parkinson's disease. They comprise a dysexecutive syndrome that includes attentional and working memory impairment with secondary deficits of internal representation of visuospatial stimuli, and in the use of declarative memory storage. Skill and habit learning are also impaired in these patients. Near one-third of patients may eventually progress to dementia. Since in Parkinson's disease, acetylcholine, noradrenaline and serotonin neurons, besides the dopaminergic neurons, are reported to degenerate, animal studies have been helpful to reveal the contribution of each specific neurotransmitter to specific cognitive impairments. Below, we will detail some of these relevant studies.

Executive Functions

A dysexecutive syndrome is in the core of the cognitive impairments and dementia observed in Parkinson's disease, and it appears even in early stages of the disease. Executive function describes a wide range of cognitive functions required for goal-directed, adaptive behavior in response to new, challenging environmental situations, including planning, task management, attention, inhibition, monitoring and coding. All these functions are attributable to the prefrontal cortex and therefore, Parkinson's disease cognitive disabilities resemble cognitive deficits found in frontal cortex patients.

Failure of the Parkinson's disease patients in the execution of tasks planned to test executive functions, even when the motor impairments are taken into account, support the idea outlined in the precedent paragraph. One example is the Wisconsin card sorting test in which the subjects are required to sort cards according to categories (i.e., color, figure shape, etc.). The categories change without warning, according to an internal sequence unknown to the subject, that can succeed only by using his error feedback. Parkinson's disease patients need more trials to complete the first category, and achieve fewer categories, as compared to control subjects. This deficit is suggestive of an inability to initiate concepts. By the end of the test session, they usually can verbalize the correct response, like saying "it must be the color". However, they keep on following a random response, suggesting that they present a difficulty in organizing appropriate concepts into coherent actions. Further evidence that they have difficulties in inhibition, task management, and attention, is their difficulty in the execution of simultaneous and competing motor tasks.

Working Memory

Working memory is a kind of short-term memory we use to maintain information online while using it in a mental work. Working memory is composed by a central executive that manages attention to the relevant stimuli or evocates the necessary memories to the mental task that is being processed at that specific time. The central executive is fed by two slave systems that instantly store visuospatial or phonological information. The visuospatial loop of the working memory seems to be the most affected trait in Parkinson's disease.

In a study of spatial working memory, each subject had to touch 4 to 8 boxes that appeared on a computer screen. When touched, the boxes opened-up revealing what was inside them and then closed-up. The goal was to collect blue tokens that were hidden inside the boxes. The key was that a blue token appeared only once in a particular box. In order to avoid opening the same box twice, the subjects had to store in their working memory, the place of the boxes they had already searched. Mild and severe non-demented Parkinson's disease patients looked again for the blue tokens in the same boxes they had already opened. In similar verbal or visual versions of this working memory task in which monosyllabic surnames or simple colored shapes replaced the boxes, respectively, only severe but not mild Parkinson's disease patients were impaired. In another study, the subjects were shown six figures at the top and six at the bottom of a computer screen. One of the figures of the top series was highlighted and they were instructed to point with the mouse, the correspondent figure of the bottom series, by trial-and-error guessing. Each correct or incorrect response was respectively signaled by specific visual and sound stimulus. All Parkinson's disease patients, even those in an early phase of the disease, could not maintain in their working memory the places of the matching figures and returned to a previously selected incorrect figure. For this test of spatial working memory all the figures of the top series (cartoon light bulbs) and of the bottom series (cartoon playing cards) were the same. Therefore, the subjects had to remember the location of the matching figures. In an object version of this working memory task, different shapes of black figures were used. The scores of control subjects and Parkinson's disease patients did not differ in this object version of the task.

The two studies described above are examples of how working memory, especially spatial working memory, fails in non-demented Parkinson's disease patients. The articulatory (verbal-phonological) component of the working memory is usually preserved, but when a verbal working memory task demands more attention, a deficiency is also observed in these patients. These impairments are possibly consequent of failure of the central executive component that manages the short-term memory stock. Thus, these impairments appear when the working memory tasks present a higher demand on executive functions such as planning and attention shifting.

Visual Deficits

Is it possible that someone, while looking to a picture of the Amazon forest, see the trees but not the forest? It is what a study suggests that parkinsonians do. In this study, 4 different large letters, each composed of 4 different medium-sized letters, each of them composed of 4 different small letters printed in sheets were presented to the subjects. Parkinson's disease patients could name as many small and medium-sized letters as control subjects did. However, they named fewer large letters. How do they process visual information in a way that does not appear to produce a purely sensorial deficit, but result in a deformed cognitive use of this information? Other examples of cognitive-visual defects in Parkinson's disease include deficits in orientation-dependent visual tasks, such as line orientation discrimination and visuospatial orientation.

These visual alterations in Parkinson's disease have been receiving different explanations that range from impairments in the retinal to cortico-basal ganglia processing caused by dopamine deficiency. Furthermore, an apparent neglect of the contralateral visual field and other sensory stimuli modalities has been reported for animals with unilateral lesion of the SNpc. Some authors interpret this apparent sensory neglect as a defect in the initiation or execution of contralesional motor acts, instead of a deficit to detect visual stimuli per se. Others sustain that these sensorial neglects result of an aberrant mental representation of the space.

Non-Declarative Memory: Skill and Habit Learning

The first report of an independent non-declarative memory system was that of a patient known as H.M. that became amnestic after a surgery to extirpate his medial temporal lobes. After surgery he conserved his capacity to improve the skill of drawing a line between the drawings of two concentric stars, while looking at its image in a mirror. This kind of learning and memory that one proves to have, not by a declaration (non-declarative), but through a procedure (procedural), and that is acquired unconsciously (implicit), was proposed to be mediated by the striatum.

Many studies have tested whether Parkinson's disease patients, known to have a striatal depletion of dopamine, present non-declarative learning and memory deficits. In one of these studies, non-demented Parkinson's disease patients were trained in reading words by their inverted mirror images. Some words were repeated throughout the trials. After seeing these words, these patients could improve their mirror reading by using their declarative memory that was relatively preserved. However, they did not improve their reading of words that appeared only once during the test. Therefore, this impairment can be attributable to a skill learning deficit. Variations of these tests using words made of non-inverted letters that had to be read from the right to the left, and horizontal lines of dots that had to be counted from the right to the left also confirmed that Parkinson's disease patients are impaired in this kind of right-to-left reading visual skill. Parkinson's disease patients were shown to present impaired skill learning not only for visuoperceptual but also for motor skills tasks, as for puzzle assembly, pressing specific keys in a computer keyboard in response to stimulus presented on the computer screen, and drawing lines in hidden mazes.

It is not consensual that Parkinson's disease spares declarative memory. Part of the discrepancies can be explained by cortical degeneration due to co-morbidity with Alzheimer's disease and Body Lewy disease, observed in some demented patients. However, the non-intentional and automatic nature of a non-declarative task, such as learning a list of words or matching pairs of words, may also determine whether it can be learned normally or not by Parkinson's disease patients. Some studies showed that they are impaired to remember well-known words that can be automatically retrieved without an attentional effort. On the other hand, they are unimpaired to learn and retrieve new words that require a purposeful effort from them. Therefore, in those cases, their deficits rely more in the unconscious (implicit) than in the non-declarative nature of the learning and memory task.

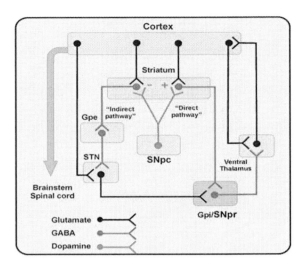

Figure 9.5. Alexander and Crutcher's model for the "direct" and "indirect" pathways from the striatum to the GPi. Glutamate acts on excitatory receptors, while GABA acts on inhibitory receptors. Dopamine acts either on excitatory (D1-like) and inhibitory (D2-like) receptors. See the text for a description. GPe – globus pallidus, external part; GPi – globus pallidus, internal part; STN – subthalamic nucleus; SNpc – substantia nigra pars compacta; SNpr – substantia nigra pars reticulata.

Habits are by definition stimulus-response (S-R) associations that are unconsciously learned though repetitively rewarded experiences. The main difficulty to model a habit task is to guarantee that the subjects will not respond consciously in order to receive the reward. One of the most well designed studies planned to test whether non-demented Parkinson's disease patients are impaired in S-R habit learning, used a probabilistic classification task. Three groups of subjects of both sexes, matching in age were tested: non-demented Parkinson's disease patients, Alzheimer's disease patients and healthy subjects. The task consisted in seeing a combination of up to 3 decks of 4 cards in a computer screen. Each card had a particular pattern and appeared randomly. After the subject had seen the cards cue, he/she had to predict raining or shining by pressing the correspondent key in the computer keyboard. Each card determined independently and probabilistically, what outcome would appear on the screen, immediately after the subject's response, followed by a high-pitched (correct) or low-pitched (incorrect) tone sound. The probabilistic structure of the task made that the subjects learned it unconsciously by trial-and-error. Parkinson's disease patients scored worse than Alzheimer's disease patients and healthy subjects, but when asked about it, they remembered to have participated in the previous training sessions. Alzheimer's disease patients, on the other hand, learned this task like healthy subjects, but barely remembered the training episode. This study supports the double dissociation proposed for the respective medial temporal and basal ganglia mediation of declarative (episodic) and non-declarative (implicit habit learning) memory systems.

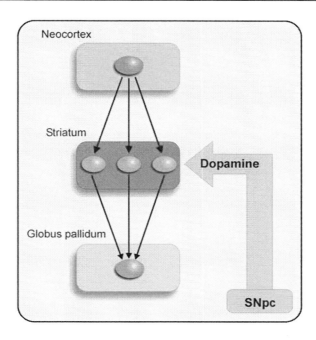

Figure 9.6. Cortico-basal ganglia circuits encode engrams for skill and habit learning through divergent and convergent neocortical remapping. Dopamine release from striato-nigral neurons is critical for the plastic events that occur during this process. Adapted from Graybiel, A. The Basal Ganglia and Chunking of Action Repertoires. Neurobiol Learning Memory, 70, 119–136, 1998.

Dementia

The risk of developing dementia in Parkinson's disease patients is up to six times higher than in healthy subjects of the same age. Different studies reported different incidence and prevalence of dementia in Parkinson's disease. In most cross-sectional studies, prevalence of dementia in Parkinson's disease varies from 10 to 40%. The discrepancies can be explained by the use of different diagnostic tests. Furthermore, the prevalence of dementia in Parkinson's disease is a function of the patients' age, age at the disease onset, severity and duration, and co-morbidity with Alzheimer's disease and Lewy body disease. A prospective study has revealed that 78% of Parkinson's disease patients became demented in 8 years' time. In other prospective studies the cumulative incidence of dementia in Parkinson's disease varied from 20 to 50%. Parkinson's disease dementia is characterized by a worsening of the same cognitive impairments observed in non-demented patients.

The core of the impairments is in executive functions (e.g. set-shifting). Mood (e.g. depression), and psychotic (e.g. visual hallucinations) symptoms are also common in demented Parkinson's disease patients. Other common impairments include visuospatial and visuoconstructive skills. Speech and language difficulties, such as naming and sentence comprehension, are also common. Furthermore, poor verbal fluency would be predictive of dementia in Parkinson's disease. However, aphasia, apraxia or agnosia is more common in Alzheimer's disease than in Parkinson's disease dementia. Declarative memory impairments are present, but are less severe, as compared to Alzheimer's disease. There is a deficit in free recall, but it can be compensated by semantic cueing. Furthermore, Parkinson's disease patients have more problems to recall than to encode declarative memories, that is, their impairment relays on difficulties in activating processes involved in the functional use of memory storages, probably consequent on the dysexecutive syndrome. Recognition memory is relatively intact. Some of these cognitive impairments, especially attention impairment, are aggravated by a degeneration of cholinergic neurons of the nucleus basalis of Meynert and of noradrenaline neurons of locus coeruleus that also occur in Parkinson's disease. Impairments in declarative memory, aphasia and apraxia, on the other hand, when occur are related to cortical pathology indicative of Alzheimer's disease or Lewy body dementia. Regarding the last co-morbidity, it is noteworthy how the characteristics of Parkinson's disease dementia are similar to Lewy body dementia. Additionally, *postmortem* studies revealed that many Lewy body disease patients were wrongly diagnosed in life as being Parkinson's disease patients and many Parkinson's disease patients undergo Lewy body disease, later on.

Interventions

In medicated Parkinson's disease patients, the non-motor symptoms that include cognitive deficits can be more important than the motor deficits to determine the patients' quality of life. Furthermore, dementia is associated with increased mortality and is an important factor to determine the need of nursing home placement, besides the distress it causes the caregivers. In spite of that, most of the drugs available to treat Parkinson's disease nowadays are more efficient to alleviate motor than cognitive impairments.

The most efficient treatment for the motor disabilities of Parkinson's disease is based on the replacement of dopamine through the administration of its precursor, levodopa. However, many studies have shown that most of the cognitive impairments persist in Parkinson's disease patients medicated with levodopa. This fact has led many researchers to postulate non-dopaminergic mechanisms for the cognitive symptoms of this disease. It is possible that failure in other neurotransmitter systems contribute to these cognitive impairments, especially in demented patients. However, a study carried out in our laboratory has suggested how the beneficial effect of the levodopa therapy can be overwhelmed by a misbalance between the dopamine levels in the striatum and the prefrontal cortex. In this study SNpc lesioned rats were treated with levodopa/benserazide and tested in the two-way active avoidance memory task. Instead of improving, the levodopa treatment worsened the impairment of these rats in learning the memory task. Post-mortem analysis revealed that the dose of levodopa that had restored the striatal level of dopamine, had caused an increase higher than 10 fold, of the dopamine level in the frontal cortex. Therefore, it is possible that the levodopa therapy may also cause an abnormal increase of the dopamine level in the frontal cortex of Parkinson's disease patients, thus resulting in other cognitive impairments, similar to those observed in psychotic patients. Such impairments possibly overwhelm the cognitive benefit of restoring the dopamine level in the striatum. In this sense, it is noteworthy that visual hallucinations and vivid dreams are the most common psychotic symptoms that occur in Parkinson's disease patients treated with levodopa. It is possible that the addition of atypical dopamine receptor antagonists with higher affinity for the frontal cortex, as compared to striatal dopamine receptors would alleviate the cognitive symptoms of Parkinson's disease patients under levodopa therapy. However, such clinical studies are not yet available.

Motor disabilities in Parkinson's disease patients improve with pallidotomy and bilateral chronic high frequency deep brain stimulation of the subthalamic nucleus. However, most of the cognitive symptoms seem to be refractory to these treatments. Moreover, subthalamic stimulation has been reported to cause moderate worsening on executive and language functions, and declarative memory. Attempts have been made to adjust the parameters of deep brain stimulation in order to avoid these adverse cognitive responses while maintaining the motor symptom efficacy. Besides, an improvement of non-declarative memory and time perception in Parkinson's disease patients under subthalamic stimulation has been reported.

Independently of the low potential of subthalamic stimulation and dopaminergic drugs to treat the cognitive symptoms of Parkinson's disease, other approaches have been under study. In our laboratory, we have discovered that the treatment of SNpc lesioned rats with the adenosine receptor antagonist, caffeine, has reversed their deficit to learn the two-way active avoidance task. Another study has also reported a cognitive enhancing effect of the A2A receptor antagonist, ZM241385, in a further animal model of Parkinson's disease. The A2A receptors are known to be co-expressed with the D1 dopamine receptors in the striatum. The activation of these receptors causes opposite effects, and the A2A receptors also inhibit the release of dopamine from the striatal synaptic terminals. The α2 agonist, clonidine, has also been reported to alleviate spatial working memory impairment in Parkinson's disease patients, without affecting the performance in tests of attentional set shifting or visual recognition memory. However, to our knowledge, none of these drugs are yet in clinical use for Parkinson's disease cognitive disabilities.

Acetylcholine replacement therapy, based on treatment with cholinesterase inhibitors, has been used to treat attentional and declarative memory deficits in Parkinson's disease patients with dementia. Psychiatric symptoms, such as hallucinations, apathy and anxiety, have also been reported to improve with this treatment. As mentioned above, degeneration of the cholinergic neurons in the nucleus basalis of Meynert is commonly found in these patients. The cholinesterase inhibitor, tacrine, showed a beneficial effect in Parkinson's disease demented patients. However, this drug must be used with caution due to hepatic complications. Modest benefits have been reported for the treatment of Alzheimer's disease patients with the cholinesterase inhibitors rivastigmine, galantamine, and donepezil. Galantamine and donepezil also stimulate nicotinic receptors and proved to improve cognitive and hallucination symptoms. The dual acetyl and butyryl cholinesterase inhibitor, rivastigmine, presented similar results in demented patients with Parkinson's disease and Lewy Body disease. Given the improving effect of muscaric receptor inhibitors on motor disabilities of Parkinson's disease, it would be expected that cholinesterase inhibitors would worsen such motor disabilities. However, they have not worsened motor impairments and even improved them, with the exception of rivastigmine that has tended to increase tremor.

Box 1

An Animal Model of Memory Deficits Associated to Parkinson's Disease

Parkinson's disease symptoms result not only from the loss of SNpc dopamine neurons, but also from the loss of cholinergic, noradrenergic and serotonergic neurons. Animal models have been useful to study the contribution of each of these neuromodulatory systems to the cognitive impairments of this disease.

In our laboratory we have validated a rat model of an early phase of Parkinson's disease. The animals were submitted to a partial lesion of the SNpc induced by the perinigral infusion of the neurotoxin MPTP (Figure 9A). After a 3-week recovery, the animals did not present motor impairments that would confound the scoring of real cognitive impairments. It may seem contradictory that in a model of Parkinson's disease the animals have presented no gross motor impairment.

However, human studies have shown that the motor symptoms of Parkinson's disease appear only 5 years after the onset of the process of losing dopamine neurons. Even so, the cognitive impairments arise in these patients before the appearance of the motor disabilities. Therefore, rats treated with intranigral MPTP have shown to be a good model of the early phase of Parkinson's disease, adequate for the study of cognitive impairments associated to it.

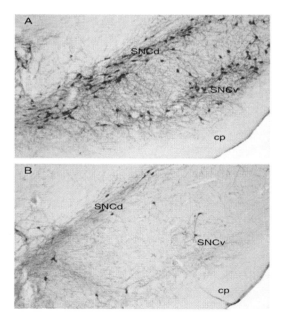

Figure 9A. Brightfield photomicrographs of a tyrosine hydroxylase immunostained section illustrating the appearance of a control (A) and a MPTP SNpc-lesioned rat (B). SNCd = Substantia Nigra, compact, dorsal part; SNCv =Substantia Nigra, compact, ventral part; cp - cerebral peduncle.

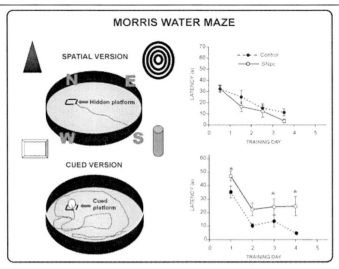

Figure 9B. SNpc-lesioned rats showed to be impaired to learn the cued, but not the spatial version of the Morris water maze task. In both versions of this memory task, rats had to find a hidden platform oriented by spatial cues placed in the room (spatial version) or by an internal cue – a ball attached to the platform. In the spatial version the platform was maintained in the same location throughout the many trials. In the cued version the position of the platform varied along trials. The figures represent a typical swimming path of a SNpc rat in the last trial and the average latencies of rats to find the platform during 4 training days. * $p < 0.05$, as compared to the control group.

The performance of these SNpc-lesioned rats has been studied in three versions of the Morris water maze task. In this task the rats swim in a round pool to find a hidden escape platform (Figure 9B). In the spatial working memory version, the platform was maintained in the same place during 4 consecutive trials. However, in the following training days, it was moved to another place in the pool. Therefore, the animals could not use the previous day memory to find the platform. Since they had found it in the first trial of the day, they had to use their spatial working memory to find it again in the subsequent trials. It always took longer to the SNpc-lesioned rats to find the platform than the control rats. However, when the platform was maintained in the same location throughout the trainings days, allowing the animals to use their long-term spatial memory to locate it, no impairment was observed in the SNpc rats (see Figure 9B, top).

In a third version of the water maze task, called cued version or S-R habit version, the platform is randomly placed in one of the quadrants of the pool and is cued by a ball that is attached to it and protrudes above the water surface. Here, the animals must learn a stimulus-response (S-R) association in order to find easily the escape platform. They must learn that where the ball is, there will be the platform. It took longer to the SNpc rats to find the cued platform, as compared to the control rats (Figure 9B, bottom).

Another S-R habit learning task in which the SNpc rats were impaired was the two-way active avoidance. In this task the animals were placed in a two compartment shuttle-box and were trained to run to the opposite compartment, when they heard a sound cue, in order to avoid a footshock. After a series of 30 sound cue-footshock pairings, control rats avoided the shock by running to the other side of the box, 8 times in average. However, the average number of avoidances of the SNpc rats was near 2. When the same rats were re-trained under the same condition the next day, control animals improved their average avoidance scores to 14, while the average score of the SNpc rats was only 4. Therefore, even a partial lesion of the SNpc could impair the learning and memory of the association of a sound stimulus with a motor response in order to avoid a punishment.

The studies reported above substantiate the conclusion that the loss of SNpc dopaminergic neurons in Parkinson's disease is sufficient to cause impairments in spatial working memory and S-R habit learning, while sparing long-term spatial-relational (declarative) memories. Therefore, the impairments of declarative memories observed in demented Parkinson's disease patients are probably due to depletion in neurotransmitters other than dopamine (i.e. acethilcholine), or to associated Lewy body disease.

Acknowledgements

The thoughtful comments of Dr. Heiko Braak, MD, are acknowledged.

References

[1] Alegret M, Valldeoriola F, Marti MJ, Pilleri M, Junque C, Rumia J, Tolosa E. Comparative cognitive effects of bilateral subthalamic stimulation and subcutaneous continuous infusion of apomorphine in Parkinson's disease. *Movement Disorders* 19:1463-1469, 2004.

[2] Baddeley A. Working memory: Looking back and looking forward. *Nature Rev Neurosci* 4:829 -839, 2003.

[3] Barrett AM, Crucian GP, Schwartz R, Nallamshetty H, Heilman KM. Seeing trees but not the forest - Limited perception of large configurations in PD. *Neurology* 56:724-729, 2001.

[4] Bellissimo MI, Kouzmine I, Ferro M, Oliveira BH, Canteras NS, Da Cunha C. Is the unilateral lesion of the substantia nigra pars compacta sufficient to induce working memory impairment in rats? *Neurobiol Learning Memory* 82:150-158, 2004.

[5] Bodis-Wollner, I. Visual deficits related to dopamine deficiency in experimental animals and Parkinson's disease patients. *Trends Neurosci* 13: 269-302, 1990.

[6] Bondi MW, Kaszniak AW. Implicit and explicit memory in Alzheimer's disease and Parkinson's disease. *J Clin Exp Neuropsychology* 13:339-358, 1991.

[7] Bosboom JLW, Stoffers D, Wolters EC. Cognitive dysfunction and dementia in Parkinson's disease. *J Neural Transm* 111:1303–1315, 2004.

[8] Braak H, Del Tredici K, Rüba U, de Vos RAI, Ernst N.H. Jansen Steur EMHJ, Braak E. Staging of brain pathology related to sporadic Parkinson's disease. *Neurobiol Aging* 24: 197–211, 2003.

[9] Braak H, Ghebremedhin E, Rüb U, Bratzke H, Del Tredici K. Stages in the development of Parkinson's disease-related pathology. *Cel Tissue Res* 318:121–134, 2004.

[10] Braga R, Kouzmine I, Canteras NS, Da Cunha C. Lesion of the substantia nigra, pars compacta impairs delayed alternation in a Y-maze in rats. *Exp Neurol* 192:134-141, 2005.

[11] Carbon M, Marie RM. Functional imaging of cognition in Parkinson's disease. *Current Opinion in Neurology* 16:475-480, 2003.

[12] Czernecki V, Pillon B, Houeto JL, Welter ML, Mesnage V, Agid Y, Dubois BTI. Does bilateral stimulation of the subthalamic nucleus aggravate apathy in Parkinson's disease? *J Neurol Neurosurgery Psychiatry* 76:775-779, 2005.

[13] Da Cunha C, Angelucci MEM, Canteras NS, Wonnacott S, Takahashi RN. The lesion of the rat substantia nigra pars compacta dopaminergic neurons as a model for Parkinson's disease memory disabilities. *Cel Mol Neurobiol* 22:227-237, 2002.

[14] Da Cunha C, Gevaerd MS, Vital MABF, Miyoshi E, Andreatini R, Silveira R, Takahashi RN, Canteras NS. Memory disruption in rats with nigral lesions induced by MPTP: A model for early Parkinson's disease amnesia. *Behav Brain Res* 124:9-18, 2001.

[15] Da Cunha C, Wietzikoski S, Wietzikoski E, Ferro M, Miyoshi E, Anselmo-Franci JA, Canteras NS. Evidence for the substantia nigra pars compacta as an essential component of a memory system independent of the hippocampal memory system. *Neurobiol Learning Memory* 79:236-242, 2003.

[16] Del Tredici K, Rüb U, De Vos RAI, Bohl JRE, Braak H. Where does Parkinson disease pathology begin in the brain? *J Neuropathol Exp Neurology* 61:413-426, 2002.

[17] Drapier S, Raoul S, Drapier D, Leray E, Lallement F, Rivier I, Sauleau P, Lajat Y, Edan G, Vérin M. Only physical aspects of quality of life are significantly improved by bilateral subthalamic stimulation in Parkinson's disease. *J Neurol* 252:583–588, 2005.

[18] Dubois B, Pillon B. Cognitive deficits in Parkinson's disease. *J Neurol* 244:2-8, 1997.

[19] Faglioni P, Botti C, Scarpa M, Ferrari V, Saetti MC. Learning and forgetting processes in Parkinson's disease: A model-based approach to disentangling storage, retention and retrieval contributions. *Neuropsychologia* 35:767-779, 1997.

[20] Faglioni P, Scarpa M, Botti C, Ferrari V. Parkinson's disease affects automatic and spares intentional verbal learning a stochastic approach to explicit learning processes. *Cortex* 31:597-617, 1995.

[21] Ferro M, Bellissimo MI, Anselmo-Franci JA, Angelucci MEM, Canteras NS, Da Cunha C. Comparison of 6-hydroxidopamine and 1-methyl-4-phenyl-1,2,3,6-tetrahydropyridine (MPTP) -lesioned rats as models of memory deficits associated to Parkinson's disease. *J Neurosci Methods*, 148:78-87, 2005.

[22] Flaherty AW, Graybiel AM. Corticostriatal transformations in the primate somatosensory system. Projections from physiologically mapped body-part representations. *J Neurophysiol* 66:1249-1263, 1991.

[23] Flaherty AW, Graybiel AM. Two input systems for body representations in the primate striatal matrix: Experimental evidence in the squirrel monkey. *J Neurosci* 13:1120-1137, 1993.

[24] Francel P, Ryder K, Wetmore J, Stevens A, Bharucha K, Beatty WW, Scott J. Deep brain stimulation for Parkinson's disease: Association between stimulation parameters and cognitive performance. *Stereotactic Functional Neurosurgery* 82:191-193, 2004.

[25] Funkiewiez A, Ardouin C, Caputo E, Krack P, Fraix V, Klinger H, Chabardes S, Foote K, Benabid AL, Pollak P. Long term effects of bilateral subthalamic nucleus stimulation on cognitive function, mood, and behaviour in Parkinson's disease. *J Neurology Neurosurgery Psychiatry* 75:834-839, 2004.

[26] Gerschlager, Alesch F, Cunnington R, Deecke L, Dirnberger G, Endl W, Lindinger G, Lang W. Bilateral subthalamic nucleus stimulation improves frontal cortex function in Parkinson's disease: An electrophysiological study of the contingent negative variation. *Brain* 122:2365-2373, 1999.

[27] Gevaerd MS, Miyoshi E, Silveira R, Canteras NS, Takahashi RN, Da Cunha C. Levodopa treatment restores the striatal level of dopamine but fails to reverse memory deficits in rats treated with MPTP, an animal model of Parkinson's disease. *Int J Neuropsychopharmacol* 4:361-370, 2001.

[28] Gevaerd MS, Takahashi RN, Silveira R, Da Cunha C. Caffeine reverses the memory disruption induced by intra-nigral MPTP-injection in rats. *Brain Res Bull* 55:101-106, 2001.

[29] Gironell A, Kulisevsky J, Rami L, Fortuny N, Garcia-Sanchez C, Pascual-Sedano B. Effects of pallidotomy and bilateral subthalamic stimulation on cognitive function in Parkinson disease - A controlled comparative study. *J Neurology* 250:917-923, 2003.

[30] Graceffa AMS, Carlesimo GA, Peppe A, Caltagirone C. Verbal working memory deficit in Parkinson's disease subjects. *Europ Neurology* 42:90-94, 1999.

[31] Graybiel A. The Basal Ganglia and Chunking of Action Repertoires. *Neurobiol Learning Memory*, 70:119–136, 1998.

[32] Growdon JH, Kieburtz K, McDermott MP, Panisset M, Friedman JH, Parkinson Study Group. Levodopa improves motor function without impairing cognition in mild non-demented Parkinson's disease patients. *Neurology* 50:1327-1331, 1998.

[33] Halbig TD, Gruber D, Kopp UA, Scherer P, Schneider GH, Trottenberg T, Arnold G, Kupsch A. Subthalamic stimulation differentially modulates declarative and nondeclarative memory. *Neuroreport* 15:539-543, 2004.

[34] Klockgether T. Parkinson's disease: clinical aspects. *Cell Tissue Res* 318:115–120, 2004.

[35] Knowlton BJ, Mangels JA, Squire LR. A neostriatal habit learning system in humans. *Science* 273:1399-1402, 1996.

[36] Koch G, Brusa L, Caltagirone C, Oliveri M, Peppe A, Tiraboschi P, Stanzione P. Subthalamic deep brain stimulation improves time perception in Parkinson's disease. *Neuroreport* 15:1071-1073, 2004.

[37] Koenig O, Thomas-Antérion C, Laurent B. Procedural learning in Parkinson's disease: I Intact and impaired cognitive components. *Neuropsychologia* 37:1103-1109, 1999.

[38] Lakke JPWF, Wilhelm von Humboldt and James Parkinson. An Appraisal of Observation and Creativity. *Parkinsonism Related Disorders* 2:225-229, 1996.

[39]   Lange KW, Robbins TW, Marsden CD, James M, Owen AM, Paul GM. L-Dopa withdrawal in Parkinson's disease selectively impairs cognitive performance in tests sensitive to frontal lobe dysfunction. *Psychopharmacology* 107:394-404, 1992.

[40]   Le Bras C, Pillon B, Damier P, Dubois B. At which steps of spatial working memory processing do striatofrontal circuits intervene in humans? *Neuropsychologia* 37:83-90, 1999.

[41]   Levin BE, Liabre MM, Weiner WJ. Cognitive impairments associated with early Parkinson's disease. *Neurology* 39:557-561, 1989.

[42]   Lewis SJG, Cools R, Robbins TW, Dove A, Barker RA, Owend AM. Using executive heterogeneity to explore the nature of working memory deficits in Parkinson's disease. *Neuropsychologia* 41:645–654, 2003.

[43]   Loeffler DA, LeWitt PA, Juneau PL, Camp DM, Arnold LA, Hyland K. Time-dependent effects of levodopa on regional brain dopamine metabolism and lipid peroxidation. *Brain Res Bull* 47:663-667, 1998.

[44]   Lozza C, Baron JC, Eidelberg D, Mentis MJ, Carbon M, Marie RM. Executive processes in Parkinson's disease: FDG-PET and network analysis. *Human Brain Mapping* 22:236-245, 2004.

[45]   Maguire-Zeiss KA, Shortb DW, Federoff HJ. Synuclein, dopamine and oxidative stress: co-conspirators in Parkinson's disease? *Mol Brain Res* 134:8–23, 2005.

[46]   Malapani C, Pillon B, Dubois B, Agid Y. Impaired simultaneous cognitive task performance in Parkinson's disease: A dopamine-related dysfunction. *Neurology* 44:319-326, 1994.

[47]   Marié RM, Barré L, Dupuy B, Viader F, Defer G, Baron JC. Relationships between striatal dopamine denervation and frontal executive tests in Parkinson's disease. *Neuroscie Letters* 260:77-80, 1999.

[48]   Miyoshi E, Wietzikoski S, Camplessei M, Silveira R, Takahashi RN, Da Cunha C. Impaired learning in a spatial working memory version and in a cued version of the water maze in rats with MPTP-induced mesencephalic dopaminergic lesions. *Brain Res Bull* 58:41-47, 2002.

[49]   Moreaud O, Fournet N, Roulin J-L, Naegele B, Pellat J. The phonological loop in medicated patients with Parkinson's disease: presence of phonological similarity and word length effects. *J Neurology Neurosurgery Psychiatry* 62:609-611, 1997.

[50]   Morrison CE, Borod JC, Perrine K, Beric A, Brin MF, Rezai A, Kelly P, Sterio D, Germano I, Weisz D, Olanow CW. Neuropsychological functioning following bilateral subthalamic nucleus stimulation in Parkinson's disease. *Archives Clin Neuropsychol* 19:165-181, 2004.

[51]   Nagano-Saito A, Kato T, Arahata Y, Washimi Y, Nakamura A, Abe Y, Yamada T, Iwai K, Hatano K, Kawasumi Y, Kachi T, Dagher A, Ito K. Cognitive- and motor-related regions in Parkinson's disease: FDOPA and FDG PET studies. *Neuroimage* 22:553-561, 2004.

[52]   Oeppen J, Vaupel JW. Broken limits to life expectancy. *Science* 296: 1029, 2002.

[53]   Owen AM, Iddon JL, Hodges JR, Summers BA, Robbins TW, Spatial and non-spatial working memory at different stages of Parkinson's disease. *Neuropsychologia* 35:519-532, 1997.

[54] Owen AM. Cognitive dysfunction in Parkinson's disease: The role of frontostriatal circuitry. *Neuroscientist* 10, 525-537, 2004.

[55] Pascual-Leone A, Grafman J, Clark K, Stewart M, Massaquoi S, Lou J-S, Hallett M. Procedural learning in Parkinson's disease and cerebellar degeneration. *Ann Neurol* 34:594-602, 1993.

[56] Passingham D, Sakai K. The prefrontal cortex and working memory: physiology and brain imaging. *Current Opinion Neurobiol* 14:163–168, 2004.

[57] Pillon B, Dubois B, Bonnet A-M, Esteguy M, Guimaraes J, Vigouret J-M, Lhermitte F, Agid Y. Cognitive slowing in Parkinson's disease fails to respond to levodopa treatment: The 15-objects test. *Neurology* 39:762-768, 1989.

[58] Pillon B, Ertle S, Deweer B, Bonnet A-M, Vidailhet M, Dubois B. Memory for spatial location in ´de novo` parkinsonian patients. *Neuropsychologia* 35:221-228, 1997.

[59] Pillon B, Ertle S, Deweer B, Sarazin M, Agid Y, Dubois B. Memory for spatial location is affected in Parkinson's disease. *Neuropsychologia* 34:77-85, 1996.

[60] Postle BR, Locascio JJ, Corkin S, Growdon JH. The time course of spatial and object learning in Parkinson's disease. *Neuropsychologia* 35:1413-1422, 1997.

[61] Prediger RDS, Da Cunha C, Takahashi RN. Antagonistic interaction between adenosine A2A and dopamine D2 receptors modulates the social recognition memory in reserpine-treated rats. *Behav Pharmacol* 16:209-218, 2005.

[62] Ramírez-Ruiz B, Martí MJ, Tolosa E, Bartrés-Faz D, Summerfield C, Salgado-Pineda P, Gómez-Ansón B. Junque C. Longitudinal evaluation of cerebral morphological changes in Parkinson's disease with and without dementia. *J Neurol,* 252:1345-1352, 2005.

[63] Riekkinen M, Jäkälä P, Kejonen K, Riekkinen Jr P. The α2agonist, clonidine, improves spatial working memory performance in Parkinson's disease. *Neuroscience* 92: 983-989, 1999.

[64] Roncacci S, Troisi E, Carlesimo GA, Nocentini U, Caltagirone C. Implicit memory in parkinsonian patients: Evidence for deficient skill learning. *Europ Neurology* 36:154-159, 1996.

[65] Samii A, Nutt JG, Ransom BR. Parkinson's disease. *Lancet* 363 (9423): 1783-1793, 2004.

[66] Schulz JB, Falkenburger BH. Neuronal pathology in Parkinson's disease. *Cell Tissue Res* 318:135–147, 2004.

[67] Smeding HMM, Esselink RAJ, Schmand B, Koning-Haanstra M, Nijhuis I, Wijnalda EM, Speelman JD. Unilateral pallidotomy versus bilateral subthalamic nucleus stimulation in PD - A comparison of neuropsychological effects. *J Neurology* 252:176-182, 2005.

[68] Soukup VM, Ingram F, Schiess MC, Bonnen JG, Nauta HJW, Calverley JR. Cognitive sequelae of unilateral posteroventral pallidotomy. *Archiv Neurology* 54:947-950, 1997.

[69] Stebbins GT, Gabrieli JDE, Masciari F, Monti L, Goetz CG. Delayed recognition memory in Parkinson's disease: a role for working memory? *Neuropsychologia* 37:503-510, 1999.

[70] Tamaru F. Disturbances in higher function in Parkinson's disease. *Europ Neurology* 38:33-36, 1997.

[71] Taylor AE, Saint-Cyr JA, Lang AE. Frontal lobe dysfunction in Parkinson's disease. *Brain* 109:845-883, 1986.

[72] Thomas V, Reymann J-M, Lieury A, Allain H. Assessment of procedural memory in Parkinson's disease. *Prog. Neuro-Psychopharmacol Biol Psychiat* 20:641-650, 1996.

[73] Zgaljardic DJ, Foldi NS, Borod JC. Cognitive and behavioral dysfunction in Parkinson's disease: neurochemical and clinicopathological contributions. *J Neural Transm* 111:1287–1301, 2004.

Index

C

E

F

G

H

N

O

P

S

T

X

Y

Z